Homemade:

MADE HEALTHY & WHOLE

A Flavor of Lebanese Cooking
and Other Healthy Recipes

Homemade:
MADE HEALTHY & WHOLE

A Flavor of Lebanese Cooking and Other Healthy Recipes

Written and Photographed by
Sara Farhat Jarrar
MS, LDN

HOMEMADE:
MADE HEALTHY & WHOLE
A Flavor of Lebanese Cooking and Other Healthy Recipes

Disclaimer Note: All nutrition and health-related information presented in this book is not intended as a substitute for nutritional and medical advice by dietitians and physicians. Readers should consult with a dietitian and/or physician in matters relating to their health, especially with respect to any symptoms that may require diagnosis or nutritional and/or medical attention.

Cover Photos and Interior Book Photos by:
Sara Farhat Jarrar

Book Design by:
ZeinDesign
www.zeindesign.me

Book Index by:
Amy Hall
amy.hall@amethystharbor.com

ISBN: 978-1-7377530-7-0

First Edition

DEDICATION

To my dearest mother, Martha,
and my sweet daughters, Julia and Diana.

Wishing you much love and good health, always!

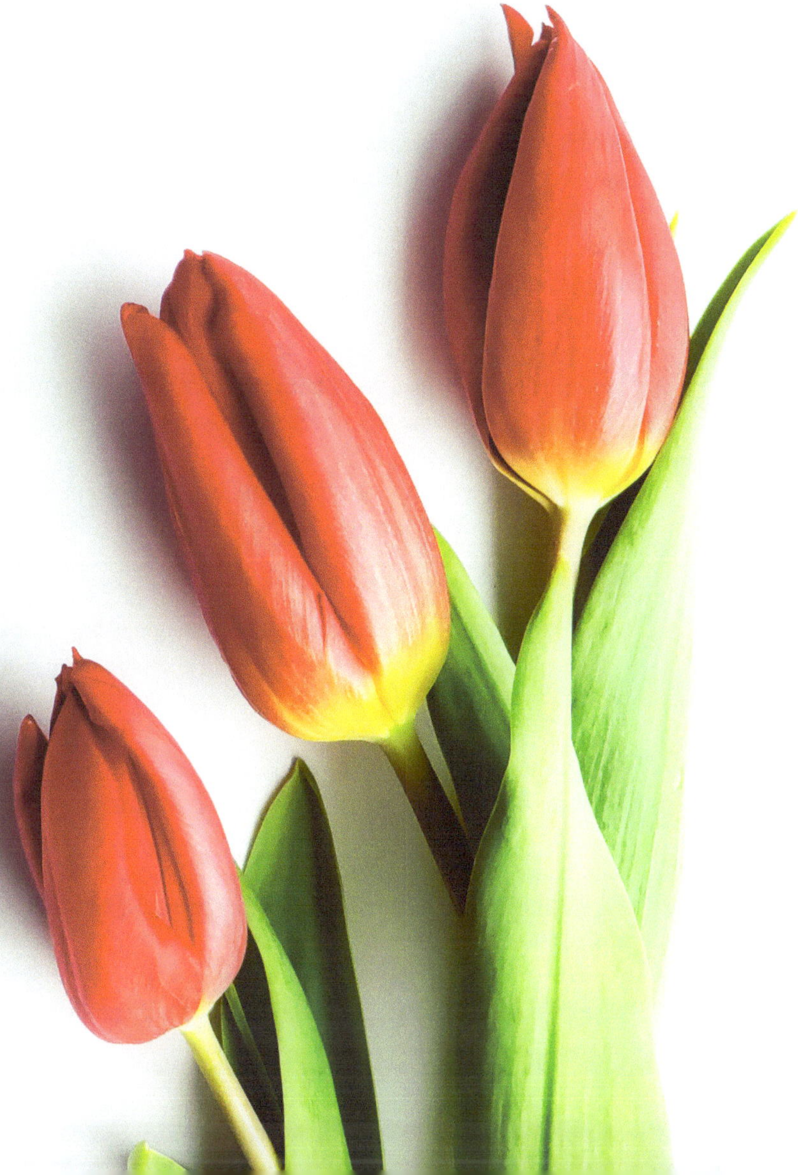

ACKNOWLEDGMENTS

I thank my lovely mother for instilling in me the love of cooking and baking. I can't thank you enough for teaching me and guiding me in everything I do! And thank you so much for helping in the editing of this book.

Thank you to my parents for inspiring my brother and me to be health-conscious individuals and for guiding us towards being healthy and conscientious eaters.

I thank my loving husband for all the support and encouragement he has offered over the years and continues to offer.

Thank you to my sweet daughters for being patient with me and tolerating all the extra hours I spent in the kitchen working on recipes and cooking, as well as all the time spent in styling the cookbook dishes and doing the photography work. I hope this cookbook becomes your favorite guide in your healthy cooking and baking journey when you are older!

Thank you to my husband and daughters combined for loving my cooked food and baked goods! You have been the biggest encouragement ever for me to recreate my recipes in an even healthier way!

Thank you to all our family members, friends, and neighbors who joined us at so many occasions to sample and enjoy my food and criticize it when needed. That's what made my recipes even more perfect!

I extend a warm thanks to my Lebanese aunts and uncles' wives for doing such a great job at teaching my mother and me the art of Lebanese cooking.

A big thank you to my dear sister-in-law Layal, a nutritionist as well, who offered her nutritional advice and feedback for my various inquiries along the way of writing my book and analyzing the nutritional data of the recipes.

Thank you to my good school friend Farah, a great cook and a talented interior architect, who guided and inspired me along my food styling and photographing journey, and who gave me some advice and insight on certain traditional Lebanese recipes and cooking techniques.

Thank you as well to my dear friend Dana, a great cook and a talented painter, for her frequent feedback and advice on my food photography.

And thank you to my creative and hard-working school friend and graphic designer Zein, as well as her talented colleague Malak, for the beautiful graphic design work they did for this book all the way from Beirut, Lebanon!

Finally, thank you to Ms. Amy Hall for the thorough indexing work she did to this book.

ABOUT THE AUTHOR

Sara Farhat Jarrar (MS, LDN)

Born in Minnesota, USA, to an American mother and Lebanese father, Sara ended up growing up in Lebanon where she attended both school and university. After graduating from high school, she followed her nutrition passion and completed her undergraduate studies in Nutrition and Dietetics at the American University of Beirut (AUB), receiving her dietetics and nutrition license afterwards. She then continued on to pursue her graduate studies in Nutrition and Dietetics at the AUB, after which she was recruited as a nutrition research assistant by the former Dean of the Faculty of Agriculture and Food Sciences at the AUB. During her four years of work at the AUB, Sara's research revolved around several projects, including coordinating a national study that investigated the nutritional status and dietary intake of the Lebanese population. She also contributed to the development of food-based dietary guidelines for the Lebanese people, as well as the development and dissemination of a nutrition education manual for pregnant women and mothers of young children.

In 2014, Sara moved back to the USA and settled in Minnesota with her husband. Since then, she has turned to becoming a proud stay-at-home mom of two daughters. Still a nutritionist at heart, she has done some freelance nutritional counselling over the past years, while focusing her remaining free time on the research, write-up, and photography of this book.

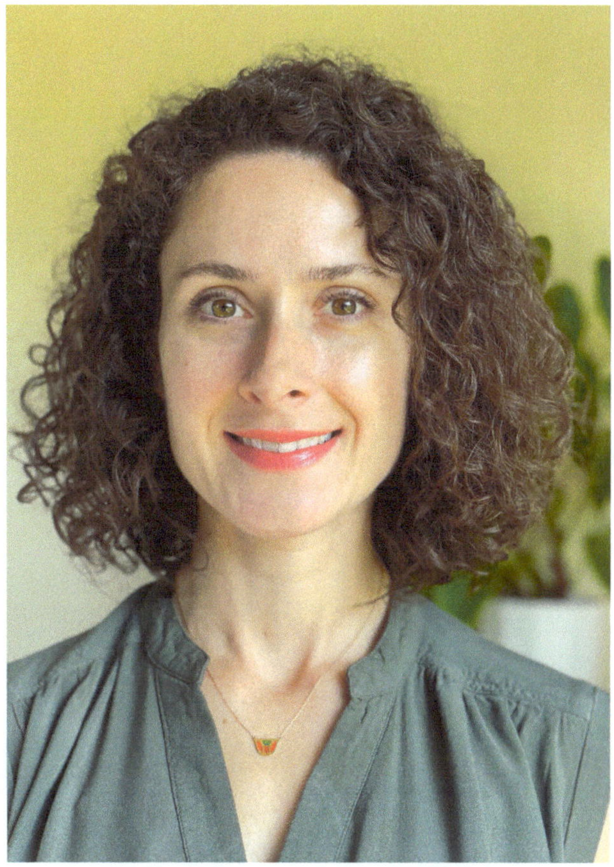

To connect with Sara for comments or questions, follow her on Instagram (homemade_healthyandwhole) or on Facebook (Sara Farhat Jarrar), or email her at sarafarhat85@gmail.com.

CONTENTS

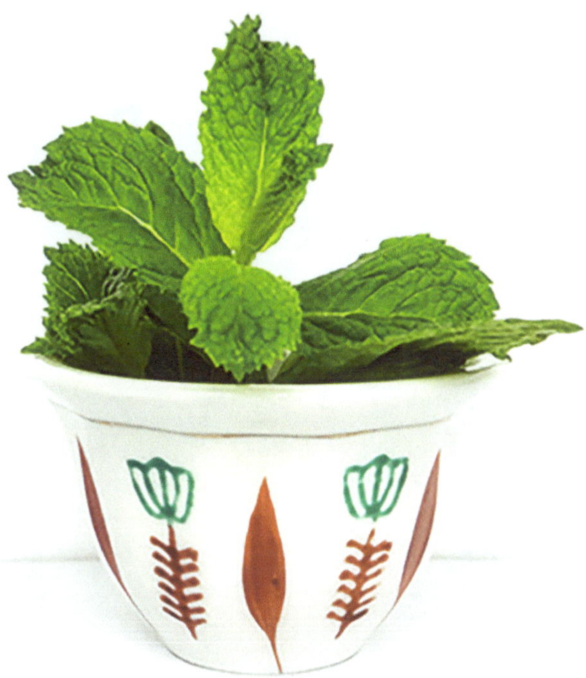

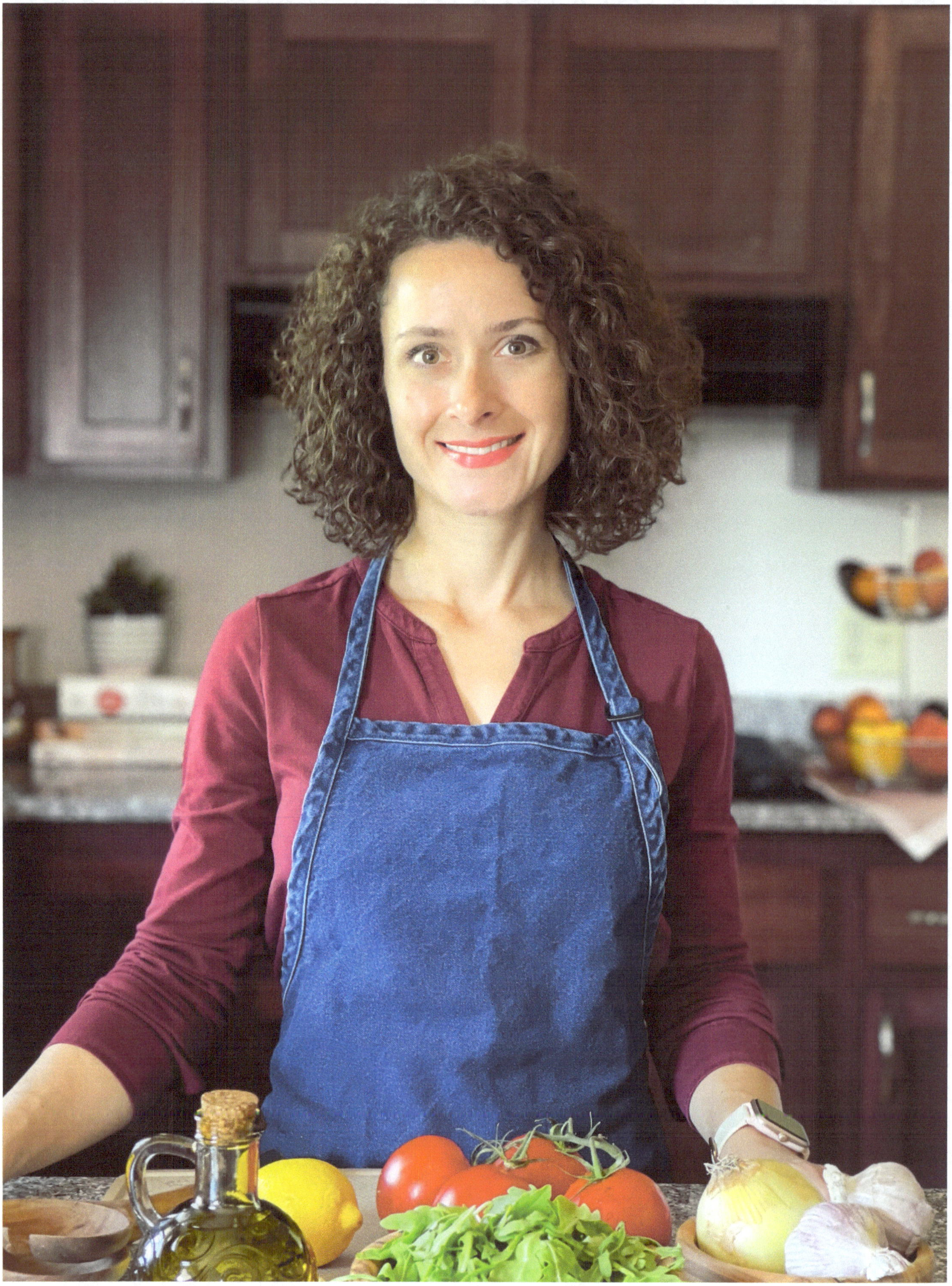

Chapter 1

INTRODUCTION

This cookbook was inspired by my long-time love for eating healthy food and being healthy. From a very young age, I spent a lot of time in the kitchen watching my mother cook and would love to join in helping her chop and mix ingredients. Though my mother was American from European decent, she was quick to learn the art of Lebanese cooking from my Lebanese aunts and uncles' wives after she married my father and they moved to Lebanon in the early 1980s. For myself, growing up in Lebanon in a household with health-conscious parents, I was spoiled by the abundance of healthy Lebanese food, and it was from there that I came to learn and love the many dishes of the Lebanese cuisine. Cooking in general, however, never became a big enough passion for me to pursue culinary school and become a chef. Nutrition turned out to be my calling, and since majoring in nutrition and dietetics and working in the field for several years, my love for eating healthy has grown even stronger.

Stemming from the Mediterranean diet, the Lebanese cuisine is rich in colorful and varied healthy plant-based ingredients, from fresh fruits and vegetables, to legumes (beans), lentils, some whole grains, nuts, seeds, herbs, spices, and native virgin olive oil. Lebanese food is full of wonderfully attractive displays, enticing aromas, mouth-watering flavors, and a multitude of health benefits. Well-known dishes may differ slightly between areas in Lebanon, and even between families, relying on some different ingredients or cooking methods. For as heathy as it is, however, the Lebanese cuisine relies heavily on some refined and processed foods (such as refined flour, rice, pasta, sugar, and refined vegetable oils), as well as some unhealthy cooking methods (such as the frying of certain food ingredients). It, thus, became a goal for me to modify my all-time favorite Lebanese dishes in ways that would make them healthier and more whole. I ultimately took on the task of modifying quantities and substituting different ingredients for others, and following better cooking methods to come up with the same tasty dishes that I was used to eating while growing up. As a nutritionist and a health-conscious person, I have made these dishes healthier and more whole in many and different ways than were their traditional versions. It is from this standpoint that this cookbook was inspired and thus created, reproducing the fabulous flavors of my favorite Lebanese dishes and desserts while enriching them with a healthier profile. My cookbook also contains several modified recipes which were handed down to me mostly by my mother and maternal grandmother and great-grandmother, as well as some family and friends. It also contains some healthy dishes and desserts of my very own creation, many of which contain a Middle Eastern touch to them.

I have to admit that the Lebanese cuisine contains some of the best dishes one could eat anywhere in the world, and I am not saying that just because I have Lebanese genes in me; it is truly a fact. I would like to stress that my modified Lebanese dishes in this cookbook are by no means meant to replace any of the traditional Lebanese recipes out there. They are meant to offer healthier and more whole alternatives for those who are interested, and to act as proof that healthy and whole don't mean less flavorful and less delicious. I like to see myself as a humble and health-conscious nutritionist and person who loves to cook and eat healthy, while offering her family the best of food options. I am happy to finally be able to share with you this cookbook of healthy and whole recipes, and I hope the food it teaches you to cook offers you and your families the same comfort, joy, and better health it does for my family and me.

و صحتين.

Sara

و صحتين : and *sahtein.* The word *sahtein* in Arabic literally means "two healths." It is used in Levantine dialects as the French use the expression 'bon appétit.' It is usually said when food is offered to someone or after one is done eating. It can also be used (as I have done so above) to wish someone good health through the enjoyment of a meal (even prior to cooking and/or consuming the meal).

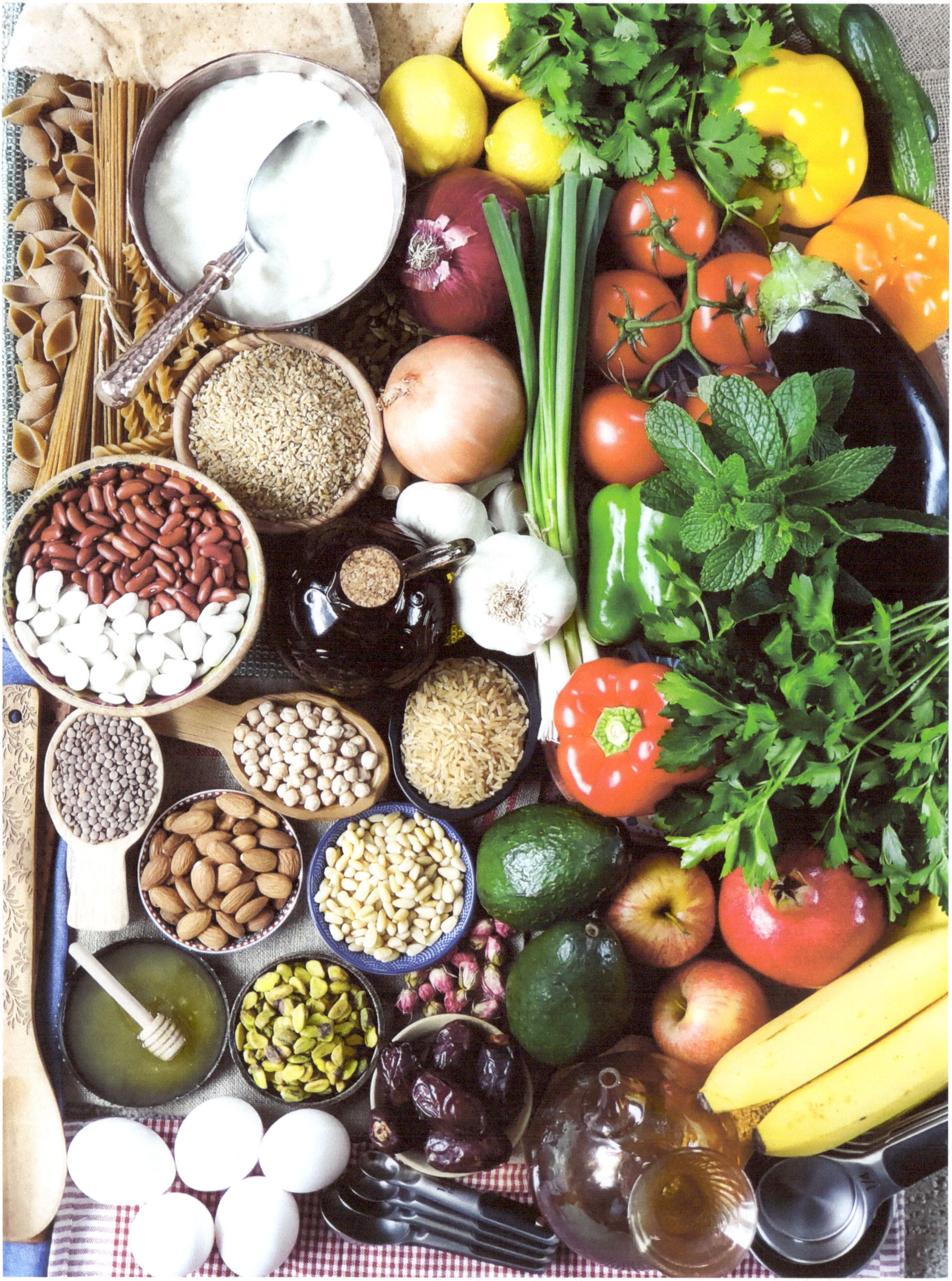

Chapter 2

ABOUT THIS COOKBOOK

No single food or lifestyle behavior can make one healthy. It is a combination of many factors together that counts the most: starting with eating mindfully, following a healthy way of eating that is food-based rather than nutrient-based, drinking plenty of water, engaging in regular exercise and physical activity, maintaining a healthy body weight, and limiting or omitting smoking as well as alcohol.

I truly believe that nutrition is not about overwhelming oneself with the mathematics of food by fretting about counting calories, fat, and carbohydrates, nor is it about always trying to lose that extra weight by following some weird dietary restraints. Eating healthy involves choosing healthy ingredients and following healthy cooking methods, combining them together to give a healthier dish or dessert. Many may jump to the conclusion that healthier food simply translates into less calories, less fat, and less carbohydrates or sugar. This may be the case for some dishes or desserts, but sometimes, a healthier dish may provide similar amounts of calories, fat, and sugar, with the health aspects/benefits coming from the different healthier ingredients used, as well as the healthier alternative cooking methods involved.

Thus, as a nutritionist, I have never been an advocate for any diet fads or nutritional dogmas, but I am a big advocate for simply following a healthier and more whole way of eating. And from here, I was inspired to create this cookbook, reproducing the fabulous flavors of many of my favorite dishes and desserts, while enriching them with a healthier and more whole profile. Research supports the idea that whole foods help in improving health and preventing chronic disease over time. Whole foods are simply foods closest to their natural form and contain very minimal or no amounts of processing (processing that can range from the refining of whole grains, to the addition of sugar to food products, to the smoking of meats), thus retaining their natural nutritional portfolio of beneficial antioxidants, phytochemicals, vitamins, minerals, and fiber. Whole foods include fresh fruit and vegetables, fresh herbs, whole grains including whole wheat products and brown rice, legumes, lentils, raw nuts, fresh eggs, unsweetened milk, unprocessed meats, and natural sweeteners (like pure raw honey). Minimal processing methods that allow for a food to remain under the umbrella of whole foods include freezing, boiling, canning, drying, roasting, crushing, milling, or pasteurization, in order to make the food suitable for storing and safe for consumption. Highly processed foods, or ultra-processed foods, often have many ingredients added to them such as salt, sugar, or fat, as well as artificial preservatives, flavors, or colors.

The various healthy and whole features of my recipes are described in the sections below.

Contain Mostly Whole Grains. Traditionally, the Lebanese cuisine incorporates many whole grain ingredients such as bulgur and whole wheat kernels. However, there is a heavy reliance on refined white flour in the making of breads and desserts, as well as a widespread consumption of refined white rice, not to mention refined pasta products. Bread and rice are staple foods in the Lebanese diet, and while whole wheat bread is gaining popularity little by little, the use of white rice as a staple ingredient for many dishes and as a side for traditional stews is still common. General recommendations advise that individuals consume more than half their grain servings as whole grains, but given the increasing health benefits associated with whole grain consumption, it is best to consume mostly whole grains instead of refined grains. As such, I have turned to using whole brown rice (mainly parboiled brown rice, as it cooks up faster and is more tender in texture once cooked than non-parboiled versions) instead of refined white rice. I have also incorporated barley and quinoa, as two protein-rich and fiber-rich whole grains, into some of my dishes. Additionally, I have completely shifted over to using whole-wheat pastas, from whole wheat spaghetti, linguini, and even lasagna in my dishes. For dishes that may call for flour as a thickening agent, to desserts and sweetbreads that use flour as a main ingredient, all flour used for recipes in my cookbook is fiber-rich and nutrient-rich whole-grain flours, including whole wheat flour as well as brown rice flour. I have, however, used some semolina flour (read more on page 17) in just a few traditional desserts that call (either completely or partially) for this kind of refined flour, as the total omittance and substitution with whole wheat flour often yielded undesired texture outcomes.

Contain Healthier Types of Fat and Less Fat. Although generally labelled as a healthy cuisine, many Lebanese dishes and desserts are notoriously high in fat, and many times, high in unhealthy fats, namely saturated fats coming from non-lean meats and full-fat dairy products, as well as added fats rich in saturated fat such as butter, ghee, and palm oil. There is also a heavy reliance on refined vegetable oils, including corn oil and sunflower oil. General recommendations advise individuals to limit their intake of high saturated fat containing foods, while incorporating heart-healthy minimally processed plant oils instead.

❋ Red Meat: is commonly added to many Lebanese dishes. Although beef is highly consumed, some like cooking with the less lean meat, lamb. I avoid cooking with lamb, and instead, turn to using extra lean and lean beef cuts. For recipes calling for beef strips, I use sirloin or round cuts which are both extra lean (at least 95% lean). For all other recipes calling for a red meat, I use extra lean ground beef. Lean beef (at least 90% lean) is also healthy to consume and includes tenderloin, flank, shank, brisket, and chuck cuts of meat. For those who enjoy cooking with lamb once in a while, aim for lean cuts of loin and leg meat (read more on page 26).

❋ Chicken: is also a common ingredient in many recipes, and although chicken is way leaner than red meat, chicken breasts are lowest in fat as compared to other parts of the chicken. As such, I mostly rely on chicken breasts in my cooking, but will use whole chickens for some dishes, namely chicken-based soups and stews. However, I always remove the skin off the white meat before serving and will skim off as much of the fat that floats to the top of the chicken broth as possible (read more on page 26).

❋ Fish: is also a healthy meat ingredient common to the Lebanese cuisine. As long as it is not fried, fish offers a very lean source of protein and healthy fats, namely the well-known omega-3 fats eicosapentaenoic acid (EPA) and docosahexaenoic acid (DHA). It is recommended to eat a variety of fish and other seafood twice a week, while limiting the consumption of contaminated seafood (read more on page 34) .

❋ Dairy Products: whether milk, yogurt, or cheese, these are commonly consumed and used as ingredients in many Lebanese dishes and desserts. Many people rely on full-fat products, but I have resorted to using skim milk and yogurt, as well as lower fat cheeses (such as part-skim mozzarella cheese and parmesan), since these offer similar amounts of protein and calcium, but much less total and saturated fat. There has been a lot of recent debate and controversy over which types of milk are best to consume: dairy (cow) milk or plant-based milks. I still prefer cooking and baking with cow milk, for reasons being the more complete nutritional profile as well as the higher versatility in both cooking and baking (read more on page 32).

❋ Added Fats: Although many Lebanese dishes contain the healthy fat, olive oil, some recipes tend to simply have too much of it. Very traditional recipes may also call for the use of unhealthy fats such as animal ghee, butter, or palm oil, and some dishes call for the frying (often deep frying) of food ingredients, such as eggplant, cauliflower, or onions. In my cooking and baking, I have limited the quantity of added fat that traditional recipes (being sweet or savory) may call for, as well as turned to using healthier types of fats. I completely rely only on vegetable oils in my cooking and baking. Many vegetable oils are available for consumption, differing mostly in their fat profile (unsaturated vs saturated fat composition), how stable they are to high temperatures of heat during cooking and baking (determined by an oil's smoke point), and how they have been extracted from their plant source (cold-pressed versus mechanically expeller pressed which often subjects the oil to high heat, versus chemically extracted with hexane usually). Oils highest in unsaturated fats remain liquid at room temperature and include oils such as olive oil, avocado oil, sunflower oil, safflower oil, corn oil and canola oil, among others, while oils rich in saturated fats solidify at room temperature and include palm oil and coconut oil. It is oils highest in unsaturated fats (polyunsaturated and monounsaturated fats) that have been consistently associated with decreased risk of chronic disease, namely cardiovascular disease, and thus are the healthiest to consume as compared to oils rich in saturated fats. Cold-pressed versions of oils are by all means the healthiest form of an oil, as the natural composition of the oil with its flavors and aromas has been preserved the most. However, these oils are often more expensive and for some types of oils (like sunflower or safflower) are not very easily available in the market. Olive oil, rich in unsaturated fats, is widely available and is always cold-pressed, making it one of the healthiest oils to consume raw and cook with, as long as no frying or high baking temperatures are followed. Refining oils makes them more stable to heat, so lightly refined olive oil (as compared to virgin and extra-virgin versions) is also good, especially for high-temperature cooking (such as roasting of vegetables). For my cooked dishes, I have resorted to using extra-virgin olive oil, since most of my cooking involves only low or medium heat. For my dessert recipes that call for a fat, I use extra-virgin olive oil or cold-pressed avocado oil, since avocado oil has a similar heart-healthy fat profile as olive oil, while being stable to higher heat temperatures (read more on avocado oil and olive oil on pages 20 and 23, respectively).

❋ **Rely on Natural Sweeteners and Contain Less Sugar.** In all my baking (as well as in my cooking), for recipes calling for a sweetener, i.e. a source of sugar, I have substituted all processed and refined sugar (whether white cane sugar, brown sugar, coconut sugar, etc.) with natural sugar sources such as fiber-rich fruit, namely dates, as well as natural sweeteners such as pure raw honey, maple syrup, and carob molasses. These natural sweeteners are rich in antioxidants and phytochemicals which are preserved if the product is raw and pure, i.e. has not been boiled or chemically treated. One should make sure to read the ingredient list to make sure it only contains honey or maple syrup or carob molasses, without any added sugar. Although these natural sweeteners contain roughly the same number of calories per teaspoon as refined sugar, they are sweeter than sugar, thus allowing to cut down on the quantity of sweetener used per recipe, hence translating into less sugar content per serving, and thus less calories. Regarding dates, I prefer using medjool dates as they are very plump, moist, and soft (thus ideal for mashing up and using whole with the skins) (read more on dates and honey on pages 21 and 22, respectively).

❋ **Contain Less Salt.** Salt is one of the most important ingredients in cooking and baking. It plays a big role in bringing out the flavor of main ingredients in savory dishes, while balancing out the sweetness in sweet dishes and desserts. It is also an ingredient added to many processed food products for enhanced flavors, preservation, and other properties. Salt, however, provides our body with sodium, which is a mineral that our body does not need a lot of, and thus, overconsumption may lead to undesirable health outcomes over the long run (namely high blood pressure, kidney disease, and stomach cancer). It is good to know that the craving for salt in food is an acquired taste, so gradually cutting down on salty food ingredients as well as added salt in cooking (and at the table) will eventually decrease one's craving over time. In my cooking, I tend to go lighter on salt and let the flavors of main seasoning ingredients such as onions, garlic, lemon juice, vinegar, spices, and/or herbs present in a certain dish to dominate. I also always chose no- or low-salt versions of processed food products such as tomato paste and soy sauce.

❋ **Contain Minimally Browned Ingredients and Rely on Healthy Cooking Methods.** Browning food ingredients (such as onions, nuts, or bread) through the practice of frying in oil is common to several Lebanese dishes. While browning any food in general often imparts a desired distinct color and delicious flavor, one should be aware that harmful food compounds are produced as a result of chemical reactions taking place inside the food, especially during cooking with higher temperatures (>120 °C or >250 °F), for extended periods, and with low moisture (as is the case of frying). Such compounds include acrylamides, advanced glycation end products, and heterocyclic amides, all of which are considered to be possibly toxic/carcinogenic to humans. Unfortunately, some of these compounds can be obtained from regular intake of certain foods (such as French fries, potato chips, toasted breads, breakfast cereals, crackers, biscuits, coffee, or processed meats), or from exposure to cigarette smoke. Thus, adopting healthier cooking methods can play a big role in decreasing our bodies' exposure to these harmful substances. Boiling, steaming, and stewing have been recommended by the American Cancer Society to be more preferable cooking methods as compared to frying, roasting, grilling, toasting, or baking. Obviously, one may need to turn to one of the latter cooking methods in the preparation of a certain food or ingredient, so let moderation guide one's cooking choices. Onions for my recipes, for instance, are often cooked with a bit of oil on low heat for about 15 to 25 minutes (depending on the dish), being mostly steamed by the vapors arising in the closed pot during cooking. If one desires to caramelize their onions, aim to stop cooking them as soon as they turn a light golden color. For browning nuts as a garnish for certain dishes, follow dry roasting in the oven until the nuts have just turned golden. When roasting or grilling food, aim for lighter brown colors. And try to limit as much as possible the scorching/burning of food, as well as frying of any food ingredient! Certain Lebanese dishes require that some vegetables, such as eggplant, cauliflower, or potatoes, be fried before incorporating them with the rest of the ingredients. I have turned to baking all ingredients (which would otherwise have been fried) and will simply add some raw olive oil to the dish, giving the same great flavor to the food, but with avoiding the unhealthy practice of frying.

Some other features of my recipes in this cookbook include the following:

❋ **Convenient to Prepare and Cook.** All my dishes call for ingredients that are mostly conveniently available. For my Lebanese dishes, one will find needed ingredients in a basic Lebanese or Middle Eastern grocery store, while all other dishes of mine will require ingredients most probably already stored in one's refrigerator or food pantry, or readily available at one's local grocery store. Depending on where you live, some ingredients, may not be currently available but always keep your eyes open, since with globalization and open trade markets, one never knows which items will become available and when.

To further add convenience to my cooking, I have turned to using a few alternative ingredients for certain recipes, such as using ready-to-buy ground beef for many of my dishes that call for red meat (thus, minimizing on preparation time of the meat, and keeping the total amount of meat minimal in a dish by having it scattered around enough for picky eaters not to mind eating. Not to mention that ground meat is faster to cook up and more easily chewable by young children and the elderly). I have also resorted to using a few frozen vegetables (mostly frozen green beans, peas, okra, and Jew's mallow), since the fresh versions of these vegetables are often very time consuming to prepare, with a lot of work needed to sort out the bad vegetables, wash, drain, rewash, and eventually chop. Having said this, fresh vegetables are by all means healthier, as frozen vegetables may lose some vitamins, minerals, and antioxidants in the process of being frozen and over time, especially if they were not immediately frozen after harvest. But if the methods of freezing were properly followed by the manufacturer, frozen vegetables can offer almost as many nutrients as their fresh counterparts. And once one starts looking through my recipes, one will find that I use plenty of fresh vegetables such as onions, garlic, tomatoes, carrots, sweet peppers, coriander, parsley, zucchini, eggplant, and lemons, striking a balance I believe in the use of fresh versus frozen vegetables in my cooking.

To save time when cooking, I recommend preparing ingredients beforehand, such as weighing, measuring, and/or washing ingredients then setting aside in the refrigerator/on the countertop when needed. I am, however, still traditional when it comes to food mixing, blending, and processing, preferring to rely on my hands for the most part. As such, you will not find me calling for the use of electric whisks when mixing dessert batters for instance. And I only call for the use of a basic blender or food processor for only certain dishes that really require a thorough blend up of ingredients.

Give a Large Yield and Are Mostly Freezer Friendly. To add convenience to my life and help myself manage my time better, I have followed my mother's way of 'cooking for a crowd'. Not only does this save me from having to cook every single day of the week, but it offers my family and me leftovers for a couple of days at least. My recipes are therefore big, yielding many servings, thus lasting a family of 3 to 5 individuals at least 2 to 3 days. This won't really help if one has got picky eaters who will not eat leftovers, but thankfully this has worked wonders for me as my husband and daughters don't mind leftovers at all. I personally prefer day-old dishes as I feel the flavors in the food get enhanced the more the food ingredients sit and marinate together with the spices and sauces. Many of my recipes are great to freeze as well, thus offering a quick home-made dish a couple of weeks or months later, while still maintaining perfect flavor and texture (freezer friendly dishes have been identified by the 'FF' symbol at the top of each recipe page).

Do Not Display 'Prep Time' and 'Cooking Time'. A feature of my cookbook that is worth noting is the absence of the summed up 'preparation time' (prep time) and 'cooking time' at the top of each recipe page. Like many, but not all, cookbooks, and unlike many online recipes, I do not present these summed up times for the following reasons. I believe each person has a certain pace at which one feels comfortable preparing food prior to cooking, such as in the process of chopping, peeling, mixing, etc. Thus, 'prep time' can be highly variable and quite relative to how one goes about doing things in their kitchen. Also, since becoming a mom, I have frequently struggled with time management, since caring for young ones is very time consuming. I have often found myself pausing several times during the preparation of a dish, due to interruptions from my children for this and that. Additionally, during the process of cooking, one can often be carrying out two cooking steps simultaneously, if one is using multiple pots on the stove for example, or deciding to start the cooking of the onions while the chopping of another vegetable is under way. Therefore, this variability can highly affect both preparation time and cooking time of a certain dish. And to add convenience to my cooking, I will often prepare various ingredients for a given dish a day in advance, thus getting straight to the cooking of the dish on the next day. Another time variable is that some people like their vegetables in certain dishes to be sautéed or stir-fried until just cooked, while others may want them cooked further until more tender. I personally rarely sauté or stir-fry my vegetables, as my family and I prefer tender (but not overcooked) vegetables that have been cooked in a pan or pot, covered, over low heat for a time period longer than that called for by sautéing and stir-frying.

Having said this, I assure you that all the recipes in this cookbook should not take up more time to prepare or cook than any other similar recipe. In my opinion, scanning the ingredients of a recipe as well as the instruction steps will give one an idea of the time it will take to prepare and cook up a dish. I will say that the cooking time of different ingredients in my cookbook is, however, clearly stated in the instructions of each recipe, and for baked goods, the baking period is also clearly indicated in the final steps of the recipe instructions.

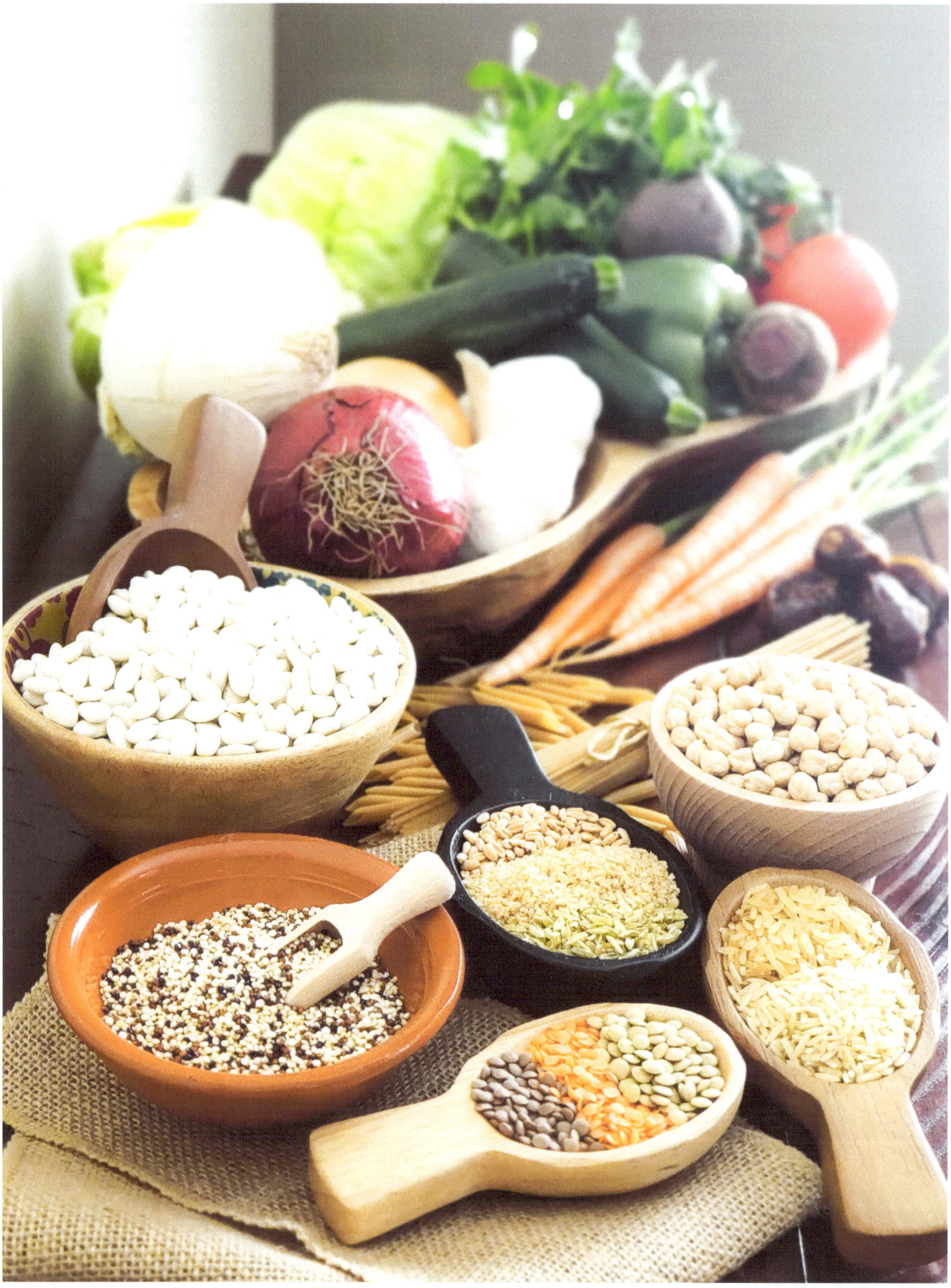

Chapter 3

FIND YOUR BALANCE

Although I am a big advocate for whole foods and I use a plentiful amount of whole ingredients in my recipes, I believe one does not need to adopt a completely whole food dietary pattern to reap health benefits and prevent chronic disease. Eliminating as many refined and processed foods from one's diet, while incorporating 'any and as many' whole foods as one can possibly find, afford, purchase, and consume is the way forward to a healthier self and healthier family. Making gradual changes to one's eating habits with time will make the transition into a healthier way of eating enjoyable and more maintainable on the long run.

You will find me calling for the use of some processed food items for some recipes (such as ketchup, tomato paste, mustard, soy sauce, or canned pumpkin), but the bottom line should not be about overwhelming oneself with only whole foods with every single ingredient or dish, but rather, to find the right balance in one's overall diet. Some processed foods can actually provide some health benefits, and are not necessarily considered 'bad' to consume. For instance, mustard products containing ground mustard seeds are also rich in antioxidants, minerals, and healthy unsaturated fats. Tomato products, such as tomato paste and ketchup, are also rich in lycopene which is a potent antioxidant present in fresh tomatoes. Reading labels for the ingredients at the back of processed food items is important because some brands contain more salt than others and some products contain high fructose corn syrup - both of which should be minimized. Additionally, choosing processed products with the least number of ingredients is recommended (i.e. closest to the natural form of the food product as possible).

With whole foods dominating a lot of dishes in this cookbook, this translates into more fiber in one's diet, coming from fruit and vegetables, legumes, lentils, whole grains, and nuts. Many high fiber foods are considered high FODMAP foods. FODMAP is an acronym that stands for: Fermentable Oligosaccharides, Disaccharides, Monosaccharides, and Polyols. These fermentable carbohydrates, found naturally in most high fiber foods, are poorly absorbed in the intestine and get rapidly fermented by bacteria in the gut. Thus, depending on how much is consumed and one's tolerance, FODMAPs can cause increased gassiness, bloating, abdominal pain, and even diarrhea for some. As such, for some individuals, too many high FODMAP foods may simply be too much for their bodies to handle, especially those who are overly sensitive to developing lose stools or bloating, and more importantly, others who suffer from more serious bowel conditions such as Irritable Bowel Syndrome, inflammatory bowel diseases, or Celiac disease. Instead of completely shying away from recipes made with whole foods and high FODMAPs, I recommend finding one's balance and experimenting to figure out the right amount of these aggravating foods that will keep one's body happy and comfortable. This may include cutting down on the quantity of onions or certain vegetables called for in a dish, or substituting part of the whole wheat flour called for in a recipe with white flour, for instance.

Eating healthy should be mindful, nourishing, enjoyable, and affordable, and I urge everyone to find the right balance that works best for one's self and family. Let balance and moderation in your food choices guide your eating habits and cooking experiences!

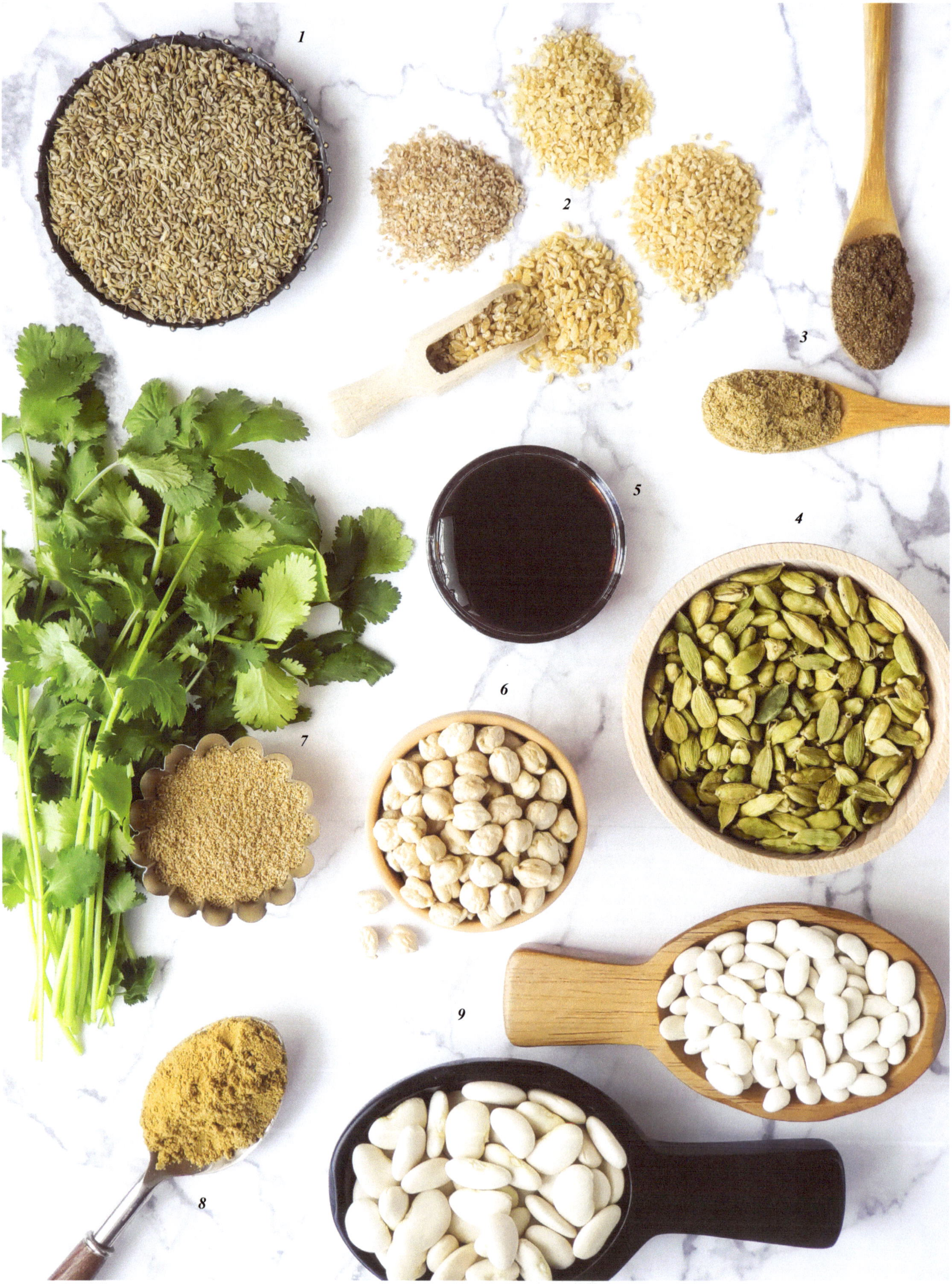
1
2
3
5
4
6
7
9
8

Chapter 4

GETTING TO KNOW SOME MIDDLE EASTERN INGREDIENTS

Below is a summary of ingredients commonly used in my recipes as well as many other recipes traditionally made in Lebanon and other Middle Eastern countries.

1. Anise Seeds. With a slight licorice flavor, these seeds are commonly used in Middle Eastern countries as an herbal tea. They are also used to flavor some desserts, added whole or ground up, or simply added as a garnish. Anise seeds are different from anise star, with the latter being stronger in flavor.

2. Bulgur. Called *burghul* in Middle Eastern countries, this common grain is a product of parboiling and then drying wheat berries that have then been ground until 'cracked'. It is a versatile ingredient of the Lebanese cuisine and is commonly consumed as a side dish with stews instead of rice (recipe on page 131). It is a famous ingredient in the world-wide known salad *tabbooli* (recipe on page 79), and is an integral ingredient for *kibbeh* dishes (recipes on pages 201 and 209). It can be purchased in different colors (light-golden or dark, based on whether it was produced from the soft lighter-colored wheat berry or the hard darker one) and textures (based on how much the berries were ground: ranging from very fine, often denoted as bulgur grade 1, to a less fine texture, grade 2, to coarser and larger textures, grades 3 and 4). All forms of bulgur are whole and are a good source of fiber, protein, and micronutrients. Cracked wheat and bulgur are often terms that are used interchangeably, although the former is produced from cracking wheat that has not been previously boiled.

3. Caraway. With a pungent flavor and aroma, this spice is used to flavor a few sweet and savory dishes of the Middle Eastern cuisine. It is most famously known for flavoring the pudding *moghleh*, traditionally made when a baby is born (recipe on page 265), as well as the savory chicken dish *moghrabiyeh* (recipe on page 191). Dark and light versions of the spice are available, based on whether the seeds were roasted prior to being ground up.

4. Cardamom Pods. Containing tiny flavorful seeds on the inside, these pods are used whole in many Middle Eastern dishes to add their wonderful flavor. Since the seeds are very pungent when bitten into and chewed, the pods are normally removed prior to serving a dish (although some people do enjoy eating them). Ground cardamom is not as commonly used in cooking, since the aromatic flavor is not as intense as that coming from the whole pods, but it is added to Turkish/Arabic coffee grounds for a different flavor.

5. Carob Molasses. Sometimes referred to as carob syrup, it is obtained from the pods of the carob tree which is native to the Mediterranean region. Lebanon is famous for the production of this nutritious dark and thick sweet syrup, which has a slight caramel-like flavor. It is traditionally mixed with *tahini* and eaten with pita bread as a dessert, and can also be used to sweeten some Lebanese desserts.

6. Chickpeas. Called *hummus* in Middle Eastern countries, these small sandy-colored legumes are commonly consumed starting with the dried (dehydrated) form of the legume, then hydrating by soaking overnight, and then boiling in water until tender. Chickpeas are the main ingredient of the famous dip *hummus bi tahini* (sometimes simply referred to as *hummus*) that has become famous all over the world (recipe on page 107). Also known as garbanzo beans in the West, they add flavor, fiber, quality protein, and iron among other nutrients to many dishes of the Middle Eastern cuisine.

7. Coriander. Commonly known as cilantro or Chinese parsley in the West, this green-leafed vegetable is a staple in many Middle Eastern stews and dishes, adding rich flavor and a boost of micronutrients and antioxidants. Dried coriander is also available and can be added to dishes, but should not substitute the fresh produce because it tastes very different.

8. Cumin. Is used in many savory Middle Eastern dishes, enriching food with flavor and aroma, while adding a boost of antioxidants and beneficial health effects.

9. Dehydrated Beans. Referred to as *fasoolia* in Lebanon, the common beans used in traditional stews include broad lima beans, cannellini white beans, and great northern beans.

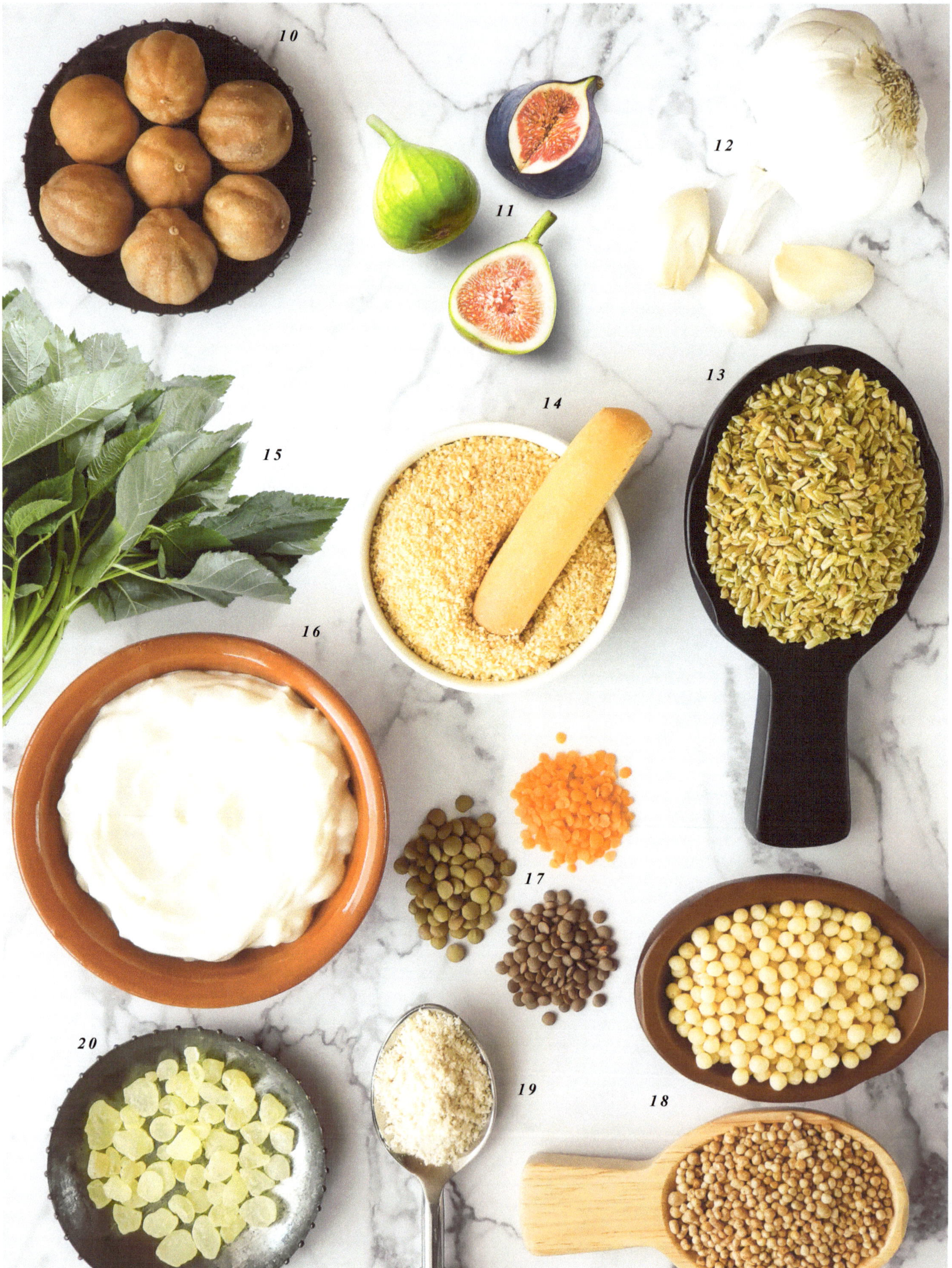
10
11
12
13
14
15
16
17
18
19
20

10. Dried Limes. Also known by the name of *loumi*, dried limes are often used whole or ground in some Middle Eastern dishes, such as *kabseh* (recipe on page 169), originally a Saudi Arabian chicken and rice dish.

11. Figs. This sweet, small, pear-shaped fruit originates from the Mediterranean region, and is available in green and black varieties that can be eaten fresh or in the dried form. In Lebanon, this fruit ripens for harvesting in the late summer months and is often turned into a jam or used in making fruit tarts.

12. Garlic. Is considered one of the most powerful, delicious staple vegetables in the Middle Eastern cuisine, taking the lead role in adding flavor and antioxidant properties to many salads, mezza foods, and dips, while often pairing up with onions to be the perfect couple of flavors in many savory dishes.

13. Green Wheat. Called *freekeh* in the Middle East, the name comes from the process by which the wheat has been harvested and processed, rather than from a specific wheat variety. Green wheat is obtained by harvesting wheat grains while still soft and green, followed by roasting and drying them. This process captures the grain at a state of high nutrition, containing a higher amount of protein, fiber and micronutrients than mature wheat. It also gives green wheat a delicious nutty flavor. Coarse cracked versions are normally used for the preparation of a main dish of the same name *(freekeh)* (recipe on page 177), while fine cracked green wheat is used in soups.

14. Ground Kaak. Common to countries of the Middle East, it is obtained by crushing *kaak*, which are simple crunchy breadsticks that are usually yeast-based and low in sugar. *Kaak* is traditionally consumed as a snack dipped in tea or hot milk, or instead of bread with cheese or *labneh* (see below). Ground *kaak* is used for breading of meats and topping savory dishes.

15. Jew's Mallow. Called *mloukhiyeh* in Middle Eastern countries, but also known as Jute Potherb or Egyptian Spinach in the West. The green leaves of this plant are commonly consumed in countries of the Middle East and North Africa, most commonly making it into a stew with the same name as the vegetable (*mloukhiyeh*) (recipe on page 187). When cooked, the leaves turn dark green and the broth can turn thick and gooey, but the flavor is quite delicious and distinct from any other vegetable. Adding lemon juice (a source of acid) to the stew decreases the viscosity produced.

16. Labneh. This tangy white paste, commonly known as yogurt cheese, is traditionally made in cheese cloths by straining yogurt of its water to reach the desired consistency. It constitutes a staple spread in a traditional Lebanese breakfast (how to make on page 29).

17. Lentils. These iron, fiber, and protein rich legumes are a staple food in the Middle Eastern cuisine. Brown, green, and red (actually orange when in dry form and yellow when cooked) versions of lentils are used, depending on the dish to be made.

18. Maftool and Moghrabiyeh. These terms refer to a wheat product that consists of small dry dough balls, somewhat like couscous, but larger, that are eaten as a side dish (recipe on page 133) with a stew of the same name (being called *maftool* in Palestine and Jordan, and *moghrabiyeh* in Lebanon and Syria) (recipe on page 191). As such, *maftool* (which translates into 'rolled'), is often referred to as Palestinian couscous, though larger in size and darker in color, and has a nutty texture given that it is made from hand rolling bulgur with whole wheat flour (although some companies may use a combination of white and whole wheat flours). *Moghrabiyeh* (which translates into 'from Morocco', possibly indicating the origin of the concept of rolled wheat balls), is often referred to as Lebanese couscous, giant couscous, or pearl couscous. It is much larger than couscous with almost a similar color, but has a softer, starchier texture as compared to *maftool*, given that it is only made from semolina flour without any bulgur. *Maftool* is therefore richer in fiber than *moghrabiyeh*, given that the fiber content of semolina flour is lower than that of whole wheat flour.

19. Mahlab. Is an aromatic spice obtained from the seeds of a species of cherry, giving a fruity but subtle flavor when added to sweets.

20. Mastic. Is an aromatic resin that comes in the form of hard and translucent droplets that are dried from the sap of the Mediterranean Mastic tree. It is crushed into smaller pieces/powder before being added to sweets and puddings for imparting an almost cedar-like flavor.

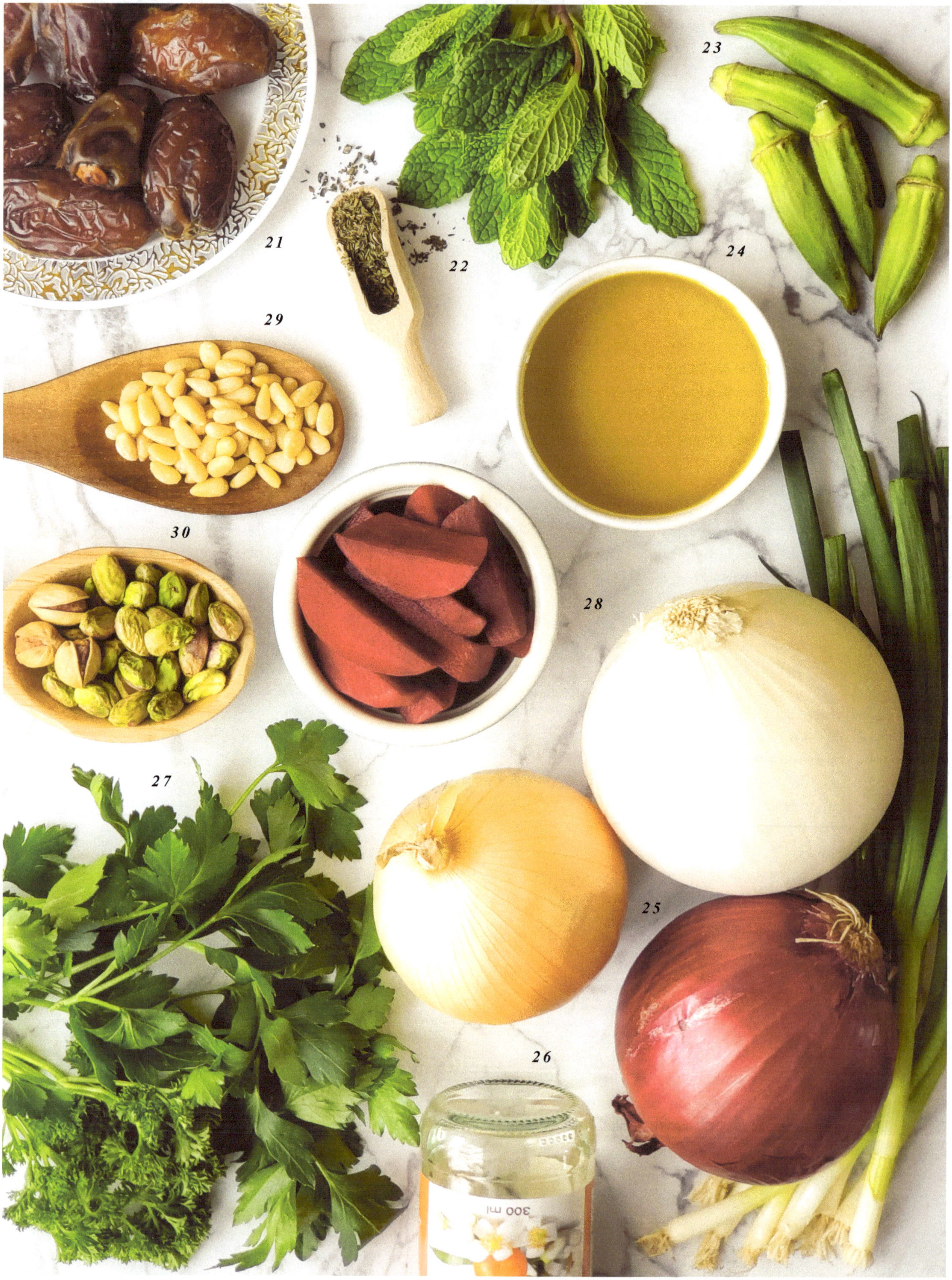
21
22
23
24
29
30
28
27
25
26

21. Medjool Dates. This nutritious fruit has been cultivated for centuries in Middle Eastern and North African countries, and was a valuable food source as well as a natural sweetener long before the introduction of cane sugar. The Medjool date variety is soft, plump and semi-dry, with a very sweet, almost caramel-like flesh, making it ideal for use as a natural sweetener in desserts.

22. Mint. Almost every household in Lebanon has a mint herb plant on their balcony or out in their garden. Fresh mint leaves are commonly eaten raw with many traditional breakfast foods, are added to salads for flavor, or are used as garnish on savory dishes. They are also often added to black tea after brewing. Crushed dry mint leaves are also highly used in the Lebanese cuisine, adding extra flavor in the absence of fresh mint leaves.

23. Okra. Low in calories and high in fiber, this vegetable (referred to in Arabic as *bamyieh*) is mostly used in two Lebanese dishes (recipes on pages 151 and 183). Like Jew's mallow, okra can turn a broth or sauce a little thick and gooey, if cut open or sliced. Traditionally, the vegetable is kept whole, and care is taken when the stem is cut off to prevent the broth from becoming viscous during cooking. If the vegetable does develop a cut, simply having lemon juice, tomatoes, or tomato paste in the dish can help prevent any sliminess from developing.

24. Olive Oil. This powerful antioxidant- and monounsaturated fat-rich oil is widely produced and consumed in Lebanon and countries of the Mediterranean region. In past generations, olive oil was largely consumed raw and in cooking. As plant-based oils started getting introduced, individuals turned to using the latter for cooking purposes, leaving olive oil mostly for raw consumption (in salads, on dips, and with *labneh*). Although years of research went by saying that olive oil should be not be used in cooking, it has now been concluded that olive oil is safe for low to moderate-heat baking and most methods of stove-top cooking except for high heat cooking for extended periods of time, frying, and deep frying (read more on page 23).

25. Onions. These antioxidant-rich vegetables are a staple in many, if not most, Middle Eastern salads and savory dishes, adding much pungent (when raw) or sweet (when cooked) flavors essential in complementing the other ingredients present in food. Onions are also the most important ingredient, alongside bay leaves and cinnamon sticks, in the making of homemade chicken broth. Green onions (also known as scallions), are also commonly added to salads and eaten with meals for adding a fresh crunch and extra flavor.

26. Orange Blossom Water. Obtained by steeping orange blossoms in boiling water, this scented water has long been traditionally used in Middle Eastern sweets to add an aromatic orange flavor. It can impart some bitterness to the food product, so care must be given with respect to the quantity added.

27. Parsley. Flat leaf parsley, also known as Italian parsley, is the common type grown in Lebanon and many other Middle Eastern countries, as compared to curly parsley (also known as French parsley), which is more common in Western countries. Both types are similar in their micronutrient and antioxidant profile. Though both can impart a strong flavor to food, curly parsley is ideal for fresh use in salads, as it is crunchier and will not wilt as fast as flat leaf parsley, which is best used for cooking purposes.

28. Pickled Turnips. Are a signature pickle in Middle Eastern countries. The beautiful dark pink color comes from beets that are pickled alongside turnips (how to make on page 30).

29. Pine Nuts. These small ivory-colored seeds are collected from the inside of pine cones, and are usually long and slender or short and plump, with very similar flavors and healthy fat profiles. The former type is native to Lebanon and countries of the Middle East, and is used to garnish and flavor sweet and savory dishes.

30. Pistachios. These healthy nuts are beloved for their striking green color and rich flavor. They are traditionally consumed in different ways: added raw or roasted in savory dishes, topping desserts or mixed into sweets, or eaten by the handful as a snack with other nuts.

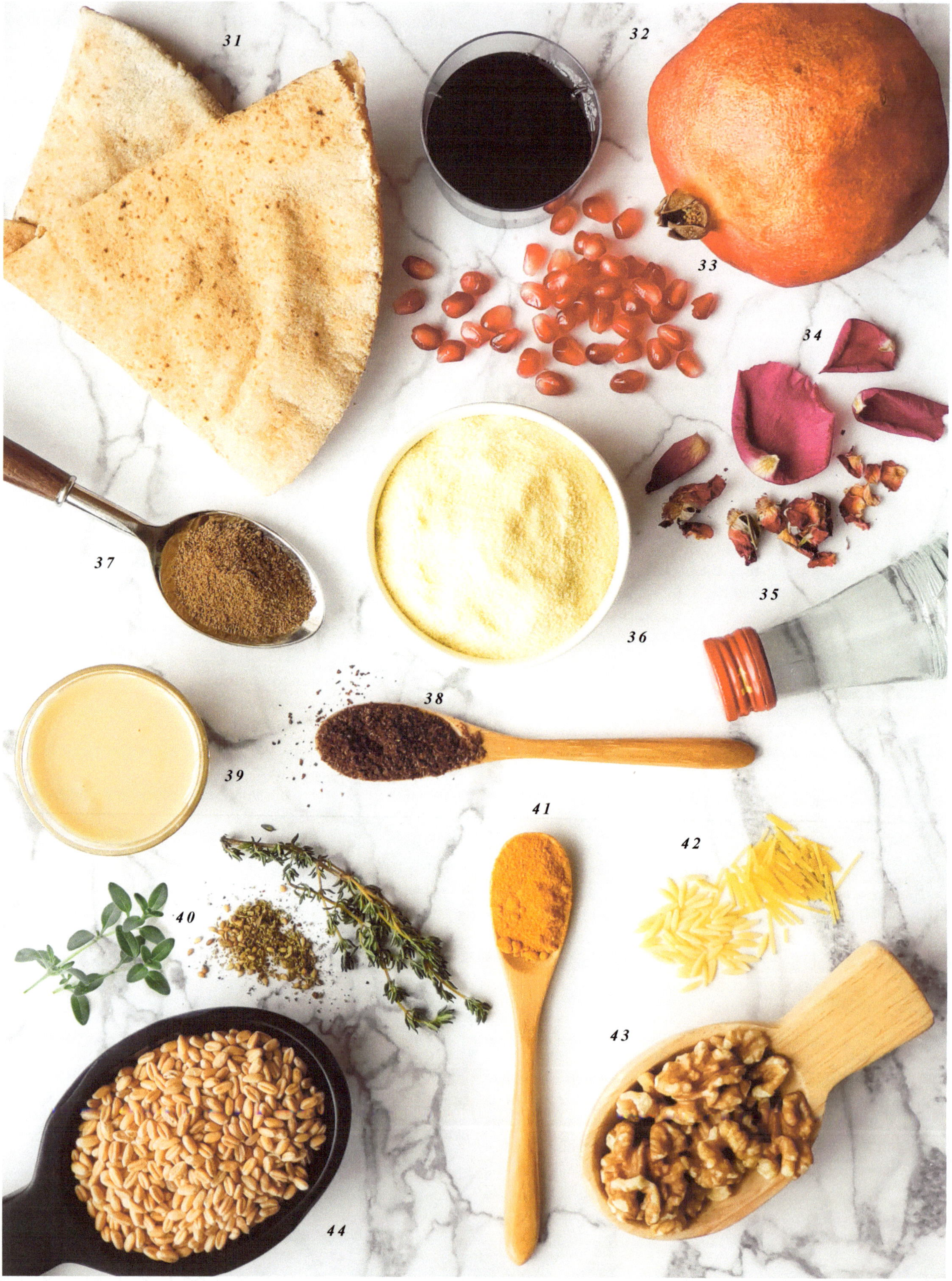
31
32
33
34
35
36
37
38
39
40
41
42
43
44

31. Pita Bread. Also referred to as Arabic bread, this circular bread with a hollow center or pocket is a staple food in Lebanon and many other Middle Eastern countries. It is commonly used to roll up sandwiches or is broken into small pieces for scooping up dips or mezza dishes. Many will also eat it instead of plain rice or bulgur alongside stews. Pita bread pieces are also traditionally fried to be mixed in with certain mezza dishes, or to top salads (namely *fattoush* on page 81).

32. Pomegranate Molasses. Is obtained from the pomegranate fruit cultivated in the Mediterranean region. The molasses is often home-made and produced by crushing the pulp-loaded seeds of the ripe red fruit, then boiling the juice for a lengthened period of time until the water evaporates, leaving behind a pungent, sour, and dark ruby red molasses ideal for use in salads and some savory dishes.

33. Pomegranate Seeds. These bright red pulp-laden seeds are commonly juiced or eaten whole, and are often added to salads or used as garnish on some dishes.

34. Rose Buds and Petals. Are dried to be used as a beautiful garnish on Lebanese sweets, especially those containing rose water. Damask roses *(joury)* are specifically used as a fragrant and flavorful garnish.

35. Rose Water. Obtained by steeping damask rose petals in boiling water, this distilled aromatic water has long been traditionally used in Middle Eastern sweets to impart a sweet rose flavor (although there is no sweetness to the water itself).

36. Semolina Flour. Is milled from the hard durum variety of wheat, which has a high protein content, but a lower fiber content (as compared to wheat varieties used for the milling of whole wheat flours). In Arabic, semolina flour is referred to as *smeed* (if it is coarsely ground) or *taheen farkha* (if it is finely ground). It is used for its slightly gritty texture and pale yellowish color in a few Middle Eastern desserts.

37. Seven-Spice Mix. Denoted as '7-Spices' mix, this is a flavorful blend of the following seven fragrant spices: black pepper, cinnamon, allspice, ginger, cloves, nutmeg, and dry coriander or mahlab (this depends on the manufacturing company). It is used in many Lebanese soups, salads, and savory dishes.

38. Sumac. A very popular spice in the Middle Eastern cuisine, non-poisonous sumac is used for its pungent tart flavor reminiscent of lemon juice. It is a nutritious spice used to flavor many salads and savory dishes.

39. Tahini. Is the paste made from ground sesame seeds, and is a vital ingredient in the making of the famous *hummus bi tahini* and *baba ghanouj* (recipes on pages 105 and 107, respectively), some Middle Eastern mezza and savory dishes, as well as *tahini* sauce (recipe on page 139).

40. Thyme. A popular plant that grows wild in the Middle East, this olive-green pungent herb is commonly consumed fresh in salads or as a garnish. The leaves dry very well, and when ground then mixed in with sesame seeds, sumac, and salt, they form *zaatar*, a traditional breakfast food eaten with olive oil and pita bread. Thyme comes in different forms, with the thin twigs and tiny leaves variety being the more common type in Western countries.

41. Turmeric. Beloved for its distinct yellow color and containing the popular antioxidant curcumin, this spice is added to savory dishes for color more than flavor. It is used for both color and flavor in the traditional Lebanese dessert *sfoof* (recipe on page 269) and some other Middle Eastern sweets.

42. Vermicelli. Is enriched semolina flour pasta rolled thin (similar to angel hair spaghetti) and cut short, that is traditionally lightly sautéed and added to plain rice or bulgur. Orzo, a rice shaped semolina flour pasta, can be used instead of vermicelli.

43. Walnuts. These nutritious nuts are traditionally consumed raw and eaten with dates and other dried fruit. They are also used to top desserts or are mixed into baked goods, as well as being used ground up for paste fillings in Middle Eastern desserts.

44. Wheat Berries. Are whole wheat kernels that have not undergone any processing or milling. Wheat berries can range from being soft white kernels to hard red versions, with various color shades of light yellow and amber between them.

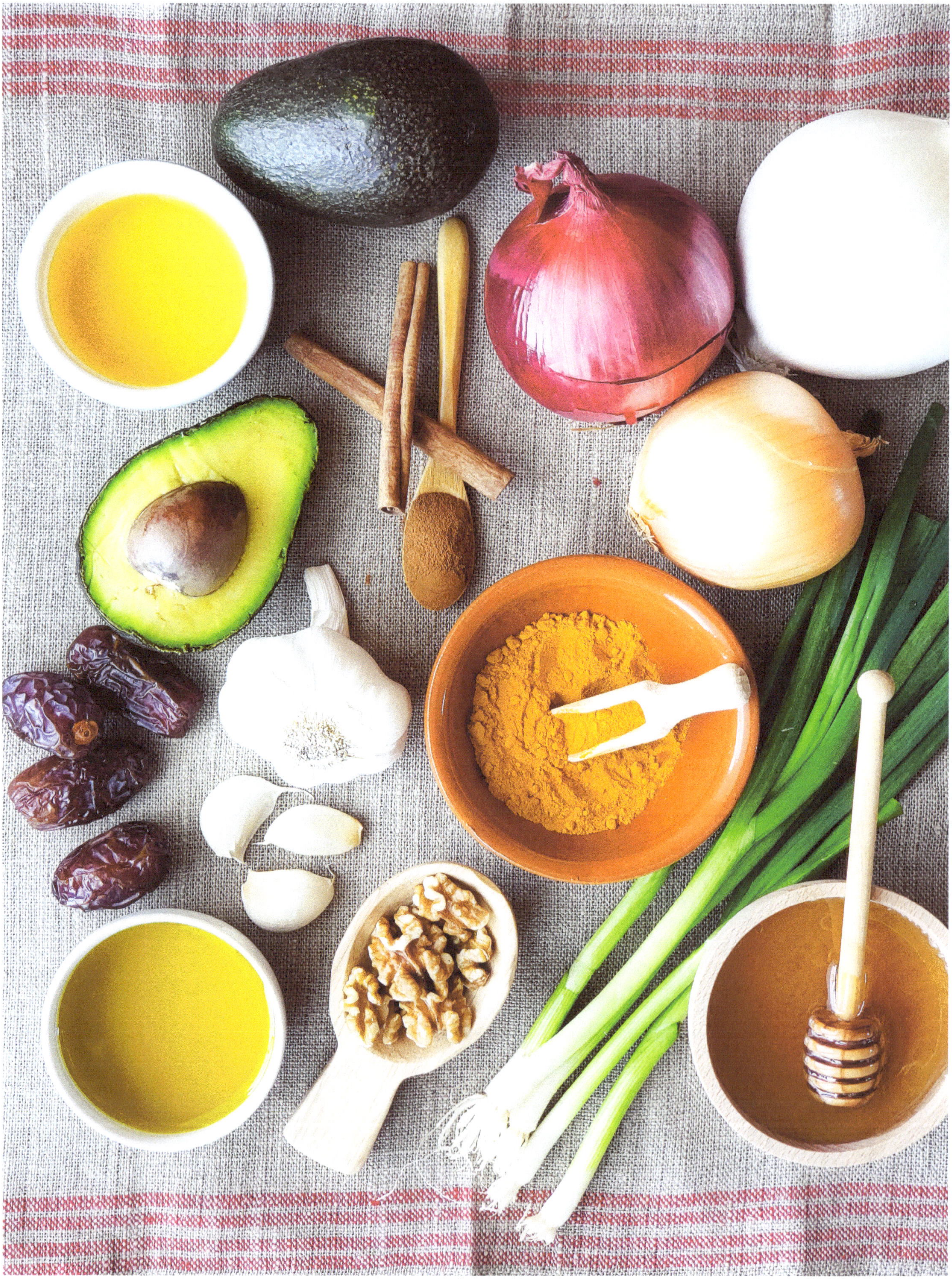

Chapter 5

MY SUPER FOODS

Many of you may have heard of or read the term 'Super Food', which actually has no scientifically-based or regulated definition. This term is, however, so widely used that the Merriam-Webster Dictionary included a definition for it, being: "a food (such as salmon, broccoli, or blueberries) that is rich in compounds (such as antioxidants, fiber, or fatty acids) considered beneficial for a person's health."

The labelling of food items or ingredients as 'Super Foods' first started long ago as a food marketing strategy and remains today a widespread means for driving sales of a specific food, more than for providing optimal nutrition recommendations. Not surprisingly though, plant-based foods often top the circulating lists of "Super Foods", given their rich nutritional profile and health-promoting benefits.

My opinion on the matter of 'Super Foods' is that one should aim for MODERATION in consuming super hyped foods, while working on including as much VARIETY in one's diet. This will ensure one is consuming all equally nutritious foods that are not as popular in the food marketing world. I could easily come up with a list of 20 or more nutritious and powerfully healthy foods that I believe should be given the "Super Foods" title, but I have narrowed the list down to 10 favorite healthy foods that I use a lot in my cooking and/or baking.

My top 10 list of 'Super Foods' includes:

1. Avocados
2. Avocado Oil
3. Cinnamon
4. Dates
5. Garlic
6. Honey
7. Olive Oil
8. Onions
9. Turmeric
10. Walnuts

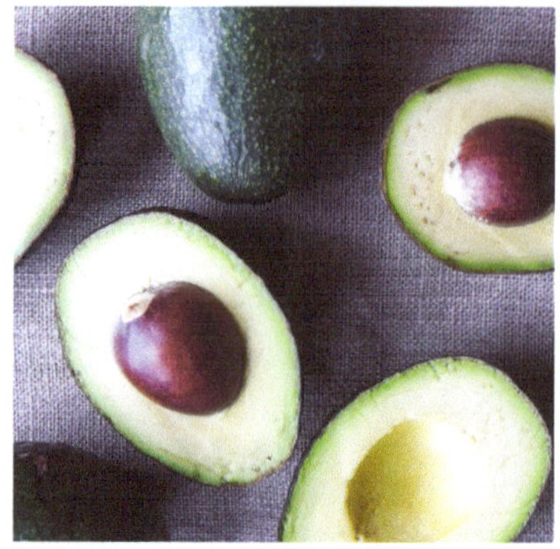

1. Avocados. Also called alligator pears, avocados were first domesticated in tropical America, but did not receive much horticultural attention until the 1990s. The avocado industry later started to flourish in Mexico and many countries of south America, before extending to other parts of the world, including California, Florida, Australia, South Africa, and recently, some Middle Eastern countries, including Lebanon and Palestine. Growing up in Lebanon, I never consumed avocados, mostly because they are not native to the Middle Eastern region. I got exposed to them as a young adult when avocados started appearing in the Lebanese market, being imported mainly from Mexico and South America. I haven't developed a taste for eating avocados plain, but once I experienced their flavor with other ingredients in salads and dips, I fell in love with them. I now use avocados in salads and in many of my desserts, for their rich and creamy flavor and texture.

Avocados are categorized as a fruit and come in many varieties, with the Californian, Mexican, and South American Hass varieties being the most common. According to the American Heart Association, avocados are now considered among the foods that may play a role in minimizing one's risk of heart disease. Research suggests that adding an avocado a day to a heart-healthy diet may decrease LDL cholesterol levels in overweight or obese people, thanks to all the heart-healthy fat present in avocados.

Regardless of the variety, one avocado on average provides around 320 calories, 30 g fats (4.3 g saturated fat, 19.7 g monounsaturated fat, and 3.7 g polyunsaturated fat), 4 g protein, 17 g carbohydrates, 14 g fiber, and minimal amounts of sugar (unlike most fruits). An avocado also provides around 20 micronutrients, including the minerals calcium (24 mg), magnesium (58 mg), potassium (975 mg), phosphorus (105 mg), sodium (14 mg), zinc (1.3 mg), iron (1 mg), and fluoride (14 μg), as well as several B vitamins (namely folate: 163 μg), and vitamin C (20 mg), vitamin E (4.2 mg alpha-tocopherol), vitamin K (42.2 μg), and vitamin A (293 IU, with 125 μg beta-carotene). Avocados also contain potent antioxidants such as xanthins and lutein.

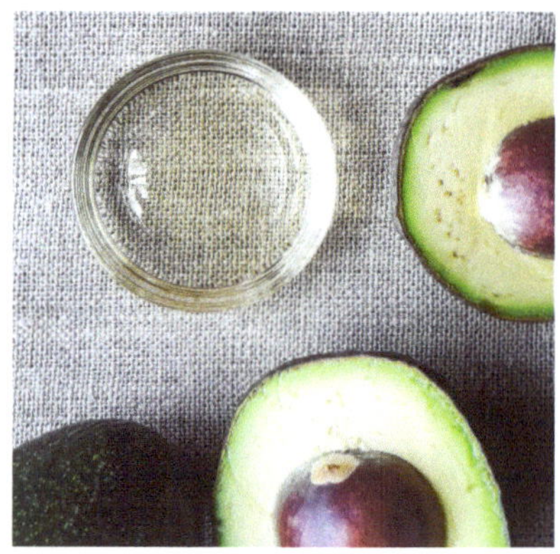

2. Avocado Oil. Since moving to the US several years ago, I came to meet this heart-healthy oil, which was first only available in specialty stores, but which is now gaining popularity on the shelves of many local grocery stores. Extracted from the pulp of the avocado fruit, this mild-tasting and light-colored oil has a very similar fat profile to olive oil, being high in monounsaturated fats, while containing some polyunsaturated fats as well. Like olive oil, it is very high in the monounsaturated omega-9 fatty acid Oleic acid, which is associated with lowering the risk of heart disease (due to its effect on lowering total cholesterol levels as well as LDL cholesterol). Aside from its healthy fat profile, one feature that makes avocado oil desirable is that it has a moderately high smoke point, which is the temperature at which an oil starts to visibly smoke when subjected to heat. When any oil reaches its smoke point, the structure of the oil starts to change, some nutrients get lost, flavor is affected, and undesirable/dangerous compounds can be formed. As such, lightly refined avocado oil is suitable for moderate-to-high heat sautéing, cooking, and/or baking (as well as frying, although I am not an advocate of frying any food).

Another reason why avocado oil is superior to other oils, is that cold-pressed versions are available in the market, as compared to the more common (and cheaper) oils on the shelves of most grocery stores which are mostly (with the exclusion of olive oil) expeller-pressed oils. As previously explained, cold-pressed versions of any oil are the healthiest, as the natural composition of the oil has been preserved the most. Other forms of oil extraction subject the oils to heat or chemicals. Extra-virgin cold-pressed avocado oil is harder to find in the market but is very similar to extra-virgin olive oil when it comes to the darker color and stronger flavor and aroma. Lightly and naturally refined avocado oils are more common and have milder sensory characteristics.

Avocado oil, like all other oils and fats, is a calorically dense food item, providing around 124 kcal per tablespoon and 14 g of fat, with a fat profile very similar to olive oil. It is low in saturated fat (1.62 g) and polyunsaturated fats (1.89 g) but rich in monounsaturated fats (9.88 g).

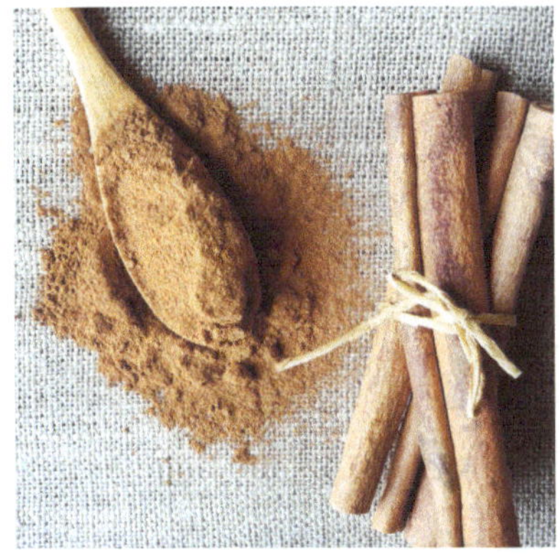

3. Cinnamon. Is a spice popularly used in Middle Eastern cuisine, and dry cinnamon sticks are traditionally used to flavor food (especially in cooking meats), or in brewing teas. I use cinnamon spice a lot, adding it to many of my savory dishes and desserts, and I always add cinnamon sticks when cooking red meat and chicken. Cinnamon comes in many types, with Cassia cinnamon (the darker-colored cinnamon native to China) being the most common type sold in the United States and Canada, while Ceylon cinnamon (native to Sri Lanka and known as "true" cinnamon) is common in other parts of the world. When purchased in grocery stores, ground cinnamon could be one of the two or a mixture of both types. Cinnamon, which is obtained from the bark of the cinnamon tree, has long been used for flavoring food, as well as for alternative medicinal purposes. Nowadays, some take cinnamon supplements to alleviate certain health conditions such as gastrointestinal problems or diabetes. Cinnamon supplements seem to be safe for most people when used on a short-term basis and in low amounts. Several reports have highlighted the numerous beneficial properties of cinnamon, including its antioxidant, antimicrobial, anti-inflammatory, anticancer, and antidiabetic properties. However, further investigations are needed before cinnamon can be prescribed for specific health conditions. Regarding diabetes management, the American Diabetes Association dismisses cinnamon's use in the treatment of diabetes, since research findings have been mixed. It is possible that cinnamon, specifically the cassia cinnamon, helps the body use insulin more efficiently, thus lowering blood sugar in people with diabetes, but further research is needed.

Cinnamon spice, like most spices, is very low in calories (19 kcal per tablespoon) and barely provides any protein or fat. It contains some carbohydrates (6.3 g) and fiber (4 g), as well as a few minerals, namely calcium (78 g), magnesium (4.7 mg), potassium (33.6 mg), phosphorus (5 mg) and iron (0.7 mg), as well as a few vitamins, mostly vitamin A (23 IU, with 8.7 µg beta-carotene), and vitamin K (2.4 µg).

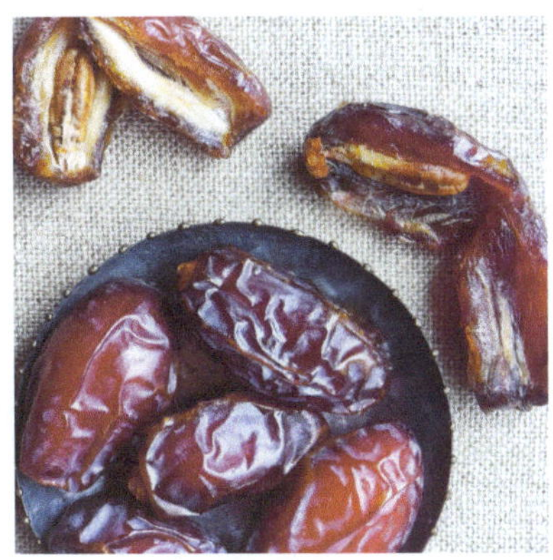

4. Dates. Date fruits are harvested from the date palm tree which is considered one of the oldest trees cultivated around the world. Dates have been a staple fruit in the Middle East and North Africa for thousands of years, and are widely grown in Egypt, Saudi Arabia, Iran, and Iraq, as well as in Algeria and Tunisia. Nowadays, dates are also grown in other countries such as India, Pakistan, Mexico, and California in the United States. The date fruit comes in numerous varieties, including medjool, deglet, khodary, and ajwa dates. I love the medjool variety for its soft, plump, and semi-dry flesh, that is very sweet and almost caramel-like, making it ideal for use as a natural sweetener in a wide variety of my desserts.

In Middle Eastern and North African culture, and specifically in Islam, dates have long been prized for their health-enhancing benefits (which have ranged from regulating bowel movement, to controlling blood sugar, aiding healthy vision, protecting against cancer, and improving cardiovascular health). Modern day science has shown that dates are indeed highly nutritious and may play a role in chronic disease prevention thanks to their healthy nutritional profile and their anti-oxidant, anti-inflammatory, and anti-bacterial properties.

Dates are energy dense fruits, with calories ranging from 20 kcal (per one deglet noor date) to 66.5 kcal (per one medjool date). Dates are generally low in fat and protein, containing varying amounts of carbohydrates (5 g for deglet noor dates and 18 g for medjool dates), and providing varying amounts of simple sugars (mostly fructose and glucose). Dates are generally regarded as low to medium glycemic index fruit. They contain a good amount of fiber (0.6 g per deglet noor date and 1.6 g per medjool date) as well as several micronutrients (values presented below are per 1 medjool date) including the minerals calcium (15.4 mg), magnesium (13 mg), phosphorus (15 mg), potassium (167 mg), and iron (0.2 mg), as well

as several B vitamins, namely folate (3.6 µg) and vitamin A (35.8 IU, with 21.4 µg beta-carotene).

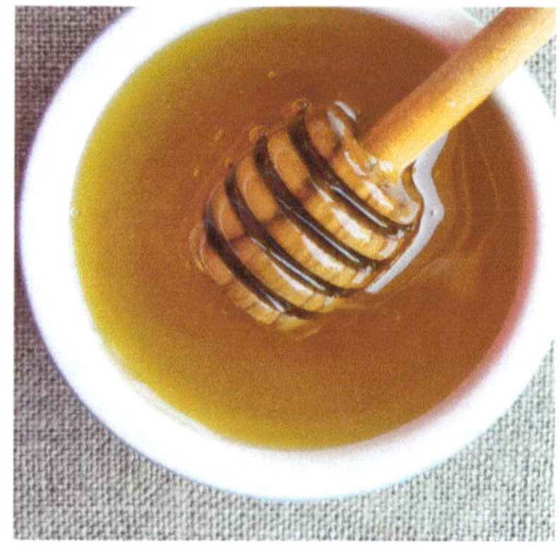

5. Honey. This sweet and viscous liquid food is one of the most valued natural products introduced to humans. Honey is made by honeybees from the nectar of flowers, and comes in many flavors, colors, and thicknesses. I rely on pure and raw honey as the main sweetener for my baked goods, eliminating the need for any refined and processed sugars. I love using wildflower honey for its milder flavor and lighter color, but one can let their personal taste guide them in their choice of honey. Almost all honey will granulate and develop sugar crystals with time, turning from a liquid to a semi-solid state, especially if pure and raw. Quite often, honey crystallization is thought to indicate poor quality, bad storage conditions, or adulteration with water and added sugar, but the opposite is true. Crystallization is a natural process that occurs in pure and raw honey (i.e. untreated and unfiltered honey). The time it takes for honey to crystallize depends on several factors, including the type of honey itself, the surrounding weather (colder temperatures favor crystallization), and the presence of pollen, beeswax, or even dust particles in the honey. I will often follow the harmless method of slowly liquefying my honey by placing the jar in a warm water bath or by placing it in the microwave for a few seconds for a faster liquefication process.

Mentioned in both the Qur'an and Bible, honey was almost the only source of sugar in ancient times and was used by many ancient civilizations, including the Egyptians, Babylonians, Greeks, and Chinese, for its nutritional and medicinal benefits. Holistic practitioners nowadays regard honey as one of nature's best remedies thanks to its antioxidant, antibacterial, and anti-inflammatory properties. In general, the darker the honey color and the stronger the flavor, the better its health powers. Honey has been shown to have mild antiseptic properties and has been used in stimulating the healing of wounds. A specific type of honey called Manuka honey, which is produced in New Zealand, is used to treat chronic leg ulcers and pressure sores. Honey has shown potential in alleviating coughs, especially among children, and may act as a prebiotic and help control certain viral infections. Much research is needed before honey can be prescribed to treat certain health conditions, but study findings are promising. It is important to note that pediatricians strongly caution against the feeding of honey to newborns and infants (below the age of 1) to avoid any risk of botulism, since this vulnerable age group doesn't have a fully developed gastrointestinal tract and a strong immunity to fight the spores of the botulism bacteria that may have found their way into the honey from dust or soil.

With respect to diabetes management, honey doesn't affect blood sugar differently than refined white sugar. However, honey has a higher sweetening power than sugar (being mostly comprised of the simple sugars fructose and glucose, the former of which is sweeter than sucrose, which is the complex sugar making up granulated sugar). This means one can use almost half as much honey as sugar, which can translate into less carbohydrates and calories.

On average, 1 tablespoon of honey supplies 64 kcal and 17 g carbohydrates (as compared to around 49 kcal and 13 g carbohydrates for white granulated sugar). Aside from being rich in carbohydrates, honey does not provide any protein, fat, or fiber. It does, however, contain some potassium (11 mg) and small amounts of calcium (1.3 mg), with trace amounts of other micronutrients.

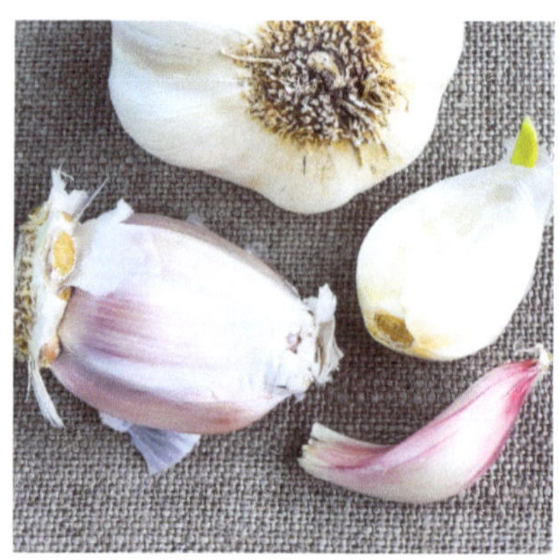

6. Garlic. This mighty vegetable is related to onions, leeks, and chives, and is a long-time kitchen staple for many cuisines, including the Middle Eastern cuisine. Possibly originating in central Asia, garlic was widely used in India and Egypt, and is currently grown around the world, being added to food for flavor but also for health benefits. Garlic contains a compound called alliin, which upon the crushing or chopping of garlic, is enzymatically converted to another compound, allicin, which is mostly responsible for the sulfurous smell and flavor of garlic. It is believed that allicin provides many of the antioxidant and anti-inflammatory properties of garlic, but many more compounds in garlic may be adding to its health benefits.

Garlic has long been consumed to boost one's immunity and treat/prevent many health conditions related to the common cold, bacterial and fungal infections, conditions related to the heart and circulatory system, as well as certain types of cancer. While claims about garlic's health-promoting benefits are not fully proven by science, garlic consumption (whether in raw or supplement form) has been shown to be possibly effective in preventing atherosclerosis with aging, decreasing blood sugar and thus controlling diabetes, reducing total cholesterol and the bad LDL cholesterol (in individuals with high blood cholesterol), lowering high blood pressure, and decreasing the risk of certain cancers especially those affecting the prostate, colon, rectum, and stomach.

Consuming garlic raw is best for maximizing its benefits, as heat and water inactivate sulfur enzymes within the garlic, but cooked garlic and supplemental powder forms still retain a lot of beneficial power.

A teaspoon of raw crushed garlic contains only 5 kcal, with barely much protein, fat, or carbohydrates, but it provides a few important micronutrients namely calcium (5 mg), phosphorus (4 mg), potassium (11 mg), magnesium (1 mg), and vitamin C (1 mg).

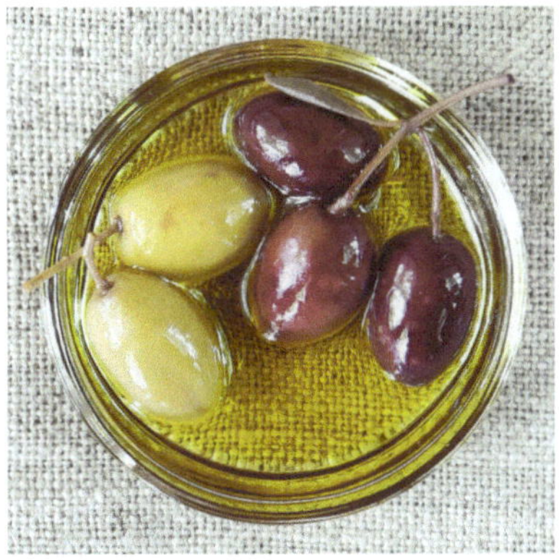

7. Olive Oil. Is the oil extracted from the fleshy part of the olive fruit. The majority of the world supply of olive oil is produced in countries of the Mediterranean region richest in olive trees, specifically Italy, Spain, Greece, and Tunisia, with some production occurring in other parts of the world including California, South America, and Australia. Olive oil is a central component of culinary cooking in the Mediterranean region and is also used in the preservation of certain foods (such as olives and *labneh*), and in the production of traditional Middle Eastern olive oil soap.

The color of olive oil varies widely, depending on whether the oil was extracted from ripe or unripe olives - ranging from clear yellow to golden for the former, with more common varieties having a greenish tinge for the latter. The flavor and odor of olive oil can vary as well, depending on where the olive trees are grown, as well as the ripeness condition of the harvested olives. Olive oil is normally classified into four grades, based on the purity of the pressed oil. Extra-virgin olive oil is obtained from the first mechanical cold pressing of olives, without further treatment, and meets a high chemical standard with a very rich flavor and odor, and has a very low free fatty acid content. Virgin olive oil is also derived from the first pressing of olive pulp, but is of a slightly lower chemical standard, possessing a less strong taste and odor, and has a bit higher free fatty acid content. Refined or commercial olive oil is obtained from subsequent pressings of residual olive pulp with hot water and have a higher acid content, and is often further refined to remove acid, color, and/or odor. Pure or edible olive oil is usually a mixture of both refined and virgin olive oils. When it comes to the use of olive oil in the kitchen, since extra-virgin olive oil has a low smoke point (the temperature at which an oil begins to smoke and breakdown, causing it to lose some of its nutritional value and impart an unpleasant flavor due to the undesirable compounds released), it is best for use in cold dishes and recipes that are prepared using low heat. Virgin and refined versions of olive oil are best for use in cooking at higher temperatures, although it is recommended to keep the heat no higher than medium to medium-high temperatures when using olive oils. For higher temperature cooking or frying, it is better to use avocado, sesame, soybean, or peanut oils, since these have very high smoke points.

Olive oil has long been used to treat many health conditions such as constipation, high cholesterol, ear infections, arthritis, and skin conditions including wounds, minor burns, and eczema. It has been used in the pharmaceutical industry for medicinal purposes and is nowadays also used in the making of supplements. It is olive oil that is at the heart of the famous Mediterranean diet which is associated with beneficial cardiovascular health. Olive oil is not only rich in heart-healthy monounsaturated fatty acids and low in saturated fats, but is also high in antioxidants, namely vitamin E, and healthy polyphenols. Studies of olive oil consumption (particularly extra-virgin oil) have shown positive associations with lowered risk of cardiovascular disease (by way of lowering cholesterol and blood pressure) and type 2 diabetes, as well as Alzheimer disease and breast cancer. It has been shown that one gains these health benefits mostly if saturated and trans fats in one's diet are replaced with olive oil and other unsaturated fat sources.

To reap the health benefits of olive oil, like most other oils, it is best to keep it stored in an airtight and dark container, away from light and humidity, in order to prevent it from going rancid (especially important for extra-virgin olive oil).

Olive oil, like all other oils and fats, is a calorically dense food item, providing around 120 kcal per tablespoon and 13.5 g of fat, with the majority being monounsaturated fats (9.85 g). Olive oil is also a source of vitamin E (1.94 mg alpha-tocopherol) and vitamin K (8.13 µg).

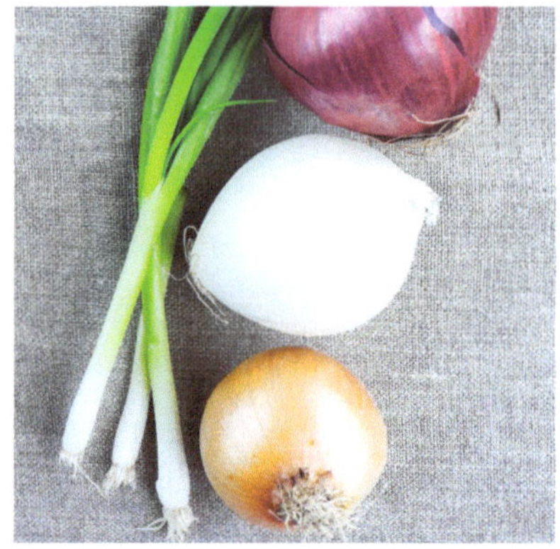

8. Onions. Onions are among the oldest cultivated vegetables around the world. They were worshiped by the ancient Egyptians and symbolized eternity because of their concentric circles on the inside. Likely native to southwestern Asia, onions are now grown all over the world. These powerful vegetables are valued for their rich flavor and are a staple in Middle Eastern cooking. There are a number of commercial onion varieties - my favorites include the strong-flavored yellow, white, and red globe-shaped onion varieties for cooking or use in salads, as well as the milder-flavored young green onions (also known as scallions or spring onions), for salads or use as a crunchy garnish.

The characteristic pungency of onions is the result of the release of sulfur-rich compounds within the onion pulp following the peeling, then slicing/chopping of the vegetable. Although there are plenty of tricks and tips to ward off tears, such as frequently wiping the knife with a piece of bread, chewing gum while cutting an onion, keeping the root ends of the onion on and intact until the rest of the onion has been sliced/chopped, the ones that work best for me are: chilling the onion in the refrigerator prior to slicing/chopping, followed by wearing sunglasses as a physical barrier for the eyes (make sure to go light on the shades so as to see properly while handling a knife).

Onions are rich in powerful phytochemicals and antioxidants, and curative properties have been attributed to these vegetables throughout the centuries. In folk medicine, onions were used for treating various health conditions such as the common cold, earaches, laryngitis, animal bites, and skin burns. Modern day science suggests that onions may play a role in reducing inflammation, improving blood pressure, decreasing blood sugar, lowering bad cholesterol, and protecting against cancer. However, more evidence is needed before onions and onion extracts can be medically prescribed for specific health conditions.

From a nutrient perspective, onions are very low in calories (40 calories per 100 g of raw onions), partly due to their high water content. Onions contain very little fat and protein, but provide some carbohydrates and fiber (around 9 g and 1.7 g in 100 g, respectively), as well some micronutrients, including vitamin C (7.4 mg), folate (19 µg), calcium (23 mg), potassium (146 mg), phosphorus (29 mg), and magnesium (10 mg).

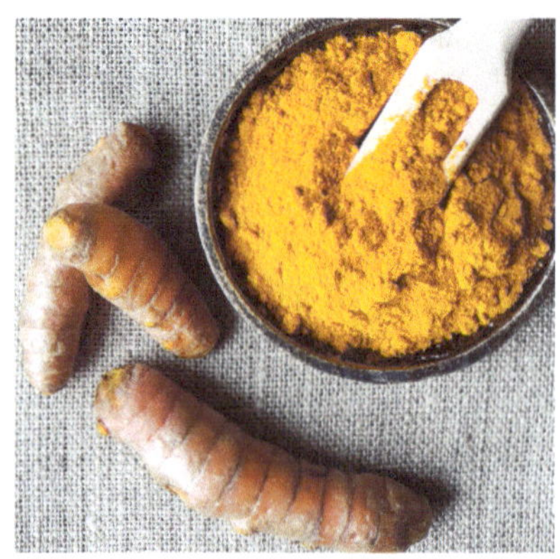

9. Turmeric. Is a spice that comes from the tuberous underground stems of the herbaceous turmeric plant which belongs to the ginger family. It is native to southern India and Indonesia, and is widely cultivated in the Indian Ocean region. In ancient times, turmeric was used as a spice and perfume, loved for its slightly bitter and warm taste, and strong pepperlike aroma. Turmeric contains compounds called curcuminoids, with curcumin being the most widely known, and these impart the strong staining yellow-orange color. It is turmeric that is added to curry powders and sometimes mustards to impart color and flavor.

Turmeric has long been reputed to have anti-inflammatory properties, and is often consumed as a spice, tea, or supplement to treat conditions such as arthritis and intestinal problems. Curcumin and other compounds in turmeric are mostly responsible for the anti-inflammatory properties of turmeric. Studies show possible benefits of turmeric in lowering blood triglyceride levels and cholesterol, decreasing non-alcoholic fatty liver disease, and minimizing symptoms of itching (in patients with long-term kidney disease), hay fever, and depression. Research continues on the role of turmeric in treating many health conditions including certain types of cancer (namely colon cancer), preventing type 2 diabetes, relieving symptoms of Crohn's disease as well as irritable bowel syndrome, and reducing pain (such as post-surgery pain and premenstrual pain).

Pairing turmeric with black pepper in cooking is ideal, as this enhances the absorption of curcumin. For those interested in turmeric supplements, make sure to choose those containing turmeric 95% curcuminoids in addition to black pepper extract (usually indicated as BioPerine).

Ground turmeric spice contains 29 calories and almost 1 g of protein per tablespoon, with around 6 g of carbohydrates, 2 g of fiber, and very little fat (0.3 g). It contains an array of minerals, namely calcium (15.8 mg), magnesium (19.6 mg), phosphorus (28.1 mg), potassium (196 mg), iron (5.17 mg), sodium (2.54 mg), and manganese (1.86 mg). It also contains some vitamins, namely folate (1.88 µg), vitamin K (1.26 µg), and vitamin E (0.42 mg alpha-tocopherol).

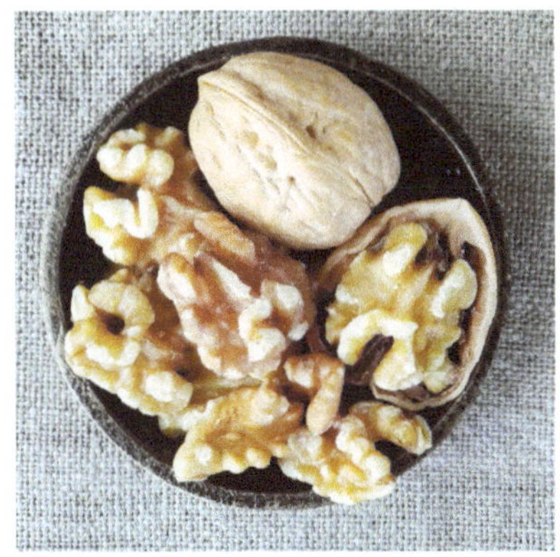

10. Walnuts. These famous bumpy golden-brown nuts, known for their brain-like shape and hard outer shell, are native to countries of North and South America, southern Europe, Asia, and the West Indies. Walnuts originated in Persia (Iran) and spread throughout Asia and Europe. There are many species of the nut, with the black walnut, native to North America, and the English/Persian walnut, native to Iran, among the most common types. The latter type of walnuts are members of the Juglandaceae family, and in ancient Rome, walnuts were referred to by their Latin name, 'Juglansregia', which translates into "Jupiter's royal acorn."

Nuts in general are an important part of the heart-healthy Mediterranean diet, and previous studies have shown that populations with higher nut consumption have lower rates of cardiovascular disease and cardiovascular risk factors, such as lower blood pressure and cholesterol levels. Walnuts particularly are among the healthiest of tree nuts, being low in saturated fat, high in polyunsaturated fats, and the richest tree nut in alpha-linolenic acid (omega-3) acid, thus imparting anti-inflammatory effects that keep blood lipids low and protect blood vessels from atherosclerosis. Studies assessing the consumption of walnuts have shown favorable outcomes in regards to lower total and LDL cholesterol, as well as lower triglycerides. Research has also shown that walnut consumption can help manage chronic diseases such as the metabolic syndrome and diabetes, improve cognitive function and memory, lower risk of Alzheimer's disease and dementia, and lower risk of certain types of cancer.

To reap the biggest heart-healthy benefits of walnuts, it is best to choose unsalted and raw or dry-roasted versions of the nut. Since walnuts have a high oil content which causes them to go rancid faster when exposed to air and heat, it is best to keep them stored in airtight containers placed in the refrigerator or freezer.

Walnuts, like most nuts, are nutritionally dense, providing per ounce of walnuts (around 14 halves or 7 whole walnuts) 185 calories, 18.5 g fat, 4.3 g protein, 3.9 g carbohydrates, and 1.9 g fiber. Walnuts are low in saturated fats (1.7 g) and contain some monounsaturated fats (2.5 g), but are highest in polyunsaturated fats (13.4 g), with around 2.6 g of omega-3 alpha-linolenic acid. Walnuts also contain an array of vitamins, namely folate (27.8 µg), vitamin A (5.7 IU, with 3.4 µg beta-carotene), and different forms of vitamin E (with gamma-tocopherol in the highest concentration: 5.9 mg). Walnuts also contain many minerals, especially calcium (27.8 mg), potassium (125 mg), phosphorous (98 mg), and magnesium (45 mg).

Chapter 6

GOOD-TO-KNOW FACTS AND TIPS

Arabic (Pita) Bread. Traditionally, the popular flour used in Lebanon and other Middle Eastern bakeries for making this flatbread was refined white flour. Nowadays, more bakeries are using whole wheat flour as well. However, some bakeries tend to 'cheat' their customers (to save on cost) by adding carob molasses to give a dark color to the bread, while using only refined flour. Many bakeries, including Middle Eastern bakeries within the US, tend to mix whole wheat flour with refined white flour in the making of their 'whole wheat' Arabic bread. Loaves of Arabic bread vary in size and thickness. The most common sizes are the small loaf (~ 18 cm in diameter) which usually is baked thick, medium loaf (~ 23 cm in diameter), and the large loaf (~ 35 cm in diameter). Traditional Lebanese loaves of Arabic bread are normally thin, and it is the thin medium-sized loaf that I use/call for in my recipes.

Baking Powder. Is a leavening agent that comes in two main types: fast, single-acting baking powder, and slow, double-acting baking powder. The latter is the more common type available to consumers in grocery stores in the US. Double-acting baking powder contains baking soda and other acids; one acid that starts reacting in the cold batter or dough in the presence of moisture, with another acid reacting once exposed to heat in the oven. Products prepared with single acting baking powder should be placed in a preheated oven right away. Some double-acting baking powders contain small amounts of aluminum (which is part of the acid ingredients), but this is unlikely to be a cause for concern. If one runs out of baking powder at home, one can mix a ¼ teaspoon baking soda, ¼ teaspoon cornstarch, and ½ teaspoon cream of tartar for each teaspoon of baking powder called for.

Baking Soda. Is a leavening agent that starts working when exposed to moisture. It works best in baked goods that contain a source of acid, such as yogurt, buttermilk, vinegar, molasses, honey, citrus juice, and cocoa. Any batter or dough that contains baking soda should be placed in the oven as soon as possible after being mixed. Baking soda is almost 4 times stronger in leavening than baking powder, which means only ¼ teaspoon of baking soda is needed in place of 1 teaspoon of baking powder to raise a batter (as long as an acid source is present).

Beef. No matter the cut of beef one is using, always try to trim off as much visible fat as possible when cutting the meat. If using ground beef that is not extra lean or lean, drain away as much of the juices as possible post-cooking to decrease the saturated fat content of the meat.

Butter. This fat has received much hype in the past years, I believe mainly because it contains 'butyric acid', a saturated fatty acid that doesn't lead to atherosclerosis like most other saturated fats do. In fact, growing research shows that butyric acid may be linked to improving intestinal health and decreasing colon cancer! However, it is important to note that butyric acid is synthesized by the good bacteria living in our intestines following the ingestion of dietary fiber. Also, the amount of butyric acid found in butter or ghee for instance is very small as compared to what our intestines make. Not to mention that butter is actually not the sole dairy product that contains butyric acid; milk and parmesan cheese contain it, too. In the end, butter remains a fat, since it is a solid at room temperature, that is mostly made up of unhealthy saturated fats, which can negatively affect cardiovascular health outcomes, as compared to heart-healthy unsaturated fats, such as olive oil or avocado oil. The American Heart Association recommends that butter (and other high-saturated fats such as ghee and lard) be used/consumed in limited amounts. If one wants to improve their gut health, simply eat healthier fiber-rich foods as well as probiotic-containing foods!

Chicken Broth. After boiling a chicken, use a broth fat separator to discard as much of the top fat layer as possible before using the chicken broth in soups, stews, or other dishes. If not using a broth fat separator, place the broth in the fridge and skim off the fat layer with a spoon once it has hardened. The simple recipe I follow for making my own no salt and low-fat homemade chicken broth is as below.

1. Ingredients: 1 small whole chicken (~ 1.5 kg, raw), 14 cups water, 2 medium yellow onions (peeled and halved), 2 celery stalks, 10 whole dry bay leaves, 8 whole black peppercorns, 6 whole cloves, 4 whole allspice seeds, 2 large rolled cinnamon sticks, 1 whole nutmeg seed, and 1 teaspoon of whole dried rosemary.
2. Discard the bag of giblets that comes inside the chicken. Place the ingredients in a large pot (making sure to place the chicken breast facing downwards), cover, and bring to a boil on high heat.
3. Turn down to low and boil for 1 hour.

4. Remove the chicken and strain away the whole spices, herbs, and vegetables (gently squeeze and save as much juice that drains away from these before discarding).
5. Separate the fat layer as much as possible and discard.
6. Divide up the broth (yield: ~ 14 cups) into separate labelled containers as desired and freeze what is not used on the spot.

Note: Bay leaves, also known as laurel leaves, are used in Middle Eastern countries when cooking red meat and chicken, as it is believed they off-set any unpleasant scent or flavor the meat could impart. Dry bay leaves are usually used and are then removed from the dish after cooking.

Chickpeas. Since there are two varieties of chickpeas (smaller, tougher, and darker skinned chickpeas versus larger, softer, and lighter skinned chickpeas), these dried legumes tend to vary in the way they absorb water when soaked and cooked. The later variety is more common among Middle Eastern countries, and it is this lighter (whiter) version that I like using in dishes that call for chickpeas. However, differences in cooked chickpea textures can be noticed as well from brand to brand, and in between countries. Thus, dishes calling for chickpeas may vary slightly in terms of yield because of this.

Coconut Oil. This fat has received much hype in the past years, mostly due to the fact that it contains some medium chain triglycerides (MCTs), which are less atherogenic saturated fats, and can actually help raise good cholesterol (HDL) levels. However, for as good as this sounds, there remain some facts that downplay this positive aspect of coconut oil. For one thing, coconut oil is very high in saturated fat (about 80 to 90%) - even higher than butter. Also, MCTs make up only a small amount of the saturated fats found in commercial coconut oils, and if one wants to reap the health benefits of MCT, one would really need to take supplements. In the end, coconut oil is a fat that can negatively affect cardiovascular health outcomes, as compared to heart-healthy unsaturated fats, such as olive oil or avocado oil. The American Heart Association recommends that coconut oil be used only sparingly. I believe if one wants to benefit from the coconut plant, it is best to eat the coconut meat or drink coconut milk/water, instead of consuming processed and refined coconut oil. I like using coconut oil only for the greasing of my baking pans as it spreads on well and prevents any sticking of the baked good. I also use it on my hair and skin for moisturizing purposes.

Coriander. When using it in cooking, make sure to retain as much as possible of the plant - only discarding the dry/damaged ends of the lower thick stems, since the stems contain almost as many healthy compounds as the leaves. However, I have noticed that within the US, grocery stores sell coriander bunches differently, with some selling it with the whole long stems intact, while others selling the bunches with half of the stems cut off. For standardization purposes, and given that a lot of the lower halves of the long coriander stems may be thick and woody, with lots of damaged dry sections, I will always cut the very long stems in half, discarding the bottom half. Fresh coriander freezes well, so I will often have chopped coriander in the freezer ready to use when needed. As most of my dishes that contain coriander call for 2 bunches, I normally prepare packages with 2 coriander bunches (washed, drained, patted dry, finely chopped) to freeze for future use.

Corn. Since fresh sweet corn is not always in season, I will often turn to using canned sweet corn. On average, 1 medium cob of corn equals 1 cup of cut boiled corn kernels. When choosing canned corn, make sure to go with brands that contain no added sugar or preservatives. Frozen sweet corn kernels are also a good replacement for fresh or canned corn kernels.

Cucumbers. When it comes to salads calling for cucumbers, I always use Middle Eastern cucumbers, also known as Persian cucumbers. They are slender and short, with a thin, smooth, and edible skin, and contain very few, if any, developed seeds. These cucumbers are rich in flavor and add a wonderful crunch to salads.

Dates. While it may not happen often, it is not uncommon for dates to attract small pests that can find their way inside the drying fruit and lay their eggs. Always check the inside of dates when opened for small brown specks and/or tiny pests (usually already dry and dead). One bad date in a batch, though, does not indicate that the rest are bad. It could be the only one or one among a couple or a few. Also, some dates may be very dusty. So, it is best to rinse, then pat dry before consumption.

Flaxseeds. These seeds are rich in fiber and heart-healthy omega-3 fats. Since flaxseeds have a very hard coat, it is best to consume them ground up, as this form is easier to digest. Whole flaxseeds may pass through our intestines undigested, which means we wouldn't be obtaining much of their nutritional benefits. Flaxseeds grind up best using a food blender (not a processor) or a coffee bean grinder.

Garlic. After crushing (pounding or pressing) garlic for stews or other dishes, set it aside for around 15 minutes before adding it to the pot, to maximize the formation of Allicin, the main biologically active component of garlic with anti-inflammatory and anti-oxidant properties. The longer the garlic sits after crushing, the more Allicin is formed by enzymatic activity inside the garlic. Always remember to scrape the garlic press very well if following this method of crushing garlic, since you don't want to lose any of the garlic flesh. Adding the called-for-quantity of salt in a recipe to the crushed garlic helps melt the garlic into a smoother paste (best to use a fork to mash up), so this step is highly recommended, especially when using garlic in salads, dips, and sauces. 2 small garlic cloves on average yield 1 teaspoon of crushed/pound garlic; 3 medium garlic cloves yield around 1 tablespoon.

❋ **Greek Yogurt.** The term 'Greek yogurt' was first popularized by a yogurt company located in Greece, but then the term became internationally used by other companies worldwide. Greek yogurt is thicker as compared to regular yogurt, since it contains less water and more protein. Depending on the brand, 1 cup of Greek yogurt can provide between 17 g to 22 g of protein, while a cup of regular yogurt normally supplies 8 g of protein. Although some companies may add dry milk powder to the liquid milk during the production of Greek yogurt to give it a thicker texture and higher protein content, most companies nowadays produce Greek yogurt by straining away some water and liquid whey to thicken the texture and bump up the protein content per volume. As such, some refer to Greek yogurt as yogurt cheese (read more below in *labneh*). Similar to *labneh*, Greek yogurt is usually lower in calcium than regular yogurt, but some commercial companies may fortify their Greek yogurt with added calcium.

❋ **Homemade Yogurt.** Growing up in Lebanon, I got accustomed to eating homemade yogurt that was tart in flavor and super delicious. Even store-bought yogurt always had that same loved sour flavor. But since moving to the US, I came to realize that most, if not all, commercial brands of yogurt miss that tartness that I was used to growing up. As such, I decided to start making my own yogurt, and realized how easy and non-complicated a process it is. To start with, I use a one gallon of skim cow milk and one cup of plain full-fat store-bought yogurt (I use the most sour brand that I have been able to find), to act as a starter. I have made sure that the commercial yogurt I buy contains live active cultures (indicated on the packaging and/or at the bottom of the nutrition label), as these beneficial probiotic bacteria (most commonly Lactobacillus and Bifidobacterium, among others) are what will cause fermentation and thickening of the milk into yogurt. I also try to avoid using yogurt brands that contain thickeners and stabilizers like gelatin, pectin, inulin, or food starch (although most commercial brands of yogurt contain at least one of these ingredients), since these may affect the texture outcomes of one's new batch of yogurt. To go about making homemade yogurt, follow these simple steps below, making sure all utensils and storage containers to be used are washed well (if not sterilized):

1. Add the milk to a large pot and heat over medium-high heat, stirring gently, but frequently, so as to prevent any scorching on the bottom.
2. Keep stirring until the milk just comes to a boil (~ 200 °F), starts forming small bubbles, and just starts to rise to the top of the pot. Turn the heat off.
3. Let the milk cool until the outside of the pot is just warm to touch (110 °F to 115 °F).
4. Remove 4 cups of the heated milk and place in a clean bowl.
5. Add the starter yogurt and whisk well.
6. Pour the mixture back into the milk pot and whisk gently until the milk is homogenous.
7. Pour the milk into the desired clean containers with covers.
8. Cover the containers with a warm blanket and let set for 24 to 48 hours (in warmer weather it will take 24 to 36 hours; in colder weather, 48 hours is best. The longer the yogurt sets, the more tart it turns out). Make sure the yogurt is not disturbed by any movement during the time it is setting.
9. Remove the blanket, uncover the yogurt containers, and wipe off any condensation on the covers, then refrigerate (uncovered) for a couple hours before consuming.
10. Cover the yogurt with the container cover once it has completely cooled in the refrigerator.
11. Do not pour off the top layer of separated whey. Gently fold the whey into each individual yogurt batch only when it is to be eaten from. Leave the other containers untouched until the time of consumption.

My closed yogurt containers can keep up to 4 weeks on the top shelf of the refrigerator. This method of homemade yogurt yields a total of 3.75 kg of yogurt. To prepare a new batch of yogurt, use 1 cup of the newly prepared yogurt batch. Continue this process for a few times before going back to using a cup of store-bought commercial yogurt to culture a new batch. This is basically because over time, the bacteria strain in one's yogurt may weaken and thus, not culture a new batch of yogurt as properly as it should. But also, because some outside bacteria may have entered one's yogurt with time, so it's better to start afresh.

❋ **Herbs.** For recipes calling for dry herbs, such as basil, oregano, mint, or marjoram, one can easily prepare them at home. I will often do so myself, especially when I have some fresh herbs in the fridge that I don't want to go to waste. All one needs to do is wash/soak the herbs in clean cold water, then proceed to let the leaves air dry on a dry towel. For a quicker drying method, one can then place the herbs in the microwave for around a minute, then let completely dry on a plate, for another 24 hours, before crushing and placing in a clean and airtight container. One can use the oven instead of the microwave, or simply leave the herbs to air dry on a towel for 48 to 72 hours.

Iodized Salt. Is table salt to which iodine has been added. Iodine is a mineral naturally present in some foods, namely seafood and vegetables which have been grown in iodine-rich soils. A main health outcome of iodine deficiency is thyroid problems and goiter. Thus, for people who are unable to get enough iodine in their regular diet, consuming iodized salt instead of regular (non-iodized) salt isan easy and inexpensive way to increase one's intake of iodine.

Iron-Rich Plant Foods. Iron is a vital mineral for preventing anemia. In food, iron is present as two different forms: heme-iron, which is present in animal sources such as red meat, chicken, fish, and eggs, and non-heme iron, which is present in iron-fortified food items and plant-based food sources such as chickpeas, lentils, beans, whole grains, nuts, and green-leafy vegetables. The body's ability to absorb heme-iron is much higher than that of non-heme iron. Generally, non-heme iron is of low-bioavailability since certain compounds naturally present in plant-based foods can decrease the absorption of iron. Examples of non-heme iron absorption inhibitors include phytates (naturally present in beans and grains) and various polyphenols (naturally present in green-leafy vegetables). As such, to maximize one's absorption of iron, it is recommended to consume iron-rich food sources with iron-absorption enhancers, while minimizing the simultaneous consumption of food items that contain additional inhibitors of iron absorption. Vitamin C is a main iron-absorption enhancer, therefore consuming vitamin-C rich sources such as citrus fruit, bell peppers, or tomatoes with non-heme food sources is recommended. Moreover, to absorb the most iron from food, it is preferable to avoid consuming foods or drinks that contain inhibitors of iron absorption, such as calcium (present mostly in dairy) as well as tannins and caffeine (present in coffee, tea, and carbonated beverages). It is a common Middle Eastern custom to consume yogurt with many traditional meat-containing dishes, and this can negatively influence one's absorption of iron (both heme and non-heme). It is also common among many cultures to drink coffee or tea right after a meal. To maximize the absorption of iron (as well as many other minerals for that matter), it is preferable that one avoids these drinks for at least 1 hour following a meal.

Ketchup. Added sugar is an ingredient in all commercial ketchup brands; those that are sugar-free contain artificial sweeteners. It is best to avoid artificially sweetened ketchup for children, and it is also important to avoid ketchup brands that contain high fructose corn syrup. Too much of this added ingredient is more harmful to everyone's health than plain sugar itself. Also, since tomatoes are considered high-pesticide vegetables (read more on page 35), it is best to choose organic ketchup (and organic tomato paste for that matter).

Labneh. Also known as yogurt cheese, *labneh* is very simple to make. One needs to start with yogurt placed inside a cheese cloth or a thin, lint-free, cotton dish cloth (also referred to as flour sack cloths/towels) lining a strainer or colander, set over a bowl (I prefer the dish cloth over the cheese cloth). Gently whisking the yogurt prior to pouring into the cloth makes for a more homogenous *labneh* paste. Add a pinch of salt to help the water drain out of the yogurt faster. Hanging the cheese cloth over the bowl helps speed up the draining process. Let strain for 8 hours. If the cheese cloth is not hanged, then place a double-layered paper towel over the surface of the yogurt and change every 2 hours (after giving the yogurt a little stir each time) during the 8-hour period. Discard the drained away liquid, which is mostly whey protein, excess water, and calcium. Although *labneh* is rich in protein, it is much lower in calcium than yogurt since a lot of the calcium drains away with the liquid. 3 cups of yogurt will yield around 1 cup of *labneh.*

Lemons Versus Limes. In Lebanon and Middle Eastern countries, people often use the word 'lemon' to refer to both the green as well as the yellow fruit. The former is actually a lime, which are more commonly grown in the Mediterranean region, and tend to be slightly smaller and more sour. Lemons are the yellow fruit, which is usually larger and a bit sweeter. In my recipes, I call for lemons/lemons juice, so make sure to adjust the quantity for flavor if limes are to be used instead.

Lemon Juice. When preparing lemon juice for a dish, squeeze the lemons right before using/serving, or make sure the lemon juice is placed in an airtight container immediately after squeezing, to be consumed within a few hours. This helps maximize the use of vitamin C and prevent/decrease its oxidation when exposed to air. One can also pour freshly squeezed lemon juice into ice cube trays to be placed in an airtight bag, then stored in the freezer for later use. I always save the pulp and add it to all my dishes that call for lemon juice, for added soluble fiber. Pre-squeezed/bottled lemon juice does not retain the full amount of vitamin C, and often contains preservatives that may affect the flavor.

Oats. These cereal grains are most prized for their nutritional and health benefits, being rich in fiber and micronutrients, and being associated with a reduced risk of heart disease. Oats come in many forms, depending on how and how much they were processed, including whole oat kernels (or oat groats), steel-cut oats, rolled (or old-fashioned) oats, and quick (or instant) oats. The processing of oats involves steps such as removing the inedible hulls, cutting the grains, stone-grinding them, or steaming then rolling and drying for better shelf life and faster cooking. The nutritional content between the different kinds of oats is fairly the same, but the more processed forms, such as rolled and quick oats, take a shorter time to digest, thus have a higher glycemic index than whole or steel-cut oats.

Parboiled Rice. Parboiling is the process of partially cooking rice in the husk. The end result after removing the husk is a rice that requires no precooking soaking and washing, cooks up faster than non-parboiled versions, and yields a more tender cooked rice. Parboiling doesn't affect the fiber and protein content of rice, but enhances the mineral and vitamin content, as it drives them deeper into the heart of the grain, preserving them against leaching out during cooking. As such, parboiled brown rice as well as parboiled white rice are higher in nutrients than non-parboiled rice varieties.

Parmesan Cheese. Is naturally lower in fat and higher in protein than other common cheeses. Real parmesan cheese is called Parmigiano-Reggiano and is of Italian origin. Many countries, including the US, imitate the cheese and produce similar versions. If the real Parmigiano-Reggiano cheese is not easily available and accessible for purchase, the best alternative version of the cheese to revert to is hard block or wedge parmesan cheese, manufactured by a reputable cheese manufacturer, and made from the following ingredients only: milk, enzymes, and salt. It is best to avoid previously grated and packaged versions of parmesan cheese, since these often contain food additives and taste different.

Parsley. Some Middle Eastern women discard the whole stems of the parsley branch, being picky about how their salads or dishes look, considering that the stems of parsley give an unattractive look and crunch to food. Since the stems contain almost as many healthy compounds as the leaves, it is recommended to retain as much as possible of the plant, only discarding the dry/damaged ends of the lower thick stems. However, I have noticed that within the US, grocery stores sell parsley bunches differently, with some selling it with the whole long stems intact, while others selling the bunches with half of the stems cut off. For standardization purposes, and given that a lot of the lower halves of the long parsley stems may be thick and woody, with lots of damaged dry sections, I will always cut the very long stems in half, discarding the bottom half.

Peanut Butter. Aside from peanuts, many commercial brands add other ingredients to their peanut butter, such as sugar and hydrogenated oils, so as to improve flavor and texture, as well as prolong shelf life. It is best to consume natural peanut butter, which only has one ingredient, peanuts. It is normal for the oil to separate in pure peanut butter as it sits; so always make sure to stir well before each use. It is best to keep natural peanut butter in the refrigerator because of its high fat content, which will allow the nut butter to go rancid faster when exposed to heat.

Pickled Turnips. To make these pickles, one will need 3 large turnips and 1 small/medium beet (the more beets used, the darker the color of the final turnip pickles); both are scraped, washed well, then sliced (slice the beets thinner than the turnips as they remain harder when pickled). I make a simple pickling brine of 4.5 cups water with 3 tablespoons of coarse salt, and 3 tablespoons of white vinegar. In a small pan, bring the brine to a boil, and let boil for 1 minute. Turn off and let cool. Pack the turnip and beet slices into 4 (500 ml) clean jars (sterilized would be best), cover with the brine, and close the lids in an airtight manner. Set aside on the countertop for 7 days. Refrigerate for at least 2 hours before consuming, then keep stored in the refrigerator.

Potatoes. When selecting potatoes, choose those that are firm to touch, have an unshriveled skin, don't have many eyes, and have little or no green sprouts. Store potatoes in a dry and cool place, away from heat and sunlight. Keep onions away from potatoes as they shorten each other's shelf life. During potato preparation, scrub the skins very well under running water with a vegetable brush to remove any attached soil that can be a carrier of harmful microorganisms, especially E-coli. Remove any green sprouts and slice off sections of a potato that have a tint of green in the skin (or discard completely if the green is all over). A greenish tint on a potato skin or sprout indicates exposure to sunlight which will produce a bitter flavor and eventually the formation of a toxic compound (solanine) which can cause poisoning if consumed in large amounts. Buying organic potatoes is recommended, especially if they are not going to be peeled (potatoes fall at number 13 after the 'dirty dozen' list of produce - read more on page 35).

Semolina. In Lebanon and other Middle Eastern countries, both coarse semolina flour (referred to as *smeed*) and fine semolina flour (referred to as *taheen farkha*) are available in the market. In the US, I have only come across the sandy-textured fine semolina (labelled as 'Semolina Flour') in local grocery stores, and it is this type of flour that I mostly use in my recipes calling for semolina flour. Middle Eastern grocery stores in the US may carry both kinds of semolina flour, though.

❋ **Tahini.** Like natural peanut butter, it is normal for the oil to separate in *tahini* as it sits. Always make sure to stir well before each use. It is best to keep *tahini* in the refrigerator because of its high fat content, which will allow it to go rancid faster when exposed to heat. *Tahini* flavors and textures can differ depending on whether it was made from hulled or intact sesame seeds, as well as whether the seeds were raw or roasted before crushing. Some brands also add vegetable oil to their *tahini* for smoother textures. Thus, different brands whether Middle Eastern, Greek or Ethiopian, will taste and look a bit different. I prefer Middle Eastern brands that contain only sesame seeds as the ingredient, but one can explore and choose the brand that best satisfies one's taste.

❋ **Vanilla.** Fresh vanilla fruits, commonly referred to as beans, undergo a lengthy curing and drying process after harvesting before the drier dark brown seed pods are ready for use. The fragrance and flavor of cured vanilla pods comes mainly from vanillin, the distinctive compound that offers the characteristic rich and sweet aroma and flavor to vanilla beans, as well as other organic compounds present inside the pod. There are many commercial vanilla products for use. Commercial pure liquid vanilla extract is made by crushing whole cured dried vanilla beans and extracting the liquid with some alcohol. Pure powdered vanilla is prepared from ground up dried beans, while other vanilla powders are derived from vanilla extracts. Imitation vanilla is produced from commercially synthesized vanillin. Liquid vanilla flavoring is the combination of pure vanilla extract and some imitation vanilla. Vanilla paste is made from ground vanilla beans mixed with vanilla extract and suspended in a thick liquid.

In the Middle East, it is common for imitation vanilla to be used given the scarcity of vanilla beans and the cheaper cost than pure vanilla extracts/powders. Below are some general substitutions to follow when using different vanilla products.

- Scraped inside of 1 whole vanilla bean = 1 tablespoon pure vanilla extract
- Scraped inside of 1 to 2 inches of a whole vanilla bean = 1 teaspoon vanilla bean seeds = 1 teaspoon pure vanilla extract = 1 teaspoon vanilla paste
- 1 teaspoon pure vanilla extract = ½ teaspoon whole ground vanilla bean powder = 2 teaspoons imitation vanilla powder

When using imitation vanilla in the place of pure vanilla extract, one should theoretically double the quantity to match the strength in flavor of pure vanilla extract. However, given that imitation vanilla often has a bitter aftertaste, it is best to cut down on the quantity used.

❋ **Water.** Is the preferred liquid to drink for optimal body hydration. Adults need at least 8 cups of water a day to be well hydrated. Higher amounts may be required for many depending on several factors, such as for those who are physically active, exposed to very hot and humid weather, and those consuming salty food. It is recommended to frequently drink small amounts of water throughout the day, and not just when one feels thirsty. Thirst is actually not a good indicator of hydration, since the feeling of thirst may mean that one is already dehydrated.

❋ **Whole Grain Flour.** Unlike white flour that can be stored for about a year in airtight containers in a cool and dry place outside of the refrigerator, whole grain flours, including whole wheat flour and brown rice flour, should be kept in the refrigerator, and preferably consumed within 3 months. This is because whole grain flours contain the fat-rich germ part of the grain, and thus can turn rancid when exposed to heat, as compared to white refined flour which has no germ.

❋ **Whole Wheat Flour.** Commonly comes in three different types. White whole wheat flour (milled from hard white wheat) and whole wheat pastry flour (milled from soft white wheat) don't contain as much gluten (protein) as regular whole wheat flour (which is milled from hard red wheat), making the former flours lighter in texture and allowing baked products to stay fluffy and moist. Thus, for many of my moist baked goods, I use whole wheat pastry flour. I turn to using regular whole wheat flour for baked goods that are drier in nature and do not require much leavening (like some Lebanese desserts), as well as in some main dishes that require flour as a thickening agent.

❋ **Zucchini.** Belonging to the squash family, zucchini, also known as courgette, is a type of summer squash. In Middle Eastern countries, the common zucchini grown and consumed is similar to the Mexican squash, which is of a light green color with white lines/specs and is fairly short as compared to the long slender dark green zucchini variety commonly available in grocery stores in the United States. Either type can be used in different dishes calling for zucchini, as they essentially have a similar flavor, texture, and nutritional value (however, one should take note of the net weight, since individual size can vary).

Chapter 7

NUTRITION AND HEALTH AWARENESS TOPICS

Arsenic in Rice. A global staple food, rice is a leading dietary source of inorganic arsenic, a compound that is associated with adverse health effects. Arsenic is a naturally occurring compound in air, water, and soil, and concentrations can increase with erosion of arsenic-containing rocks, volcanic eruptions, contamination from mining, and previous/current agricultural use of arsenic-containing pesticides. Long term exposure to high levels of inorganic arsenic is negatively associated with heart disease and certain types of cancer. Among all grains (such as wheat, barley, oats, rye, polenta, and quinoa), rice (regardless of the type, whether white, brown, basmati, jasmine, etc.) is the most highly contaminated with arsenic. This is mostly because of the way rice crops are flooded with water in order for the plants to grow, allowing the rice crop to readily absorb arsenic present in the soil and water. While national and international organizations do not recommend the elimination of rice from people's diets, working on decreasing rice consumption while increasing the intake of other grains can help limit our exposure over time. Another recommended strategy to follow is cooking rice in excess water, then draining away what water remains (this method has been shown to decrease the levels of inorganic arsenic by 40-60%, however, micronutrients present in rice are likely to also decrease by 50-70%). Bottom line, enjoy your rice with meals, but try to incorporate other healthy grains such as bulgur, quinoa, or barley in the place of rice for some dishes.

Canned and Frozen Produce. Fresh is definitely best, but lightly processed foods with no or minimal amounts of additives are okay as well. Some processed foods can actually provide some health benefits, and are not necessarily considered 'bad' to consume. For instance, tomato products (such as tomato paste and ketchup) are very rich in lycopene, which is a potent antioxidant present in fresh tomatoes. Reading ingredients at the back of these processed items is vital though, as some tomato paste brands contain a lot of salt (so it is best to go for low-salt or unsalted versions) and many ketchup brands contain high fructose corn syrup (so it is best to just go with ones that simply contain cane sugar, making sure it is not the first or second ingredient). Regarding canned items, I personally use only a few: canned corn (when fresh corn is not in season), canned tomato paste (making sure it is organic, given that non-organic tomatoes can be highly contaminated with pesticides), canned pumpkin (since pumpkin season is very short and the process of making pumpkin paste at home is very time-consuming), and canned tuna fish (which is much more convenient to consume than fresh tuna). The material from which many cans are made used to contain a harmful compound (PVC which can release BPA into our food), but many reputable companies nowadays are avoiding its use. For vegetables, I prefer frozen produce (instead of canned) as I feel texture and flavor are better maintained. However, I personally only use a few frozen vegetables, mostly green beans, peas, okra, and Jew's mallow (since the fresh versions are often very time consuming to prepare and/or are out of season most months of the year). Fresh vegetables are by all means healthier, since frozen vegetables may lose some vitamins, minerals, and antioxidants in the process of being frozen with time, especially if they were not immediately frozen after harvest. But, if the methods of freezing were properly followed by the manufacturer, frozen vegetables can offer a great amount of nutrients just as their fresh counterparts do. I generally like rinsing my canned and frozen fresh produce (except for frozen Jew's mallow), to rinse away, to some extent, any possible contaminants from the packaging or previous handling processes.

Dairy Debate. For years, the daily intake of dairy products has been stressed in guidelines and recommendations set forth by national and international agencies, including the US Department of Agriculture, the US Academy of Nutrition and Dietetics, the World Health Organization, and the Food and Agriculture Organization of the United Nations. In the past decade, some dietary guides such as the Healthy Eating Plate (developed in 2011 by the Harvard T.H. Chan School of Public Health), the Eatwell Guide (developed in 2016 by the Public Health Department in England) and the Canada Food Guide (developed in 2019 by the Canadian Government), have started calling for limiting the daily intake of milk and dairy, placing less importance on milk as a drink, and grouping other dairy products together under the general protein group. And recently many groups are starting to call for the complete omittance of dairy from people's diets and thus, from national recommendations. These movements against the consumption of dairy are driven mostly by growing health and environmental concerns. Research on whether calcium-rich cow's milk helps keep bones strong and healthy is conflicting, as some studies suggest that cow milk intake may be attributed with no decreased risk of bone fracture (while some research points towards a possible increase in fracture risk). A major cause for public concern is the potentially present levels of hormones, antibiotics, pesticides, and specific protein molecules in dairy products, with some studies suggesting a link between dairy consumption and certain types of cancer (such as prostate cancer and ovarian cancer). There is also concern that full-fat dairy increases the risk of heart disease, but this is mostly related to the saturated fat content in dairy, which further stresses the importance of consuming low-fat or skim dairy products.

Dairy is, indeed, not for everyone. With the possible link between dairy and cancer, individuals who have a family history of cancer or who have a current or previous cancer diagnosis should consult with a medical doctor as well as a nutrition cancer specialist for further advice on what foods to eat and what to avoid. Many individuals around the world also suffer from lactose malabsorption (a condition where the small intestine cannot digest or break down the lactose ingested) and/or lactose intolerance (a condition in which digestive symptoms, including bloating, diarrhea and gas, develop after the consumption of food products containing the naturally occurring milk sugar, lactose). It is estimated that 68% of the world's population has lactose malabsorption, with it being more common among people in Africa and Asia, and it being least common among Europeans. While lactose malabsorption can cause lactose intolerance, not all individuals with malabsorption of lactose develop intolerance to lactose. In fact, many people with lactose intolerance can still handle some lactose in their diet (and lactose-free cow milk is becoming increasingly more available to consumers).

Nutritionally speaking, breast milk plays an important role in early growth and development for all mammals. After infancy, dairy products (whether from cows or goats) from milk to cheese and yogurt, provide high quality protein (including both whey and casein), good amounts of calcium and magnesium, as well as other micronutrients, namely vitamin B12 and added vitamin D. While plant-based milks, such as nut milks (from almonds, cashews, or coconuts), or soy, oat, and rice milk, have a nutritious profile as well, many are much lower in protein and/or calcium, which could be a matter of concern especially for growing children and adolescents, as well as aging adults. Furthermore, many high calcium non-dairy foods don't really supply the body with good amounts of bioavailable calcium, as many are either high in oxalates (like oranges, nuts, soy, dark green-leafy vegetables) or high in phytates (like wheat bran, nuts, and legumes), as well as being low in lactose and/or vitamin D, all of which are factors that will negatively influence the absorption of calcium from these foods.

With the current scientific evidence, I believe some dairy products, especially milk, yogurt, and cheese, when consumed in moderation by the average healthy individual, will do more good than harm, especially if consumed as low-fat and skim products. Fermented dairy, such as yogurt and kefir are especially beneficial for their probiotic effects. Dairy products that are very high in saturated fat, such as butter and cream, in my opinion add no nutritional benefit and can be completely avoided.

Egg Debate. For decades, it was thought that eggs were to blame for elevating blood cholesterol levels, due to their high cholesterol content (~ 200 mg per egg yolk), and eggs were thus advised to be avoided/consumed in limited amounts, especially among individuals with high blood cholesterol levels. Decades of research now shows that cholesterol in food is not the main culprit for increased blood cholesterol levels. Current research shows that most blood cholesterol levels are made by the liver through a process mainly triggered by dietary saturated fats as well as trans fats. Therefore, for the average healthy person, an egg a day should not pose any health harm, as long as it is prepared in a healthy way and not consumed with unhealthy foods such as butter and sausages. Egg consumption is advised to be limited to 3 or less per week for those who suffer from heart disease or are at risk of heart disease, and for those who have diabetes.

Red Meat Debate. A controversial set of dietary recommendations were published in the Annals of Internal Medicine in the fall of 2019, suggesting that individuals need not reduce or moderate their intake of red meat as well as processed meat. According to the authors, these guidelines were based on results of a series of systemic review articles and meta-analyses. However, these guidelines contradict the large body of scientific evidence that indicates a higher risk of chronic disease (namely cardiovascular disease, type 2 diabetes, and certain types of cancer such as colorectal cancer), as well as premature death, associated with higher consumption levels of red meat, especially processed red meat (unfortunately, misuse of systematic reviews and meta-analyses may have accounted, for the most part, for the published contradicting recommendations).

Top organizations including the United States Department of Agriculture, the American Heart Association, the American Cancer Association, the American Academy of Nutrition and Dietetics, and the World Health Organization, have long advised individuals to limit their intake of red meat, especially non-lean and processed red meat sources, on the basis of the strong evidence associating their intake with negative chronic disease outcomes (saturated fats in red meat products as well as nitrates/nitrates and sodium in processed meat products are the main culprits). My opinion is that individuals should continue to reduce their total intake of red meat in general, while focusing on consuming lean and very lean sources of red meat, with the minimization or complete avoidance of processed meats.

❉ Farm-Raised Versus Wild-Caught Fish. Farmed seafood is that which is raised in large tanks or artificial ponds, while wild seafood is that which is caught from a natural habitat such as a lake, river, or ocean. From a nutritional quality point of view, farmed or wild seafood are pretty much the same, offering similar macro-and micronutrients. However, from a contamination point of view, farmed seafood tends to contain higher levels of contaminants, especially PCBs (polychlorinated biphenyls) and sometimes mercury (read more below), as well as some levels of antibiotics. PCBs are a big concern with regards to farmed seafood, especially fatty seafood, as it builds up in the fatty tissue and livers. Although this industrial chemical has been banned, remnants of the chemical still cycle between air, water, and soil, with traces still found all over the world. PCBs can pose a serious health concern for those who frequently consume farmed fish or wild-caught fish from contaminated lakes or rivers. Pregnant and breastfeeding women should take extra care as this chemical can pass from mother to unborn child (increasing the risk of preterm delivery and low-birth weight) and through breastmilk (increasing the risk of learning defects). In adults, PCB exposure has been associated with possible cancer risk and negative health effects on the immune, nervous, and endocrine systems.

Levels of PCBs will vary between regions and types of fish. In general, larger predator fish (such as bass, lake trout, and walleye) as well as fatty fish such as salmon, contain higher amounts of PCBs. It is advised to check local and state advisories for restrictions and avoid possibly contaminated fish and other seafood. The Food and Drug Administration as well as the Environmental Protection Agency in the US recommends the following measures to decrease one's exposure to contaminants: trimming away fatty areas of the fish before consumption, removing part or all of the skin to allow fat to drain off, and avoiding frying fish (since frying seals in chemical pollutants inside the fish's fatty tissue).

❉ Mercury in Seafood. Fish and shellfish are important food components of a healthy diet for adults and children, as they provide high-quality protein, are low in saturated fat, and contain lots of heart-healthy omega-3 fatty acids. However, almost all seafood contains traces of mercury, and for most people, the health risks of mercury from moderate fish and shellfish consumption is not a big concern. Having said this, certain fish and shellfish contain very high levels of mercury that may cause long-term harm if consumed in large amounts, and thus their consumption should be limited. The Food and Drug Administration (FDA) and the Environmental Protection Agency (EPA) advise women of childbearing age, pregnant women, and breastfeeding mothers, as well as young children, to avoid moderate to high mercury-containing seafood (including king mackerel, swordfish, marlin, tilefish, shark, seabass, some tuna types, and yellowtail fish species used in sushi). Canned tuna is a healthy and convenient way to consume tuna fish, but care must be given to choosing more of the lower-mercury containing types of tuna, referred to as light tuna, as compared to the higher-mercury containing types, referred to as white or albacore tuna, as well as bigeye tuna.

❉ Going Gluten Free. There has been an increased interest and enthusiasm in the past recent years surrounding the gluten-free food movement, because of the idea and/or claims that limiting/avoiding gluten intake can improve overall health. However, going gluten-free is not necessary for all people. To start with, gluten is a naturally-occurring protein found in the three main grains: wheat, barley, and rye. Many people cannot handle digesting gluten, and thus are defined as those with celiac disease. Even a very small amount of gluten in these individuals can trigger an undesirable immune response, leading to inflammation and damage in the lining of the small intestine, accompanied by a number of uncomfortable gastrointestinal symptoms (namely bloating, cramping abdominal pain, diarrhea, and constipation). Many individuals report being gluten-sensitive (or having non-celiac gluten sensitivity), whereby some intestinal discomfort develops following gluten-ingestion, despite the absence of celiac disease (by blood lab testing) (these individuals may have a simple wheat allergy, which can be diagnosed by skin testing).

Following a gluten-free diet, i.e. complete avoidance of gluten-containing foods and non-food items, is thus only necessary for people who suffer from celiac disease, so as to alleviate their symptoms and manage their health. Very little clinical research has been conducted to assess the benefits of a gluten-free diet in people who do not suffer from celiac disease or other gluten-related medical conditions. Completely avoiding gluten goes beyond giving up the common breads, cereals, and pastas made with the three aforementioned grains. Going gluten-free can be extremely challenging since many processed foods have been produced in facilities that may have handled wheat, and thus the slightest cross-contamination in a non-wheat product may trigger extreme gastrointestinal discomfort. Oats, while naturally being gluten-free, are often not handled well by celiac patients as they are often contaminated with some wheat residues. Since wheat or wheat gluten is often added as a thickening agent or for flavoring and/or coloring, some gluten may also be present in candy, gravies, soy sauce, soup mixes, salad dressings, and processed meats such as hot dogs, as well as non-food items such as medications, vitamin and mineral supplements, as well as toothpaste. Going gluten-free is in fact expensive, time consuming, and quite restrictive. For those who limit or omit gluten from their diet for one reason or another, care should be taken so as to ensure the consumption of a varied diet rich in the many gluten-free whole grains such as brown rice and quinoa, as well as other nutrient and fiber-rich foods including beans, lentils, nuts, seeds, vegetables, and fruit.

Going Organic. Organic food refers to food products that have been produced without the use of most synthetic additives (which include pesticides such as insecticides and herbicides, as well as fertilizers), food products that have not been exposed to radiation, agricultural crops that have not been genetically modified, and livestock that have not been exposed to antibiotics or growth hormones and have been given feed that has been organically grown.

While research shows that the macronutrient and micronutrient content of organic food is not any different from non-organic food, some plant polyphenol compounds (which basically have antioxidant and other health benefits) have been found to be higher in organic fresh produce. However, this nutritional benefit isn't sufficient enough to justify more health benefits coming from the consumption of organic fruits and vegetables. Therefore, it becomes a matter of personal choice whether people want to do a complete shift over to organic food so as to avoid all of the above mentioned unwanted and possibly harmful 'foreign' food compounds. Two factors that will highly influence people's decisions are organic food accessibility as well as affordability. From a pesticide point of view, many organically grown fresh produce (fruits and vegetables) are significantly lower in pesticide residues as compared to conventionally grown fresh produce. Pesticides, which are important in agriculture since they are used to protect crops and increase yield, are potentially toxic to humans and can impact on both acute and chronic health problems. The Environmental Working Group (EWG), a nonprofit organization that ranks fresh produce items according to their level of pesticide contamination, releases an annual list of the "dirtiest" and "cleanest" fruits and vegetables available in the US market. It is, therefore, recommended that items on the dirty dozen list be bought as organic, if of course they are accessible and affordable to individuals.

The EWG's "Dirty Dozen" list for the year 2021 includes:

1. Strawberries
2. Spinach
3. Kale, Collard, and Mustard Greens
4. Nectarines
5. Apples
6. Grapes
7. Cherries
8. Peaches
9. Pears
10. Bell and Hot Peppers
11. Celery
12. Tomatoes

The EWG's "Clean Fifteen" list for the year 2021 includes:

1. Avocados
2. Sweet corn
3. Pineapples
4. Onions
5. Papayas
6. Sweet Frozen Peas
7. Eggplant
8. Asparagus
9. Broccoli
10. Cabbage
11. Kiwi
12. Cauliflower
13. Mushrooms
14. Honeydew melon
15. Cantaloupe

A way to minimize one's intake of pesticides from fresh produce is by washing and scrubbing the edible skins with water, and possibly water with baking soda, or by peeling the outer skins (although this will minimize one's intake of insoluble fiber and some micronutrients present). Fresh produce with thick outer skins that are removed anyway before consumption are usually much lower in pesticide residues, since the outer skins act as a protecting barrier for the inner part of the fruit or vegetable. Having said this, however, care should be given to washing any fresh produce, whether organic or not, since aside from pesticides, fresh produce may be contaminated with other harmful compounds such as fertilizers, environmental pollutants, or bacteria from soil, water, or produce handling.

Safety of Parchment Paper. Parchment paper is a common companion for baking sheets and pans when one wants to minimize the added fat otherwise required for greasing the surfaces of bakeware. It removes the need for using any fat for greasing, since it has been coated with a thin layer of silicone, making the paper stick resistant, as well as heat and moisture resistant. Silicone seems to be a non-toxic compound to humans and doesn't seem to react with food when subjected to heating (or freezing), although not much research has been conducted on this matter. I personally like limiting the use of parchment paper and will only use it when baking vegetables or potato wedges, and not when baking desserts. I also recommend using the unbleached version of parchment paper, which is light brown in color, since bleached parchment paper has been treated with chlorine to turn the paper white, and thus may leach dioxins into food. According to the World Health Organization (WHO), dioxins are highly toxic chemicals that can negatively affect many of our body organs and systems. While dioxins are omnipresent in the environments we live in, they are mainly the by-products of industrial processes, including, among many other manufacturing processes, the chlorine bleaching of paper.

❁ **Storage of Spices and Dry Herbs.** It is best to keep these fragrant and flavorful ingredients in airtight containers stored in a cool and dark place, away from air, heat, and direct sunlight, as these factors can damage flavors. According to the American Spice Trade Association, spices and dry herbs should be stored at temperatures below 60 °F (16 °C) for optimal potency, and changed every 12 months. A rule of thumb I personally follow is storing my not-so-used spices and dry herbs in the freezer (while making sure to always buy these in small quantities), my moderately-used ones in the refrigerator, and the highly-relied on spices and herbs in a cool and dark cupboard, away from any direct source of heat. Make sure when needing to access a spice or dry herb previously stored in the refrigerator or freezer, to measure out the needed amount and to return the container to cold storage immediately, so as to prevent the formation of condensation on the inside of the container (as this will trigger the formation of mold over time).

❁ **Recommended Cutting Boards.** Safe materials for cutting boards include marble, safe plastic, glass, or pyroceramic. These materials clean better than wooden surfaces, and are less prone to developing grooves over time, which can harbor food and harmful bacteria if not washed properly. Cheap plastic is not a good choice as these may develop cracks and slices more easily and may contain harmful compounds such as Bisphenol A (BPA) and Polyvinyl Chloride (PVC) (discussed below in recommended food storage containers).

❁ **Recommended Kitchen Utensils.** Metal and hard plastic utensils can injure cookware by scratching the surfaces, leading to faster wearing out of the base of pots and pans. Over time, the inner surface of cookware can also start peeling off, increasing the hazard of chipped cookware material in our food. It is, thus, best to use silicone, bamboo, or wooden utensils instead. Wood utensils, however, should not be used once cracks or rough edges start forming, as harmful bacteria can start growing in those hard to clean places. One of my favorite kitchen utensils is the spatula, as these help so much in the scraping out of remnant food from a bowl or pot, minimizing any loss in food yield. From experience, I have found that soft and flexible spatulas are better than hard and rigid ones, as the later will not do such a good job scraping out food.

❁ **Recommended Cookware and Bakeware.** Many us of are often guided by cost, convenience, and durability when it comes to choosing our pots, pans, and bakeware. However, many of these are made of materials that can lead to the leaching of unwanted and often harmful chemicals into our food (even if the cookware or bakeware is not scratched or peeling). There is really no one kind of cookware or bakeware that deserves the medal for being the 'safest of them all', while also being the best of them all in terms of cost, durability, and maintenance. Below is a summary of the most common materials used in cookware and/or bakeware, and how they are rated in terms of food safety.

❁ Aluminum. Anodized, non-stick, and scratch-resistant aluminum is a popular material and is a safe choice. Unlike the common belief that old-fashioned uncoated aluminum pots and pans should be avoided since they leach a lot of aluminum into food, it seems that cooking with aluminum ware does not negatively affect one's health. However, it is best to avoid older uncoated aluminum pots as these do not tolerate high temperatures.

❁ Cast Iron. Although quite heavy, this material is safe to cook in, although some iron is expected to leach into the food (but since iron is a good mineral to consume, this is not a matter of concern for most). Both enameled (coated) cast iron and bare cast iron cookware are safe and provide non-stick surfaces, but coated cast iron should not be used for baking.

❁ Ceramic. Ceramic glazes on cookware are not advised, since these may crack easily and leach harmful metals, especially lead, into food. The amount of lead leaching out of the ceramic glazes on the inside of cookware can increase in the presence of acidic foods, as well as with hot foods, especially liquids. However, it seems that heavy-duty pure ceramic ware made by reputable companies is safe.

❁ Copper. Uncoated copper cookware can leach copper

into food, causing undesirable symptoms such as nausea, vomiting, and diarrhea. Some copper pans are coated with another metal to prevent food from coming into contact with copper. Older and cheaper copper cookware may be coated with tin or nickel (two metals one should try to avoid), and over time, these coatings are known to easily chip, causing copper to leach into food.

Glass. Glass bakeware is safe to use, however, it does not conduct heat as well as cast iron, stainless steel, or aluminum, so baking time may need to be adjusted when using it. Aim for heavy-duty glassware made from tempered glass that has been strengthened.

Stainless Steel. Is a safe material to cook and bake with. Since it is not much of a non-stick surface when used for cooking certain foods (such as pancakes, omelets, and eggs), some oil is needed to prevent food from sticking (from my experience, good quality and thicker bottomed-stainless steel cookware lead to less sticking). Care must be taken to get good quality and relatively new stainless-steel cookware, since older and cheaper brands may scratch easily and may leach nickel or chromium into food.

Stoneware. Is considered very safe and durable for baking. However, make sure you go for heavy-duty ones made by reputable companies since cheap ones may have a layer of lead-containing enamel.

Teflon. Is a world-wide known brand as a non-stick coating for cookware. Teflon has received a lot of concern over the years since it contains perfluorooctanoic acid (PFOA), also known as C8, a possible carcinogen that was used in the manufacturing of Teflon, and was thought to leach into food once the cookware and food were heated. However, based on a recent report by the American Cancer Society and on a statement by the Environmental Protection Agency (EPA), it seems that only a small insignificant amount (if any) of PFOA remains in current manufactured products (it is mostly burned off during manufacturing), and many countries are not using it anymore in any of their products. Having said this, care must be given to Teflon cookware since they should only be used at low or medium heat, given that harmful fumes are released at high heat cooking which can irritate the respiratory tracts of humans as well as household pets.

Recommended Food Storage Containers. Plastic kitchen ware or utensils may be made of Polyvinyl Chloride (PVC) and/or contain Bisphenol A (BPA), two compounds one should look out for when choosing any plastic that will come in contact with food. PVC may leach BPA and other harmful compounds into food (especially if the food is hot and the plastic container has become worn a bit), and BPA has been shown (in animal studies) to affect organs and developmental processes in fetuses, infants, and young children. It is thus best to go with glass, porcelain, or stainless-steel storage containers, especially for hot food and liquids. If using plastic, chose products labeled as BPA-free or PVC-free (if there is no label, bear in mind that some, but not all, plastic products marked on the bottom with recycle code numbers 3 or 7 may be made with BPA).

Recommended Steps for Reducing Household Foodborne Illness. An integral part of eating healthy is ensuring food is safe to consume. By following the below safe food handling practices, one can reduce food contaminants and ward off foodborne illnesses within one's household.

Wash Hands. Wash hands before and after handling food, with soap and clean running water (preferably warm) for at least 20 seconds, rubbing hands together and scrubbing in between one's fingers (and under the nails if needed). Dry hands with a clean kitchen towel (changed frequently) or disposable paper towel.

Clean Surfaces and Appliances. Keep kitchen working surfaces and appliances (especially the areas where cross-contamination to the hands may occur) clean and sanitized by frequent wipe downs with disinfectant wipes, a chlorine (bleach) solution (1 tablespoon chlorine per gallon of water), or a white vinegar solution (in a 1:1 ratio with water for mild cleaning or a 2:1 ratio for a stronger cleaning effect).

Wash Dishes and Cooking Utensils. Clean dishes and cooking utensils with a clean sponge, dish soap, and running warm water, sanitizing surfaces that were in contact with raw meats (red meat, chicken or seafood). Or place soiled dishes in a dishwasher, adding soap, and using the whole wash and dry cycle, with a warm to hot water temperature.

Keep Kitchen Sponges Clean. With time and use, kitchen sponges can harbor harmful microorganisms, including bacteria, yeasts, and mold. Since soap or bleach with water is not enough for getting rid of microorganisms growing on sponges, the United States Department of Agriculture (USDA) recommends abiding by one of the 3 strategies to maintain good hygiene with kitchen sponges:

a. Using a new sponge every week.
b. Microwaving sponges on high for one minute.
c. Washing sponges in the dishwasher (using the whole wash and dry cycle, with a warm to hot water temperature).

Before shifting over to washable and non-disposable mesh cloths for cleaning dishes, I used to follow method b, doing it at least twice a week, and then would start using a new sponge about every 2 weeks.

❊ Separate Food During Purchase and Storage. Keep purchased eggs and raw meats away from fresh produce and ready-to-eat grocery products. Always store raw meats and unwashed fresh produce on shelves below cooked and ready-to-eat food items in the refrigerator. Keep eggs in their cartons and store inside the refrigerator, preferably on a shelf and not in the refrigerator door for more stable storage temperatures and to prevent condensation formation on the eggshells.

❊ Rinse Fresh Produce. Wash fruits and vegetables very well under running water, scrubbing them as needed, even if the produce is going to be peeled (this helps minimize the transfer of microbes from the peel to the inside edible flesh). For green leafy vegetables that are heavily soiled, soaking then rinsing the produce (as many times as needed) is recommended. For extra precaution, white vinegar can be added during soaking. Avoid using soap or detergent on food items.

❊ Do Not Rinse Meats. It is a Middle Eastern tradition to rinse raw chicken and scrub the meat and skin with lemons and salt, as it is believed this kills any bacteria present and prevents any unpleasant scent or flavor from developing during cooking. This step is unnecessary, and the rinsing of red meat, chicken, and fish with water should be avoided to minimize cross-contamination.

❊ Do Not Rinse Eggs. Unless visible fecal or foreign matter is present on the outside of the eggshell, it is recommended not to rinse eggs. If need be, use only warm tap water when rinsing eggshells to prevent any shrinkage of the eggshell and suction of bacteria on the outside of the shell to the inside through the many eggshellpores.

❊ Separate Food During Preparation and Serving. Make sure to use a separate cutting board for raw meats and one for fresh fruit and vegetables or any other food items that will not be cooked prior to consumption. Avoid placing cooked food back on a cutting board or plate that held raw meat or unwashed produce.

❊ Defrost Food Properly. Thaw frozen food in the refrigerator, in the microwave, or in cold water, then cook right away.

❊ Cook Food to Safe Internal Temperatures. Raw meats should be thoroughly cooked until deemed safe for consumption. Using a food thermometer can help. For seafood and red meat pieces or chunks, an internal temperature of 145°F should be reached, while for ground meat a temperature of 160 °F should be reached. For all poultry, an internal temperature of 165 °F should be obtained.

❊ Store Food at Safe Temperatures. Keep hot food at 140 °F or above until eaten. Keep cold food at 40 °F or below. Don't let food sit outside the fridge for too long before storing it. It is recommended to let cooked food cool down for the most part inside the refrigerator, since cooked food held between 40 °F and 140 °F for more than 2 hours may pose a risk for foodborne illness.

❊ Throw Out Old and Unsafe Food. For raw meats stored in the refrigerator, cook within 2 days or discard. For cooked leftovers, be sure to consume within 4 days. For other ready-to-eat food items (in the refrigerator or in the cupboards), watch the expiration date closely and make sure to avoid consumption beyond the indicated date. Always follow the FIFA rule (First In, First Out) when arranging food items in one's refrigerator or cupboards.

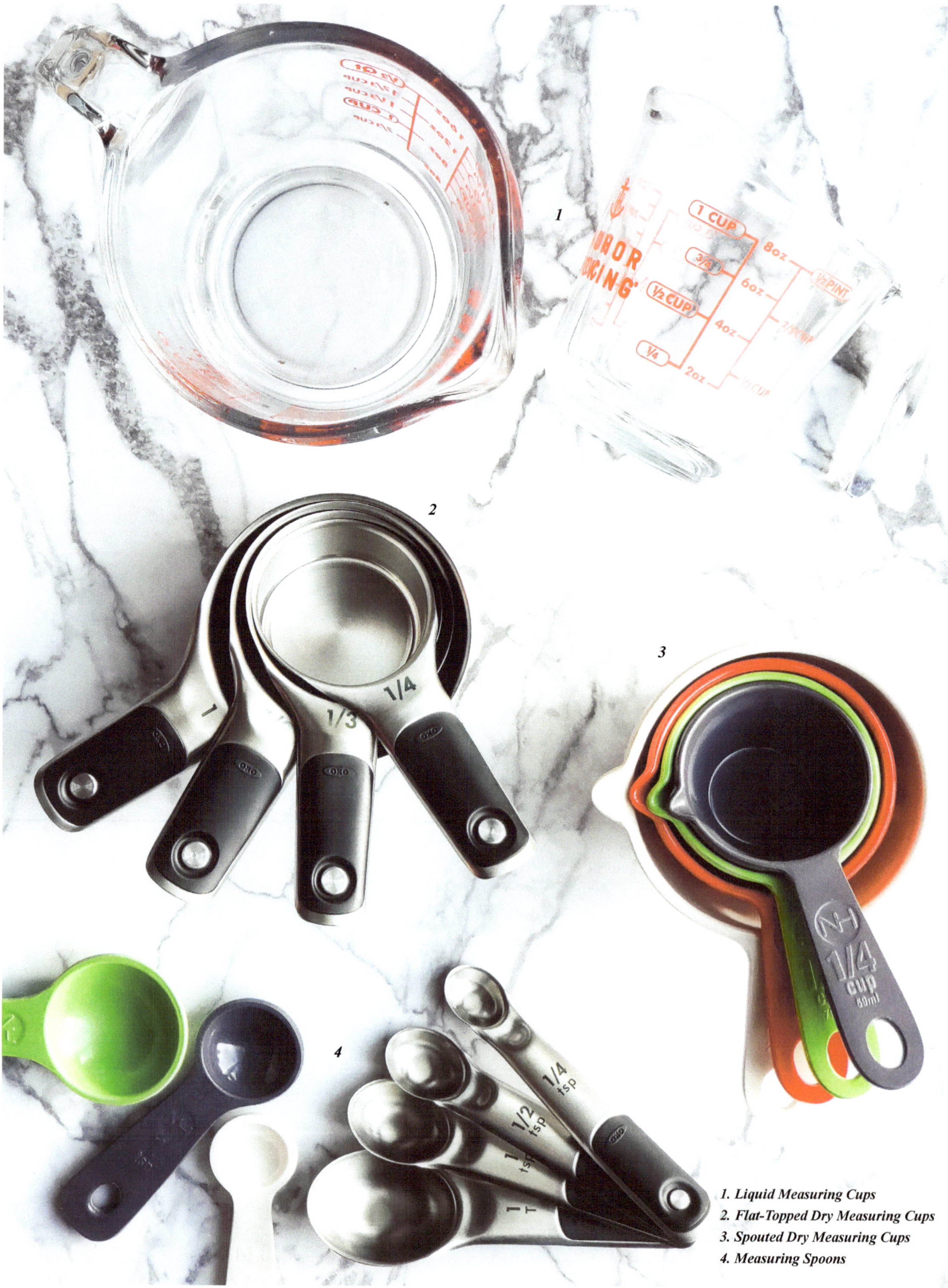

1. Liquid Measuring Cups
2. Flat-Topped Dry Measuring Cups
3. Spouted Dry Measuring Cups
4. Measuring Spoons

Chapter 8

MEASURING UTENSILS

Measuring Ingredients. Traditionally, Middle Eastern women have cooked without really following standardized recipes and exact ingredient measurements. They are experts at using a pinch of this ingredient and a handful or bunch of that ingredient, estimating the needed quantities of certain ingredients just by the feel of their hand, the look of their eyes, and most importantly, by using their expert sense of smell and taste! I personally must admit that before embarking on creating this cookbook, there were many dishes (especially savory ones) that I cooked following these traditional culinary methods, rather than following written standardized recipes. This flexible method of cooking is useful when one is in a hurry for instance, or when one is using up scraps of random ingredients to make up a new dish. But more often than not, this results in varying flavors and yields of a given dish when needing to replicate.

In terms of measuring utensils, it is traditionally common for household cooks to use common household spoons, coffee or tea cups, as well as the common household drinking glass or mug in measuring out ingredients when cooking or baking. I remember my mother telling me that she had brought over standard measuring cups and spoons with her from the US when she moved to Lebanon in the early 80s, and she may have literally been one of just a few people using standard measuring utensils at the time. While measuring utensils have become more commonly available in many convenient stores around Middle Eastern countries nowadays, some women still do simply rely on common household measuring utensils.

Accurate measurement of all recipe ingredients is actually very important in food preparation, especially if one wants to replicate the desired end flavor, texture, and yield of a dish, whether savory or sweet. It is, therefore, recommended that standard measuring cups and spoons are used, and often, a weighing scale is preferable in determining an exact quantity of an ingredient. Ingredient weighing is the most accurate method in food preparation, and is therefore used in recipe development in restaurants and food catering services. However, for as reliable as this method may be, it may be tedious and impractical for many in the home setting. I personally am not a big fan of ingredient weighing, but will rely on a weighing scale for major recipe ingredients which otherwise may not be easily and accurately measured out in terms of cups or spoons, such as meats, fruits, vegetables, legumes, and nuts. I have come to realize that for many recipes, especially desserts and sweets, weighing major ingredients is very important for replicating desired recipe outcomes.

Using standard measuring utensils can also often determine the difference between success and failure in many recipes. All my recipes in this cookbook are based on the use of US standard measuring utensils (these can differ slightly with measuring utensils used in Europe and Australia). However, there is some variation between measuring utensils of different brand names even within the US, which is not quite understandable and very frustrating, but is unfortunately nevertheless a fact. So even if one closely follows a recipe and abides by the measured amounts using measuring utensils, some slight variations in outcomes (and/or yields) may occur among dishes, depending on what brand of measuring utensils one is using. The best one can do is to choose brand names that are reputable and that cost a bit more money than the very cheap measuring utensils - the latter may be very inaccurate and thus not reliable. In the US, America's Test Kitchen has evaluated the accuracy and reliability of several brands of different measuring utensils, placing the brands OXO and Pyrex at the top of the best brands to use. According to my humble experience, commonly available and affordable brands such as Farberware and Anchor Hocking are also good brands to use, if the former two are inaccessible.

Measuring Cups

Liquid Measuring Cups. These should be transparent and graduated, with pouring lips. They usually come marked with specific measuring lines of 4 cups, 2 cups, 1 ½ cups, 1 cup, ¾ cup, ⅔ cup, ½ cup, ⅓ cup, ¼ cup (with all other quantities in between, such as 1¾ cup, 1 ⅔ cup, etc.). The US standard measuring cup measures around 240 ml (as compared to the European cup which measures at 250 ml). Use these measuring cups for measuring liquid ingredients (that easily 'pour' or 'flow' out of a container), such as water, milk, oil, honey, maple syrup, carob molasses, pomegranate molasses, orange blossom water, rose water, and soy sauce.

When measuring liquids, place the cup on a flat surface, pour in the liquid up to the desired line mark, and read the mark at eye level, with the mark of the cup displaying at the bottom of the meniscus of the liquid being measured, then adjusting as necessary. After pouring out one's liquid, always make sure to use a spatula or rubber scraper to remove any liquid sticking to the inside of the measuring cup.

Use the small 1 cup measuring cup for smaller amounts of liquid, while keeping the bigger ones (such as the 2-cup or 4-cup measuring cups) for larger quantities. If a recipe calls for 2 ½ cups of a liquid, it is best to use the 2-cup measuring cup for measuring out 2 cups, then use the smaller 1 cup measuring cup to measure the remaining ½ cup.

Glass measuring cups are generally more durable and reliable in the long run, as plastic is more prone to scratching and losing its transparency (especially when placed over and over in a dishwasher) for accurate mark reading.

Variability among brands for liquid measuring cups is common. To compare the measuring cup you have to the one I have used in my recipe development, compare the weight of water I obtained with what you obtain using a weight scale. This will give you a more accurate understanding of how your liquid measuring cups compare to mine (remember to tare your scale when measuring weights of ingredients).

1 cup water = 240 g

Variability within brands is less common, but nevertheless present. From my experience, 2-cup measuring cups often overestimate the measured liquid, compared to two full measures using the 1-cup measuring cup. As such, I personally recommend cross-checking one's 2-cup measuring cup and assessing if it is accurate. If one finds their measuring cup to be overestimating (or underestimating) liquids, it is best to resort to using a different brand that gives more accurate readings. However, if other brands are unavailable or inaccessible, one can perform the following simple technique. Fill the 1-cup measuring cup with water to the 1-cup level, then pour into the 2-cup measuring cup. Repeat this process again to obtain 2 cups of liquid inside the 2-cup measuring cup. If one has a weight scale, place your 2-cup measuring cup on the weight scale (don't forget to tare it), then fill it up slowly with water until the recorded reading is 480 g. With a black fine-point permanent marker, draw a small parallel line at the bottom of the meniscus of water. One may need to repeat this process in order to remark the line to keep it visible with time and use.

Dry Measuring Cups. Flat-topped (or flat-rimmed) measuring cups are best to be used for measuring dry ingredients, as compared to measuring cups that have a spouted tip on the top. Flat-topped cups make levelling of ingredients more accurate. Dry measuring cups usually come as 1 cup, ½ cup, ⅓ cup, and ¼ cup. The US standard measuring cup measures 16 level tablespoons. Use these cups for measuring dry ingredients, such as rice, bulgur, quinoa, semolina, flour, vegetables, fruit, nuts, wheat berries, and legumes, as well as semi-liquid ingredients (that normally 'drop' out of the container in clumps), such as yogurt, ricotta cheese, cottage cheese, ketchup, mustard, tomato paste, *tahini*, peanut butter, grated or mashed fruits and vegetables, avocado purée, and date purée.

When measuring dry ingredients in the powder form, be sure to level off the top with the back of a knife. Make sure not to pack the ingredient into the cup by shaking the cup or pressing down with one's hand or a spoon, unless otherwise specified by a recipe. This is especially important when it comes to measuring flour (the ideal method of measuring flour is by spooning the flour into the cup, then gently levelling off the top surface with a knife). When measuring grains, lentils, and legumes, press down lightly to evenly distribute the food within the cup, then level off the top with the side of a knife, pressing down lightly.

When measuring, use the largest measuring cup possible. This means that if one needs 1 cup of an ingredient, use the 1 cup measuring cup instead of using the ½ cup measuring cup, twice. Or if one needs ¾ cup of an ingredient, measure once with a ½ cup and again with a ¼ cup. Any amounts less than ¼ cup should be measured with tablespoons and teaspoons.

Metal dry measuring cups are generally better than plastic ones, since the latter are nonconductive and can hold static electricity, which can attract powdery particles, allowing certain ingredients to cling more than others. Regardless of what is used, always shake out the contents of the cup, scraping with a spatula if need be, so as not to lose any amount of the required ingredient.

Variability among brands for dry measuring cups is common. To compare the 1 cup measuring cup you have to the one I have used in my recipe development, compare the weights of the below ingredients with what you obtain. This will give you a more accurate understanding of how your dry measuring cups compare to mine (remember to tare your scale when measuring weights of ingredients).

1 cup salt (fine) = 293 g
1 cup regular whole wheat flour = 130 g
1 cup whole wheat pastry flour = 120 g
1 cup brown rice (parboiled) = 182 g

Measuring Spoons. These usually come as 1 tablespoon, 1 teaspoon, ½ teaspoon ⅓ teaspoon, ¼ teaspoon. Always level off the top smoothly with the back of a knife. Use the required measuring spoons for measuring out small quantities of ingredients, whether dry, semi-liquid, or liquid ingredients, always making sure to level off the top without packing or pressing (unless otherwise specified). When measuring, use the largest measuring spoon possible. This means that if one needs 3 teaspoons of an ingredient, it is best to use 1 tablespoon. If one needs ¾ of a teaspoon, measure once with a ½ teaspoon and again with a ¼ teaspoon.

Measuring spoons often come attached together. It is more practical to use them detached and separate from one another. As with dry measuring cups, metal spoons are generally better than plastic ones, since the former doesn't attract powdery particles, allowing ingredients to flow out easily. Regardless of what is used, always shake out the contents of the spoon, scraping with a spatula if need be, so as not to lose any amount of the ingredient.

Variability among brands for measuring spoons is common. To compare the measuring spoons you have to the one I have used in my recipe development, compare the weights of the below ingredients with what you obtain. This will give you a more accurate understanding of how your measuring spoons compare to mine (remember to tare your scale when measuring weights of ingredients).

1 tablespoon salt (fine) = 18 g
1 teaspoon salt (fine) = 6 g
1 tablespoon regular whole wheat flour = 9 g
1 teaspoon regular whole wheat flour = 3 g

Measuring Recipe Yields. Most recipes in cookbooks or online do not clarify what the yield of a recipe is in terms of an exact serving size, simply displaying the yield as '4 servings' or as 'serves 4 people' for instance. For better accuracy, I have determined the yield of all my recipes in measures of cups, to the closest approximation.

- In measuring out the yield of soups and stews, I have used liquid measuring cups to determine how many cups are yielded by one recipe.

- In measuring out the yield of recipes other than soups and stews, including mezza dips, salads, chicken or beef dishes without a broth, and puddings, I have used dry measuring cups to determine how many cups are yielded by one recipe.

Chapter 9

COMMON ABBREVIATIONS

DF	Dairy-Free (no cow milk, yogurt, cheese, cream, butter, or *labneh*)
GF	Gluten-Free (no barley, rye, or wheat, as well as no wheat products such as wheat flour, semolina, or bulgur)
EF	Egg-Free
OF	Oil-Free (no olive oil, avocado oil, or other plant oils. Does not refer to *tahini* and peanut butter)
V	Vegan (no dairy products, eggs, and meat including red meat, chicken, fish, and shellfish)
Vt	Vegetarian (no meat including red meat, chicken, fish, and shellfish)
FF	Freezer Friendly

Carbs	carbohydrates
Kcal	calories
tbsp	tablespoon
tsp	teaspoon
°C	degrees Celsius
°F	degrees Fahrenheit
IU	international unit
kg	kilograms
g	grams
mg	milligrams
µg	micrograms
lb	pounds
oz	ounces
fl. oz	fluid ounces
ml	milliliter
cm	centimeters
``	inches
~	around/about
x	by

Chapter 10

USEFUL CONVERSIONS AND ESTIMATES

1 kg	=	1,000 g = 2.2 lb
500 g	=	1.1 lb
1 lb	=	454 g = 16 oz
1 oz	=	28 g
1 fl. oz	=	30 ml
1 inch	=	2.54 cm
1 tbsp	=	3 tsp
1 ½ tbsp	=	1 tbsp + 1 ½ tsp

500 °F	=	260 °C
450 °F	=	~ 230 °C
400 °F	=	~ 205 °C
375 °F	=	~ 190 °C
350 °F	=	~ 180 °C
325 °F	=	~ 165 °C
320 °F	=	160 °C
315 °F	=	~ 155 °C

23 cm diameter round pan	=	~ 9``
25.4 cm diameter round pan	=	~ 10``
32 cm diameter round pan	=	~ 13``
23 cm x 23 cm square pan	=	~ 9`` x 9``
20 cm x 28 cm rectangular pan	=	~ 8`` x 11``
23.5 cm x 33.5 cm rectangular pan	=	~ 9.25`` x 13.25``
25 cm x 35 cm rectangular pan	=	~ 10`` x 14``
28 cm x 37 cm rectangular pan	=	~ 11`` x 14.5``
29 cm x 35 cm rectangular pan	=	~ 11.5`` x 14``
30 cm x 40 cm rectangular pan	=	~ 12`` x 16``

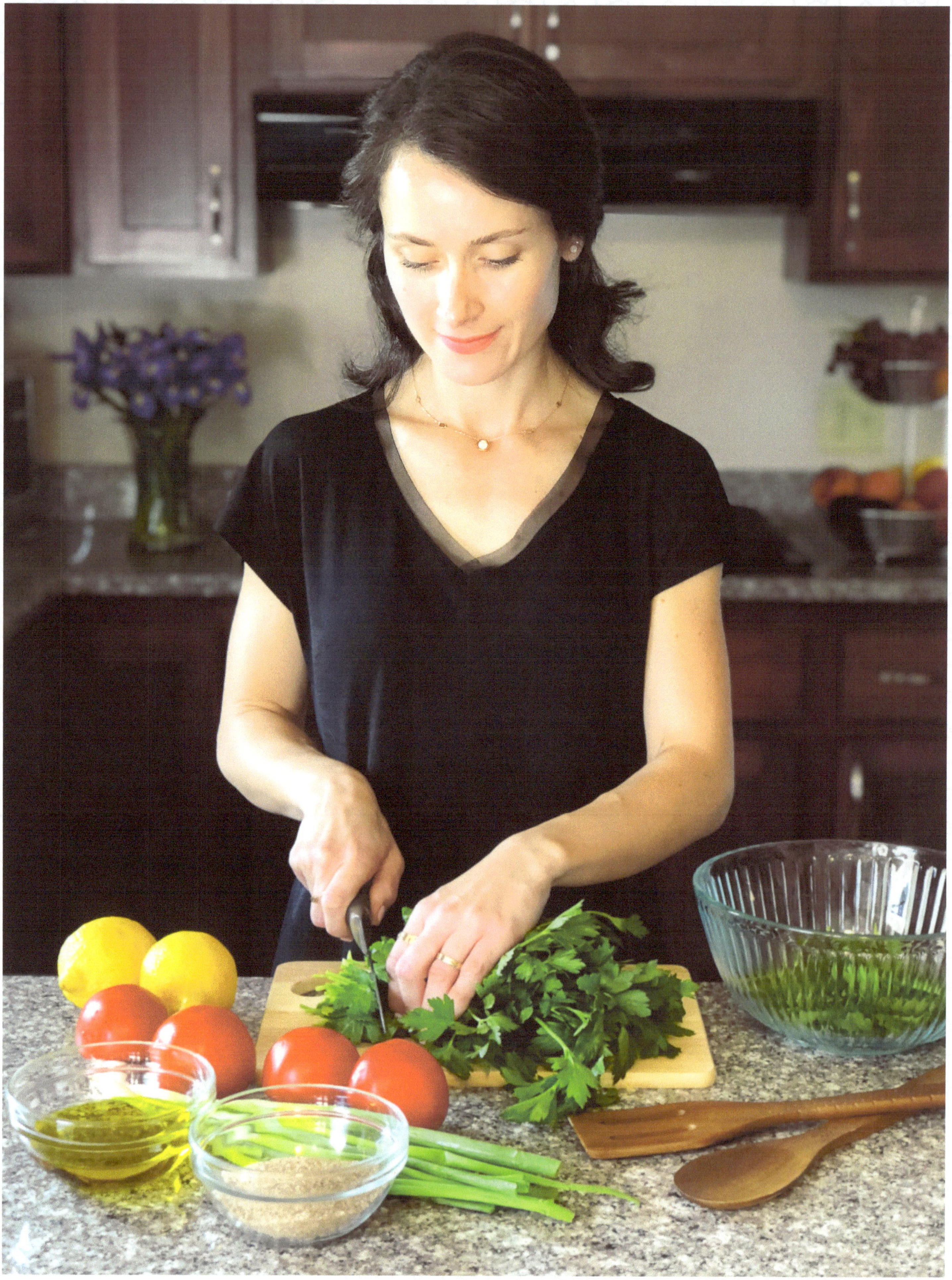

Chapter 11

RECIPES

Although reading the previous chapters in this cookbook are not a strict pre-requisite to preparing the recipes presented in the next sections, I highly recommend that one read them before starting. Alternatively, I recommend that one at least cross-check the ingredients called for in a specific recipe with relevant ingredient information presented in Chapters 4, 5, and 6.

As previously mentioned, most recipes presented in the next sections are classic Lebanese dishes modified to be healthier and more whole, sometimes with an added personal twist to the recipe. Other recipes in this book are non-Lebanese ones modified as well to be healthier and more whole, or are new healthy recipes that I developed, often with a Middle Eastern touch to them.

I always recommend reading a recipe from beginning to end (including the notes) before starting to prepare ingredients and cooking a given dish. And I always like to remind people that a cookbook is not an academic textbook, nor is it a chemistry lab manual. There is always room for personal adjustments to recipes according to preference and taste!

SOUPS

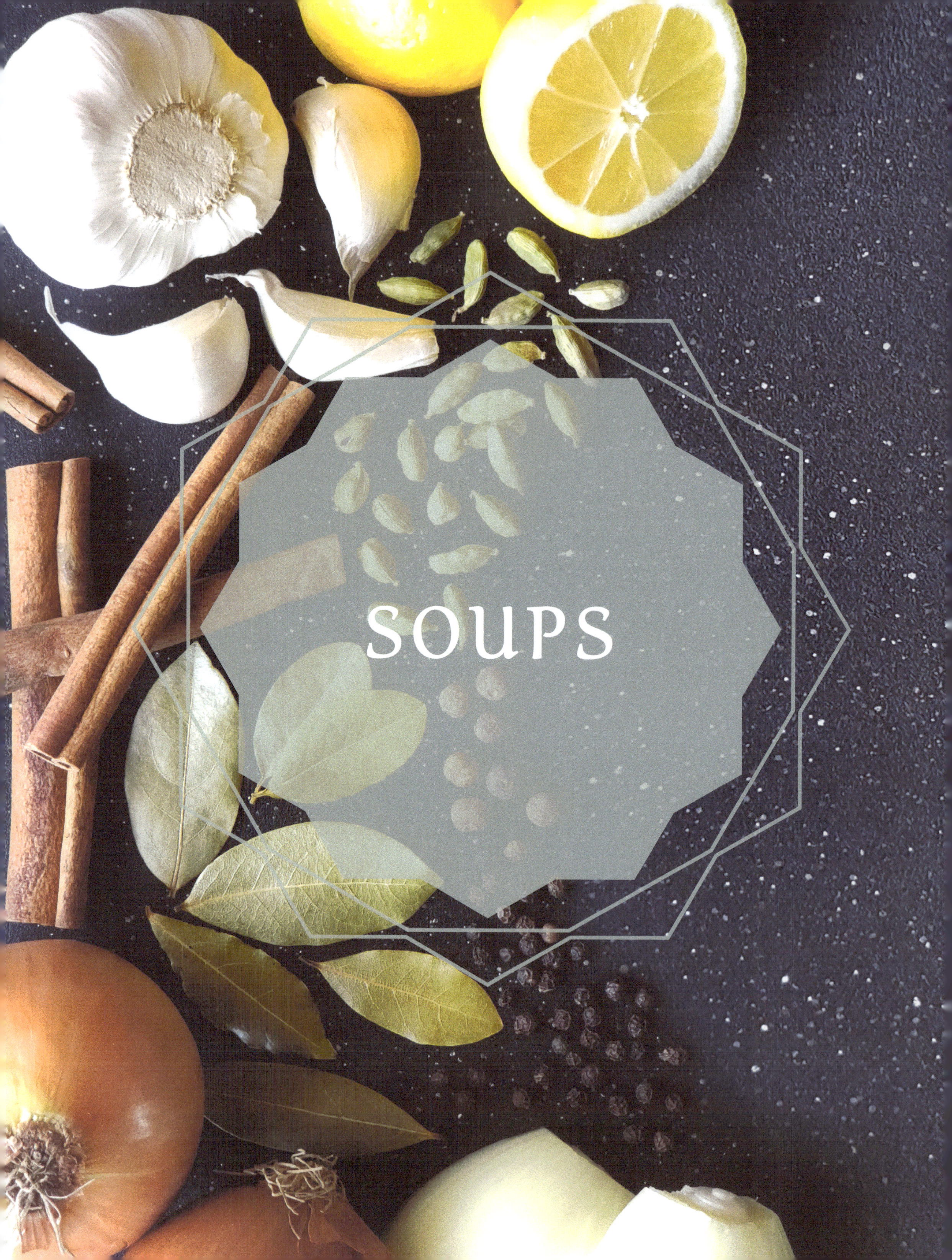

The Lebanese cuisine includes a handful of delicious soups that are considered a comfort course, mostly enjoyed during the cold winter months, but also served as a starter to meals at large gatherings or before the main dish after breaking a full-day's fast during the holy month of Ramadan. Lebanese and/or Middle Eastern soups presented in this section are named with the traditional Arabic name of the soup, along with an English transliteration of the Arabic. Soups without an Arabic name are not Lebanese/Middle Eastern. They are either recipes of my own creation or are ones adapted from recipes handed down to me by my mother.

SOME GENERAL REMARKS AND RECOMMENDATIONS

- It is very important to wash all vegetables called for in a recipe prior to starting. Vegetables can harbor soil particles from having been out in the field, and soil in turn can be the source of many harmful bacteria. Properly washing vegetables under cold running water, with scrubbing and/or quick soaking, then rinsing as many times as needed, is important. Since I do not peel my potatoes, make sure to rub the skins very well with a clean brush during washing.

- The weights presented to the right-hand side of a vegetable ingredient relate to the final net weight of the vegetable added to the pot (i.e. the net weight after peeling, removing the inedible ends or core, and chopping off bad parts of the vegetable).

- Since fresh produce can vary widely in size, shape, and weight, it is recommended to go by the presented weights of called for ingredients, in order to obtain more accurate recipe outcomes and yields.

- All spices such as cinnamon, turmeric, cumin, or ginger are called for in their ground (powdered) form, unless otherwise specified.

- I am a big fan of spices and herbs, but not a fan of salt. Thus, the salt amounts called for in my soups tend to be on the lower end, so always taste the soup once made, and accordingly adjust the salt to your taste.

- The addition of salt as an ingredient is included with the spices in the instruction steps of the recipes, unless otherwise specified.

- Whenever a cooking step calls for the addition of a main ingredient (such as water/broth, a meat source, vegetables, or rice) to a pot of soup cooking on low, follow the below steps. First turn up the heat to high, then add the ingredient(s) called for in that step, then cover. Wait until the soup returns to a rapid boil, then turn the heat back down to low. One can start timing the required cooking time from this point.

- The method I use for cooking vegetables for my soups is to boil them in a pot with the called for water or broth. I have found this method to be more convenient and dirties fewer dishes than roasting the vegetables in the oven for instance, although the latter method enhances the flavors a bit more.

- I am still traditional when it comes to soup blending. I, therefore, use a basic food blender to do the job for recipes calling for the blending of a soup. However, one can feel free to use an immersion blender instead.

- I don't like to cook with too much oil, especially since I am not fond of oily/greasy food in general. However, I make sure that the lower amount of oil doesn't negatively affect the flavor of a dish. One can definitely add more oil if desired, but this will increase the caloric and fat content of the dish.

- I like my soups on the thicker end. But to satisfy personal preferences, one can always add an extra cup or two of water or milk to the soup at the end (note that this will increase the yield, slightly influencing the nutrition facts).

- Soups containing a meat source (such as chicken or chicken broth), as well as dairy, can be made vegan by omitting the meat, replacing the chicken broth and dairy milk with water (and/or a desired plant-based milk), and omitting the called for cheese (or replacing it with vegan cheese).

- A serving of 1 cup of soup is a good serving size if the soup is to be followed by a main dish. Otherwise, a serving of 2 to 2.5 cups is a good serving size if the soup is to be enjoyed as a light meal.

- The 'sugar' value in the nutrition facts of recipes refers to the total amount of sugar (both simple and complex) that is naturally occurring in the various ingredients.

- Food items suggested as garnish are NOT included in the nutrition facts.

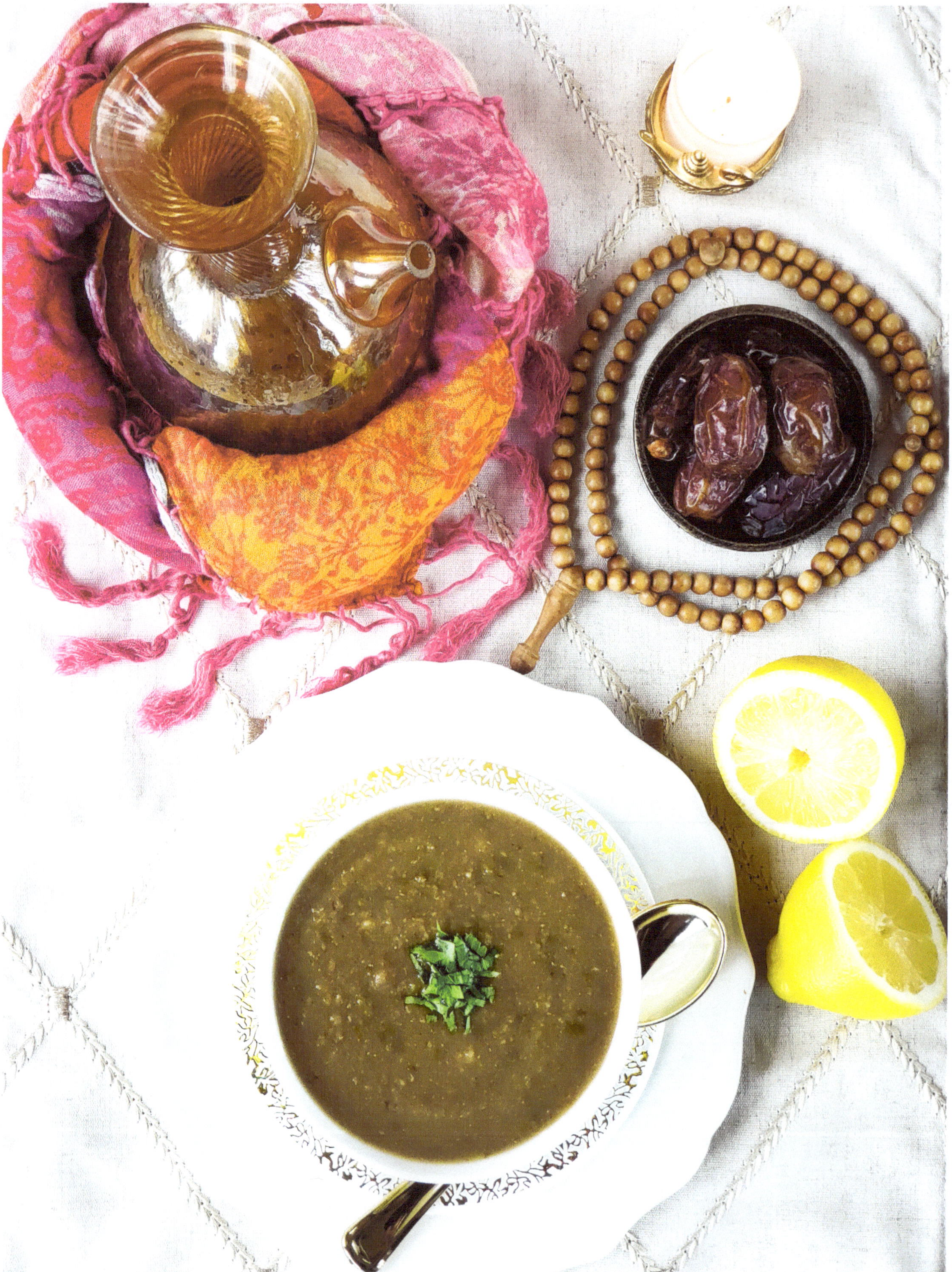

CLASSIC LENTIL SOUP

Shorbit Aadas Mamroota شوربة عدس ممروتة

This classic Middle Eastern soup is both nutritious and delicious. Lentils are a great source of fiber and protein, along with a multitude of micronutrients, namely iron. The word 'mamroota' in Arabic means blended or mashed up. Commonly made year-round, this soup is especially favored to break the fast during the holy month of Ramadan, where it is followed by a salad and then a main dish. This soup can be made with green (flat light brown) lentils or red lentils, and is traditionally made with caramelized onions that add to its flavor. Because I do not favor the process of browning onions, I compensate by adding extra cumin, and it completely makes up for the missing caramelized flavor.

RECIPE YIELD 14 cups

DF GF EF V FF

INGREDIENTS

2 ½ cups dry green lentils (463 g)
2 medium yellow onions, diced (320 g)
1 bunch Italian parsley, finely chopped (105 g)
¼ cup dry parboiled brown rice (45 g)
1 tbsp olive oil
12 cups water
⅓ cup lemon juice
4 tsp cumin
¾ tsp allspice
1 ⅔ tsp salt
black pepper, to taste

RECIPE ALTERNATIVE

For a traditional sister recipe, make the following modifications: substitute the green lentils with red lentils, omit the parsley and lemon juice, add a large diced carrot as well as ½ tsp turmeric, and decrease the cumin to 3 tsp. For this version, I like blending the whole soup together. As such, after cooking the onions, pour in only 11 cups water, add the lentils, rice, carrots, and spices, then cook all together for 25 minutes. Blend, then serve with a squeeze of lemon juice if desired.

INSTRUCTIONS

1. In a large pot, covered, cook the onions with the olive oil on low heat for 20 minutes, stirring occasionally.
2. Pick over the lentils, removing any bad pieces. Rinse well, then drain. Similarly, pick over the rice, then rinse and drain. Set aside separately.
3. Add the water and lentils, then stir to mix.
4. Bring to a boil, then cook, covered, on low heat for 25 minutes, or until tender.
5. Blend in 3 or 4 batches until smooth. Return the soup to the pot.
6. Whisk in the spices, then stir in the rice. Bring to a boil, then cook, covered, on low heat for 25 minutes, stirring occasionally (some people prefer blending the soup after this step and not earlier, so that the rice gets puréed, too).
7. Add the parsley, then continue boiling, covered, on low for another 10 minutes.
8. Stir in the lemon juice once heat is turned off.
9. Garnish with fresh parsley and add more freshly squeezed lemon juice as desired.

NUTRITION FACTS PER CUP

130 Kcal	8.4 g Protein	2 g Fat	27 g Carbs	7.5 g Fiber	1.6 g Sugar

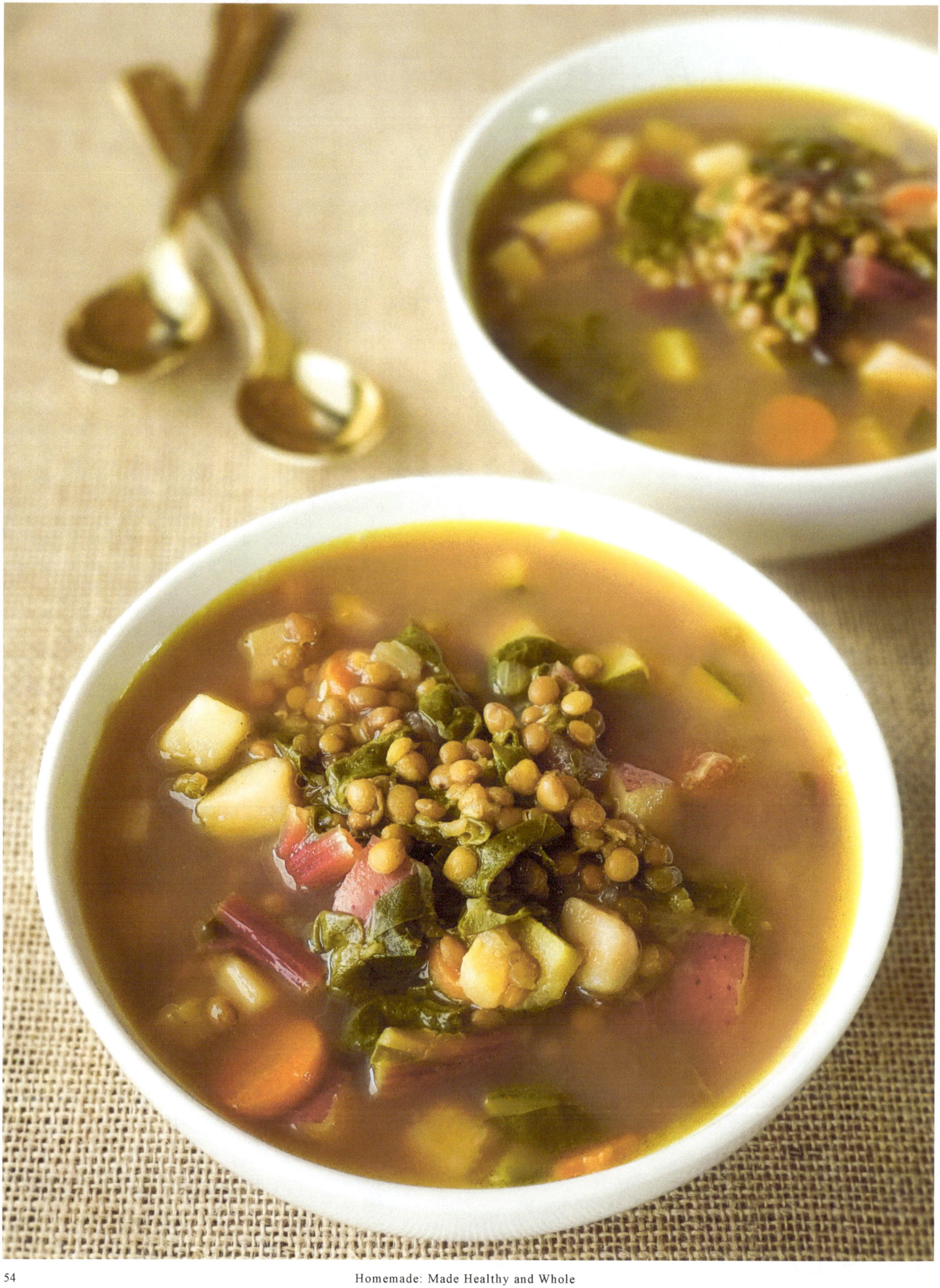

LENTIL VEGGIE SOUP

Shorbit Aadas bi Hamud wa Khudra شوربة عدس بحامض و خضرة

This is another favored Middle Eastern lentil soup, coupled with a variety of vegetables, and tasting delicious with olive oil and lots of lemon juice. Some make it with only lentils, onions, and green Swiss chard, but like many, I throw in zucchini, carrots, and some potatoes, for a variety of added goodness. Red Swiss chard is common in the US and can substitute for the green version, as they both have the same flavor. As with the classic lentil soup, this soup is also traditionally made with caramelized onions, which again I compensate for by adding some cumin.

RECIPE YIELD 18 cups

DF GF EF V FF

INGREDIENTS

2 cups dry brown lentils (390 g)
1 medium yellow onion, minced (160 g)
4 medium zucchinis, diced (450 g)
1 ½ large carrots (no skin), sliced into circles (150 g)
8 small red potatoes (with skin), diced (540 g)
6 medium Swiss chard stalks (with leaves), chopped (400 g)
2 tbsp olive oil
11 cups water
½ cup lemon juice
2 tsp cumin
½ tsp allspice
½ tsp turmeric
2 tsp salt
⅛ tsp black pepper

INSTRUCTIONS

1. In a large pot, covered, cook the onions with the olive oil on low heat for 20 minutes, stirring occasionally.
2. Pick over the lentils, removing any bad pieces. Rinse well, then drain.
3. Add the lentils, carrots, water, and spices, then stir to mix.
4. Bring to a boil, then cook, covered, on low heat for 15 minutes.
5. Add the zucchinis, potatoes, and Swiss chard, then stir to mix. Cook, covered, on low for another 15 minutes, or until the lentils and vegetables are cooked.
6. Stir in the lemon juice once heat is turned off.
7. Once served, add more freshly squeezed lemon juice as desired.

NUTRITION FACTS PER CUP

114 Kcal	6.5 g Protein	2 g Fat	23 g Carbs	6 g Fiber	2.4 g Sugar

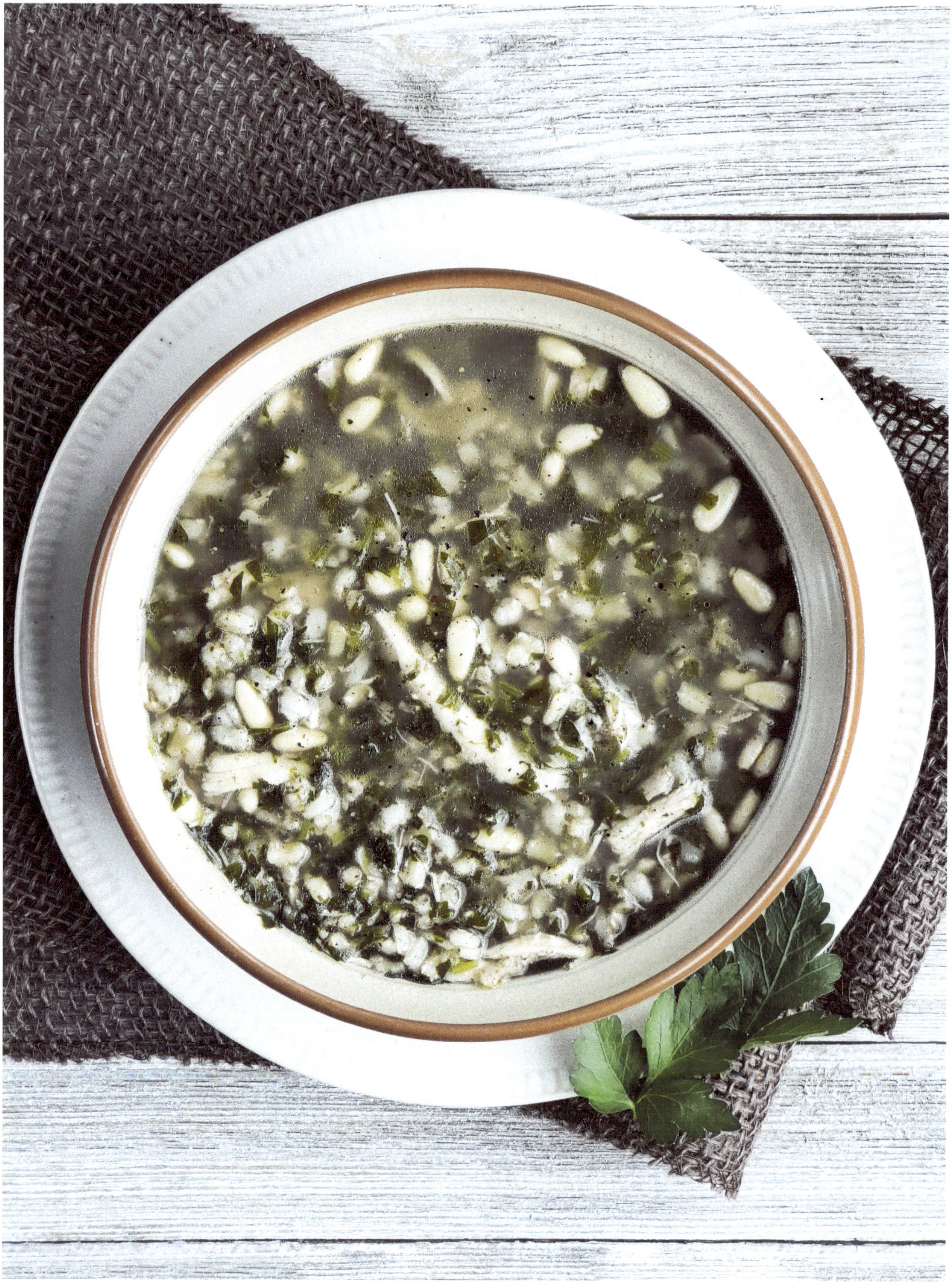

CLASSIC CHICKEN SOUP

Shorbit Djaj wa Riz شوربة دجاج و رز

This simple soup is traditionally prepared, especially in winter, to help get over a cold. Made with homemade boiled chicken and chicken broth, along with a handful of ingredients, it offers a source of protein, fiber, and micronutrients together with warmth and solace. Traditionally made with white rice and often chicken thighs, I opt for using brown rice and a small whole chicken, while making sure to create a very low-fat chicken broth.

RECIPE YIELD 15 cups

DF GF EF FF

INGREDIENTS

1 small boiled chicken (no skin, no bones), picked over by hand (500 g)
1 cup dry parboiled brown rice (182 g)
1 ½ bunches Italian parsley, finely chopped (160 g)
½ cup raw whole pine nuts (67 g)
2 tsp olive oil
13 cups unsalted chicken broth
2 tsp cinnamon
2 tsp allspice
2 tsp salt
⅛ tsp black pepper

INSTRUCTIONS

1. Pick over the rice, removing any bad pieces. Rinse well, then drain.
2. In a large pot, over high heat, whisk together the chicken broth, olive oil and spices.
3. Add the rice and pine nuts, then cover and bring to a boil.
4. Cook, covered, on low heat for 25 minutes, stirring occasionally.
5. Add the parsley, then cook, covered, on low for another 10 minutes.
6. Fold in the chicken, then stir on high heat for a few minutes.

NUTRITION FACTS PER CUP

173.6 Kcal	14 g Protein	7.6 g Fat	11 g Carbs	1.5 g Fiber	0.1 g Sugar

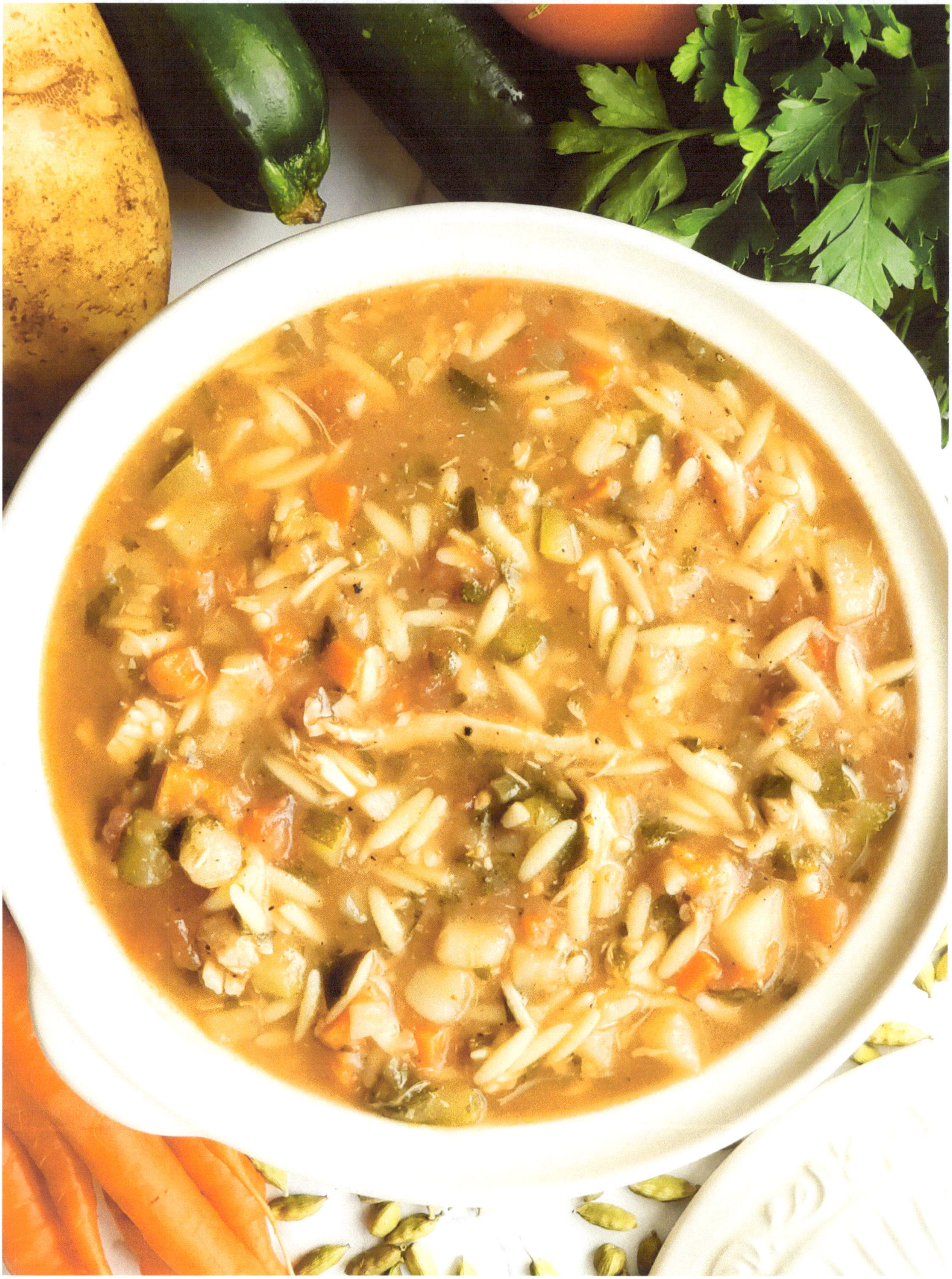

CHICKEN VEGGIE SOUP

Shorbit Djaij wa Khudra شوربة دجاج و خضرة

I have come to realize that every household in Lebanon has its own version of a chicken soup with vegetables, similar to a minestrone soup. My chicken minestrone soup with a Middle Eastern twist was adapted from the recipe of one of my Lebanese uncles' wives. One can omit the orzo (for a gluten-free version) and enjoy a lighter soup with just vegetables and chicken. This soup also tastes great with no chicken (just vegetables and orzo) and water instead of chicken broth for a vegan version.

RECIPE YIELD 18 cups

DF EF FF

INGREDIENTS

½ small boiled chicken (no skin, no bones), picked over by hand (250 g)
¾ cup orzo (126 g)
5 medium red tomatoes, diced (665 g)
4 medium zucchinis, diced (450 g)
2 large carrots (no skin), diced (200 g)
2 medium russet potatoes (with skin), diced (850 g)
1 bunch Italian parsley, finely chopped (105 g)
4 tbsp unsalted tomato paste
2 tsp olive oil
9 cups unsalted chicken broth
½ tsp cinnamon
1 tsp 7-spices
2 ¼ tsp salt
12 whole cardamom pods

INSTRUCTIONS

1. In a large pot, over high heat, whisk together the chicken broth, tomato paste, olive oil, and spices.
2. Add the cardamom pods, then bring to a boil. Cook, covered, on low heat for 10 minutes.
3. Add the tomatoes, zucchinis, carrots, and potatoes, then stir to mix. Cook, covered, on low for another 15 minutes.
4. Add the orzo and parsley, then cook, covered, on low for another 10 minutes.
5. Fold in the chicken, then stir on high heat for a few minutes.

NUTRITION FACTS PER CUP

125.5 Kcal	8 g Protein	2.6 g Fat	18 g Carbs	2.4 g Fiber	2.6 g Sugar

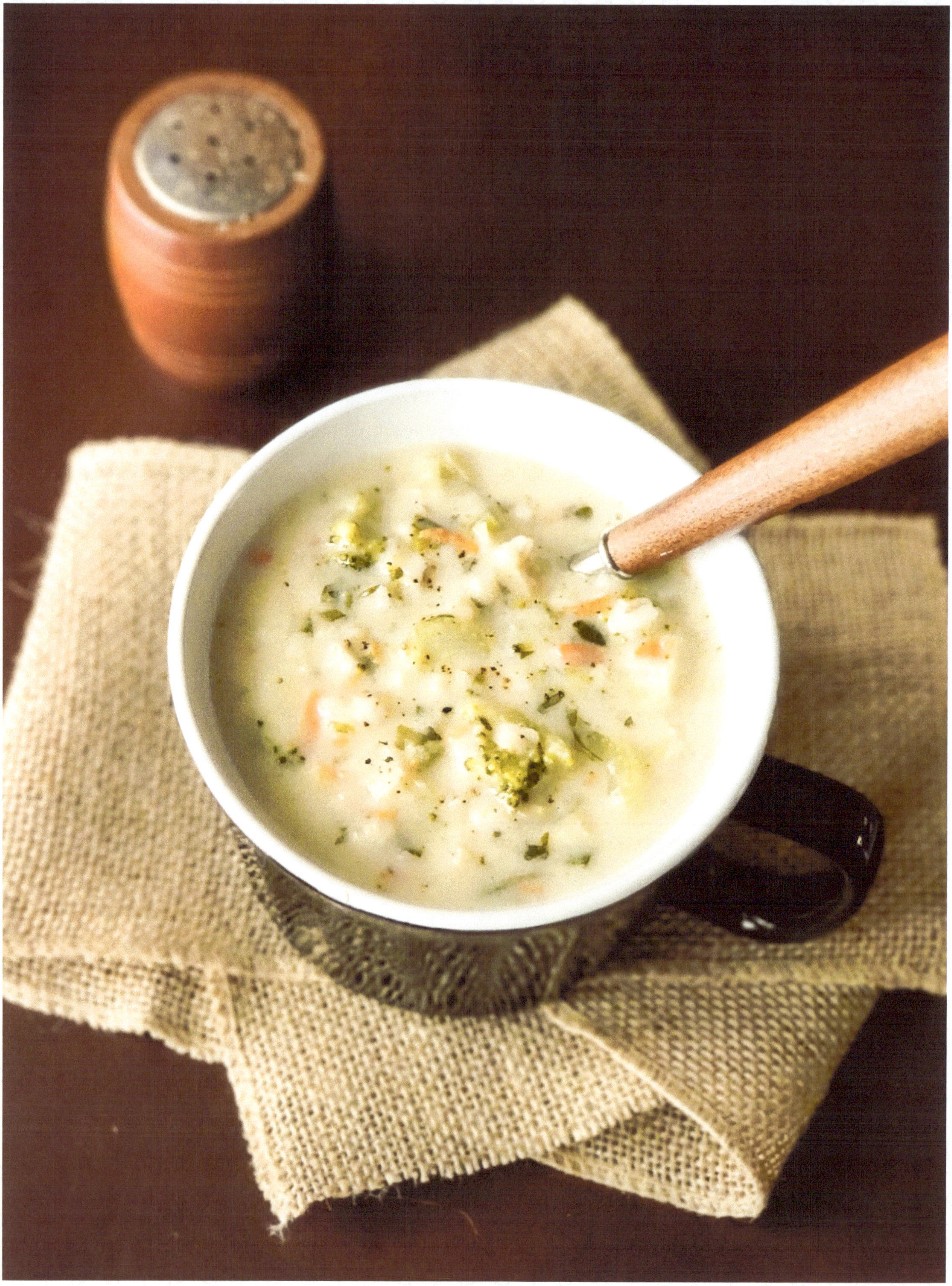

BARLEY SOUP

Adapted from a recipe of my mother's, this creamy calcium-rich soup is full of fiber and protein, and many antioxidants! I never use cooking cream in my dishes, completely relying instead on skim milk thickened with powdered skim milk, for a stronger and 'fuller' milk flavor.

RECIPE YIELD 17 cups

EF Vt FF

INGREDIENTS

1 cup dry pearled barley (194 g)
¼ medium green (white) cabbage, finely chopped (375 g)
1 medium broccoli head (no stalk), broken/chopped into small florets (175 g)
2 large celery stalks (no leaves), diced (130 g)
1 large carrot (no skin), coarsely grated (100 g)
1 medium yellow onion, minced (160 g)
½ bunch Italian parsley, finely chopped (53 g)
1 tbsp garlic, crushed
2 tbsp olive oil
7 ½ cups water
6 cups liquid skim milk
½ cup powdered skim milk (45 g)
½ cup finely grated parmesan cheese (50 g)
4 tbsp whole wheat flour
⅓ tsp allspice
¼ tsp nutmeg
2 ½ tsp salt
black pepper, to taste

INSTRUCTIONS

1. In a large pot, covered, cook the onions with 1 tbsp olive oil on low heat for 20 minutes, stirring occasionally.
2. Whisk the flour with 1 tbsp olive oil and 1 cup water in a separate bowl. Add the rest of the water and spices and whisk well. Pour into the pot.
3. Add the barley, all the vegetables (except for the carrots and parsley), and the garlic, then stir to mix.
4. Bring to a boil, then cook, covered, on low heat for 20 minutes, stirring occasionally.
5. Add the carrots and parsley, then cook for another 10 minutes.
6. Mix the powdered milk and liquid milk in a separate bowl.
7. On medium-high heat, slowly pour in the milk, then add the parmesan cheese little by little, stirring well until melted.
8. Keep stirring until the soup just comes to a boil.

NUTRITION FACTS PER CUP

131 Kcal	7 g Protein	3 g Fat	20 g Carbs	3.6 g Fiber	7.6 g Sugar

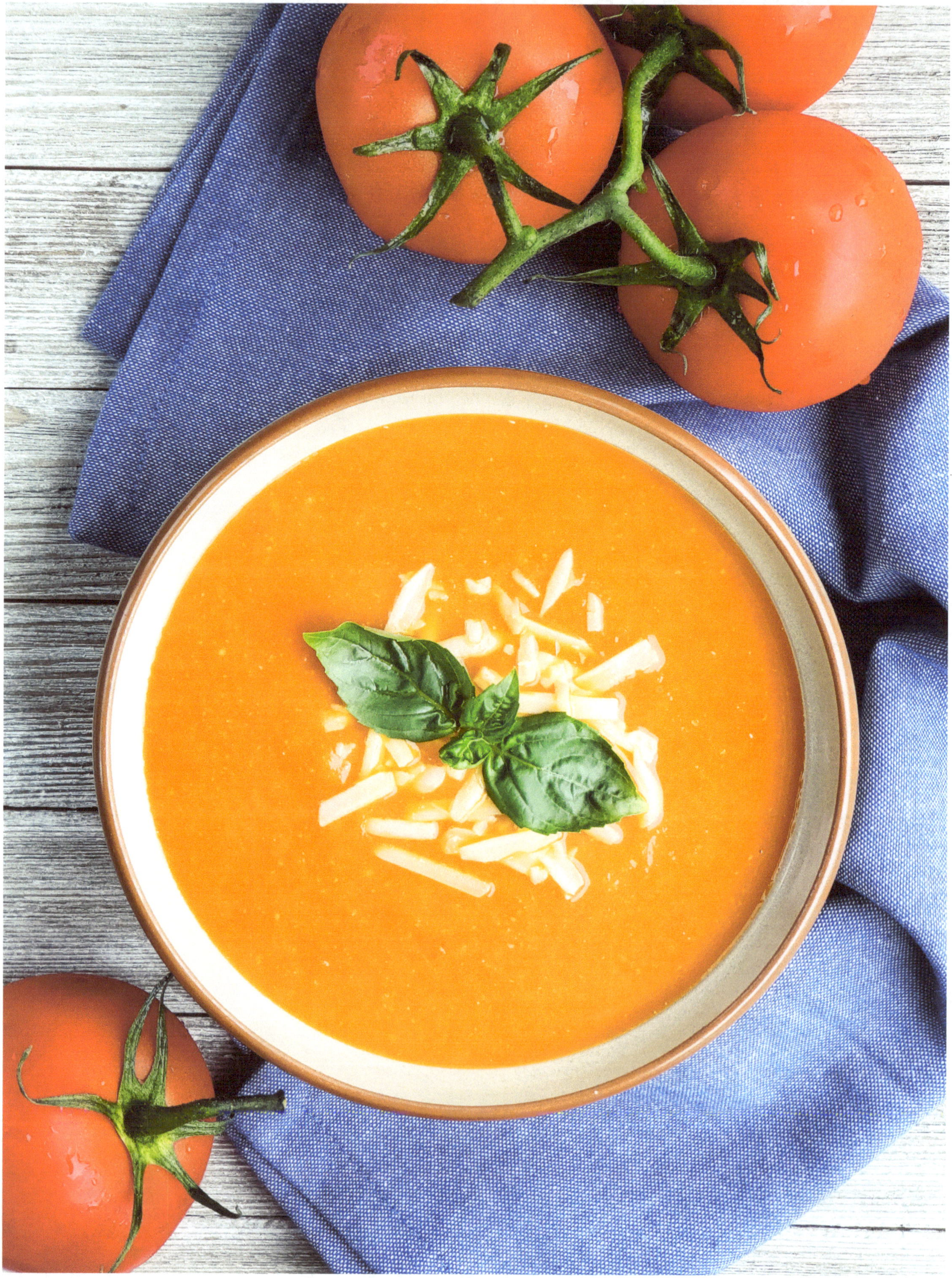

TOMATO SOUP

This is a simple nutritious soup that has a more whole and healthier take on the traditional tomato soup usually made from canned tomatoes and cooking cream. I like using fresh tomatoes which are rich in fiber and lycopene (a potent antioxidant), and skim milk thickened with powdered skim milk as a cream substitute.

RECIPE YIELD 9 cups

GF EF Vt FF

INGREDIENTS

15 medium red tomatoes, chopped (2 kg)
2 medium yellow onions, diced (320 g)
2 tbsp garlic, crushed
2 tbsp unsalted tomato paste
1 tbsp olive oil
1 cup liquid skim milk
⅓ cup powdered skim milk (30 g)
⅔ tsp salt
black pepper, to taste

INSTRUCTIONS

1. In a large pot, covered, cook the onions with the olive oil on low heat for 20 minutes, stirring occasionally.
2. Add the tomatoes, garlic, and tomato paste, then stir to mix. Bring to a boil, then cook, covered, on low for 20 minutes, stirring occasionally.
3. Blend in 2 or 3 batches until smooth. Return the soup to the pot.
4. Mix the powdered milk and liquid milk in a separate bowl.
5. On medium-high heat, slowly pour in the milk, then add the salt and pepper.
6. Keep stirring until the soup just comes to a boil.
7. Garnish with grated parmesan cheese and/or fresh basil if desired.

NUTRITION FACTS PER CUP

93 Kcal	4.6 g Protein	2 g Fat	16 g Carbs	3.5 g Fiber	11 g Sugar

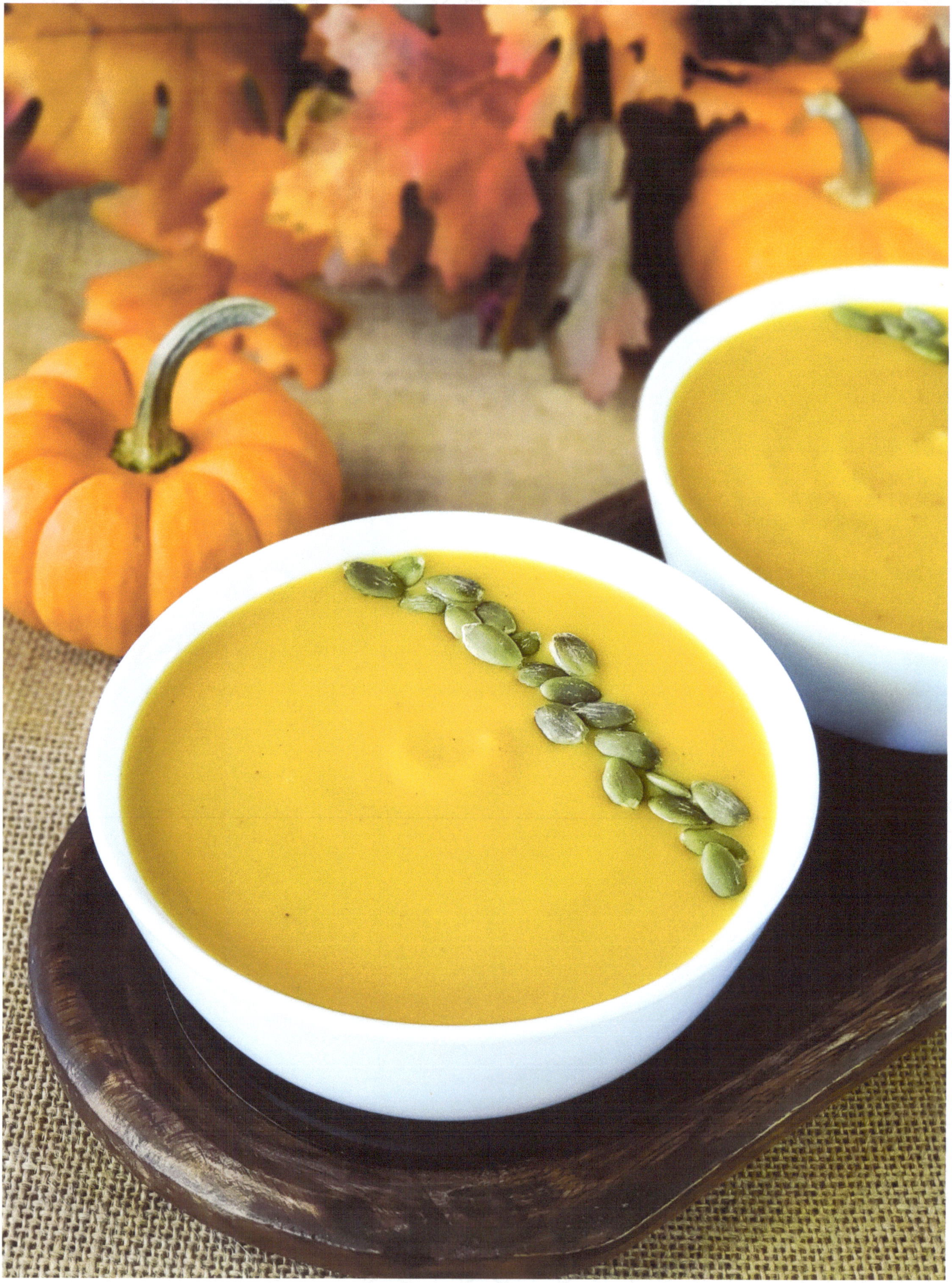

PUMPKIN SOUP

This beta-carotene and vitamin C-rich soup is a super healthy and delicious variation to the traditional pumpkin soup made with cream. Although it can be made completely with pumpkin, I like adding some sweet potatoes and carrots for additional nutritional benefits. Since I don't cook with cream, I completely rely instead on skim milk thickened with powdered skim milk to give that strong and 'full' milk flavor. In pumpkin season, it is great to make this soup from fresh pumpkins, but make sure to strain the cooked pumpkin of extra water to make a thick purée (or else the called for amount of water for the soup needs to be adjusted to account for the extra liquid from the pumpkin).

RECIPE YIELD 13 cups

GF EF Vt FF

INGREDIENTS

3 cups pumpkin purée (canned) (675 g)
1 medium orange sweet potato (with skin), diced (375 g)
1 medium carrot (no skin), sliced into circles (60 g)
1 medium yellow onion, diced (160 g)
1 tsp garlic, crushed
1 tbsp olive oil
4 cups water
4 cups liquid skim milk
½ cup powdered skim milk (45 g)
½ tsp turmeric
¼ tsp cloves
¼ tsp cinnamon
¼ tsp allspice
1 ½ tsp salt

RECIPE ALTERNATIVE

- To create an equally delicious sweet potato soup, one can use more sweet potatoes than pumpkin.

INSTRUCTIONS

1. In a large pot, covered, cook the onions with the olive oil on low heat for 20 minutes, stirring occasionally.
2. Add the water, potatoes, carrots, garlic, and spices, then stir to mix. Cook, covered, on low for 20 minutes, stirring occasionally.
3. Blend in 3 or 4 batches until smooth. Return the soup to the pot.
4. Mix the powdered milk and liquid milk in a separate bowl.
5. In 2 batches, blend the milk and pumpkin, until smooth.
6. Transfer to the pot, then on medium-high heat, whisk into the vegetable broth, stirring until the soup just comes to a boil.
7. Garnish with raw or roasted pumpkin seeds if desired.

NUTRITION FACTS PER CUP

97 Kcal	5 g Protein	1 g Fat	17 g Carbs	3 g Fiber	9.4 g Sugar

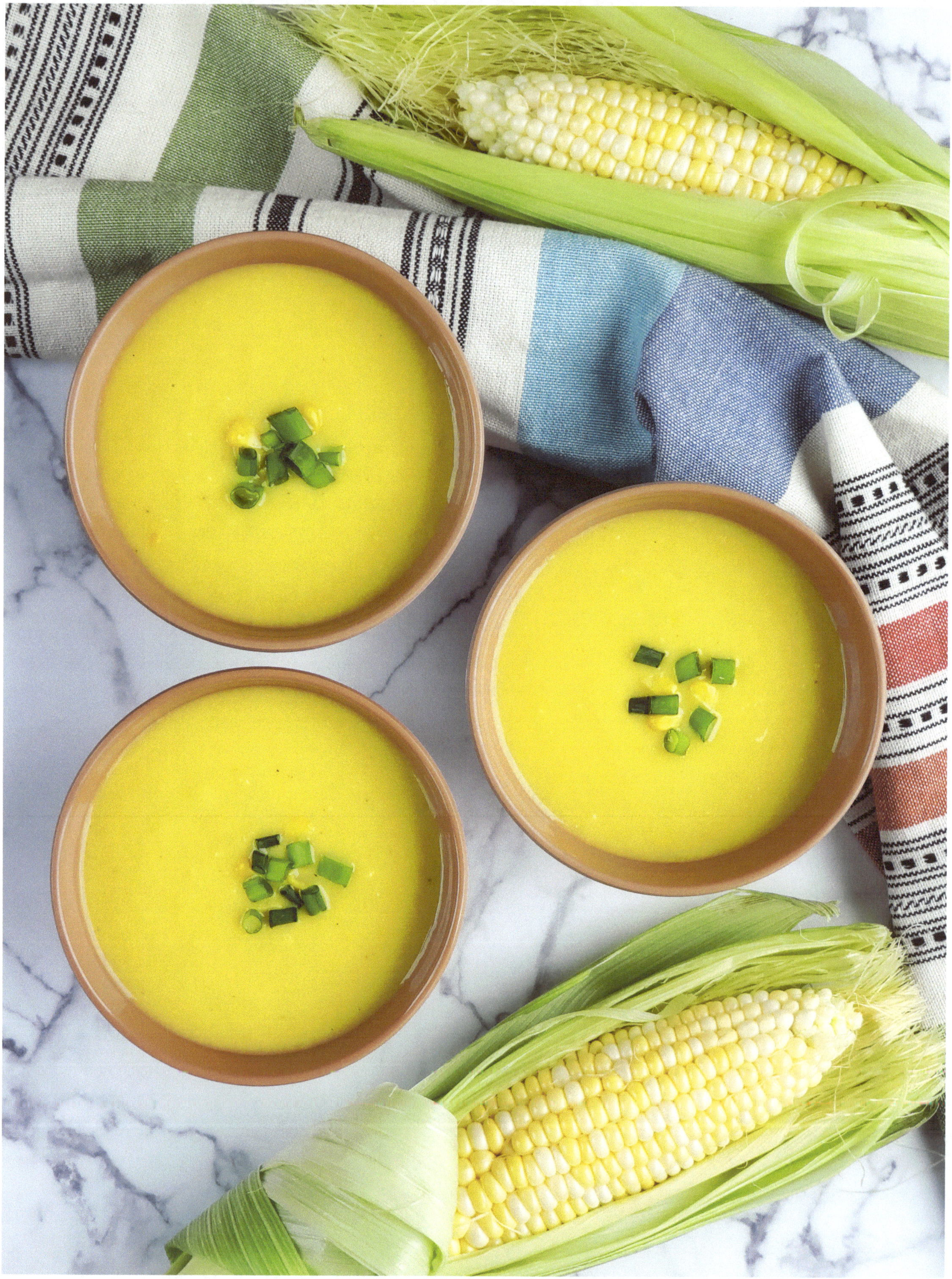

CORN SOUP

This creamy soup was inspired by traditional corn chowder soups and adapted from a recipe of one of my sisters-in-law, but made healthier with no butter or cream, and made vegetarian without chicken and/or chicken broth.

RECIPE YIELD 14 cups

GF EF Vt FF

INGREDIENTS

9 ½ cups sweet corn kernels (1.5 kg)
1 medium yellow onion, diced (160 g)
3 medium green onion stalks, diced (48 g)
1 tbsp garlic, crushed
1 tbsp olive oil
7 cups water
1 cup liquid skim milk
⅓ cup powdered skim milk (30 g)
⅓ tsp turmeric
1 ½ tsp salt
⅛ tsp black pepper

NOTE

- If using canned corn, one will need 6 (15.25 oz) cans of corn. Drain, rinse, then drain again before use.

INSTRUCTIONS

1. In a large pot, covered, cook the onions with the olive oil on low heat for 20 minutes, stirring occasionally.
2. Add the water, corn (set aside ½ cup for later; can mince if desired), green onions, garlic, and spices, then stir to mix.
3. Bring to a boil, then cook, covered, on low for 20 minutes, stirring occasionally.
4. Blend in 3 or 4 batches until smooth. Return the soup to the pot.
5. Mix the powdered milk and liquid milk in a separate bowl.
6. On medium-high heat, slowly pour in the milk, then add the ½ cup corn, stirring until the soup just comes to a boil.
7. Garnish with extra green onions or fresh parsley if desired.

NUTRITION FACTS PER CUP

101 Kcal	4 g Protein	2 g Fat	19 g Carbs	2.5 g Fiber	7.5 g Sugar

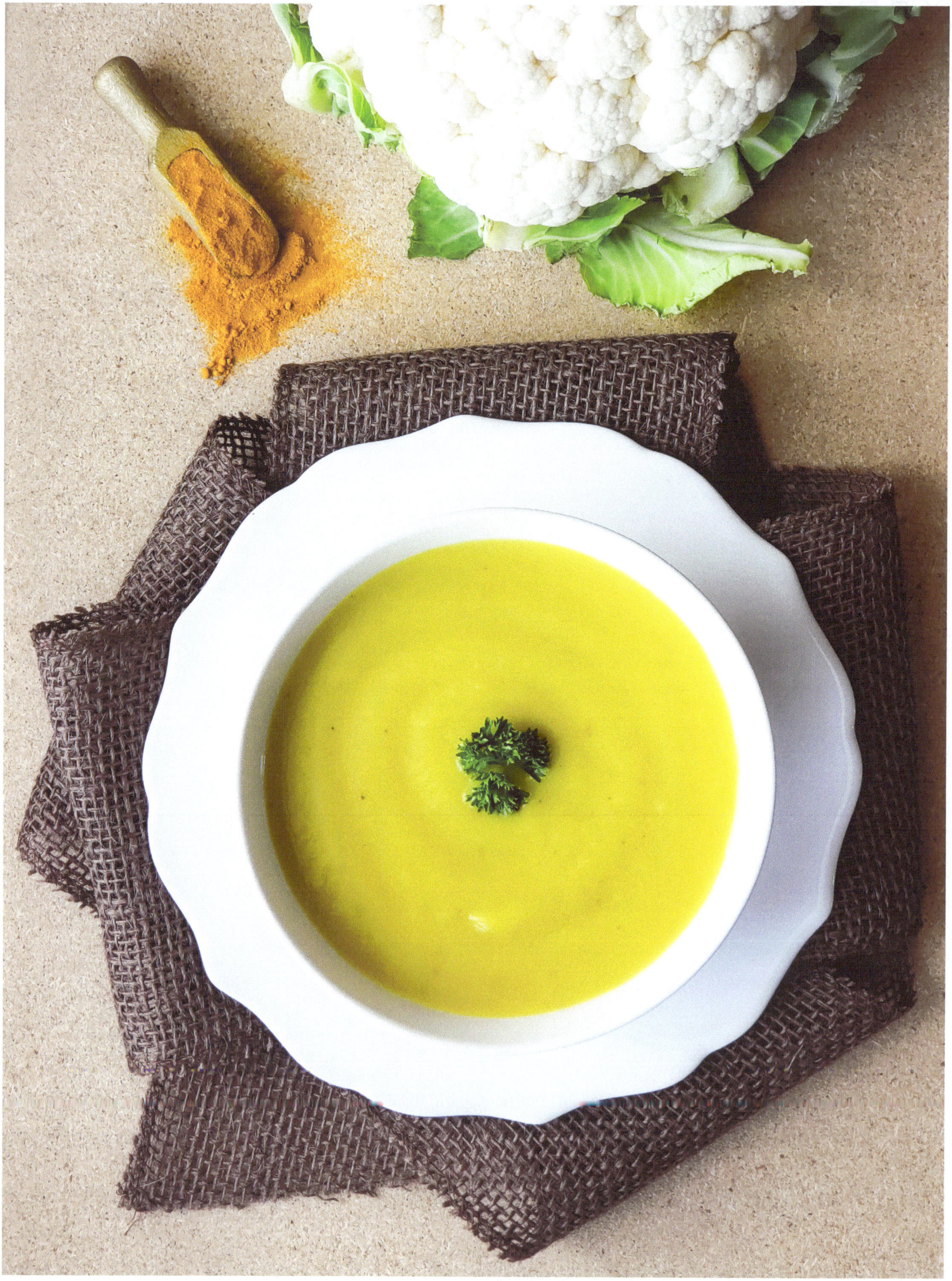

CAULIFLOWER SOUP

This creamy soup is rich in beta-carotene, vitamin C, and calcium, along with many other healthy phytochemicals. I include cabbage and sweet potatoes alongside the cauliflower in this soup for added nutrients, but one could make it with only cauliflower and sweet potatoes without jeopardizing the flavor or texture.

RECIPE YIELD 14 cups

GF EF Vt FF

INGREDIENTS

1 medium cauliflower head (no stalk), broken/chopped into pieces (800 g)
¼ medium green (white) cabbage, chopped (375 g)
2 medium white sweet potatoes (with skin), diced (750 g)
1 medium yellow onion, diced (160 g)
1 tsp garlic, crushed
1 tbsp olive oil
7 cups water
1 cup liquid skim milk
2 tsp turmeric
½ tsp curry (mild)
1 ½ tsp salt

RECIPE ALTERNATIVE

An equally delicious but simpler soup one can make is potato soup. Substitute the cauliflower, cabbage, and sweet potatoes with russet potatoes (use about 1.5 kg potatoes with skin) and add a half a bunch of Italian parsley to the ingredients. Bump up the milk to 2 cups and decrease the water to 6 cups. Decrease the turmeric to 1 tsp, eliminate the curry, increase the salt to 1 ⅔ tsp, and add 1/8 tsp black pepper. Prepare the soup as per the instructions until step 4. Add the chopped parsley to the pureed soup then boil on low for 10 min before adding the milk in step 5.

INSTRUCTIONS

1. In a large pot, covered, cook the onions with the olive oil on low heat for 20 minutes, stirring occasionally.
2. Add the water, cauliflower, cabbage, potatoes, garlic, and spices, then stir to mix (volume of vegetables will look like a lot, but the vegetables start "melting" as they cook up).
3. Bring to a boil, then cook, covered, on low for 20 minutes, stirring occasionally.
4. Blend in 3 or 4 batches until smooth. Return the soup to the pot.
5. On medium-high heat, slowly pour in the milk, stirring until the soup just comes to a boil.
6. Garnish with fresh parsley if desired.

NUTRITION FACTS PER CUP

88 Kcal	3 g Protein	1 g Fat	17.4 g Carbs	4 g Fiber	6 g Sugar

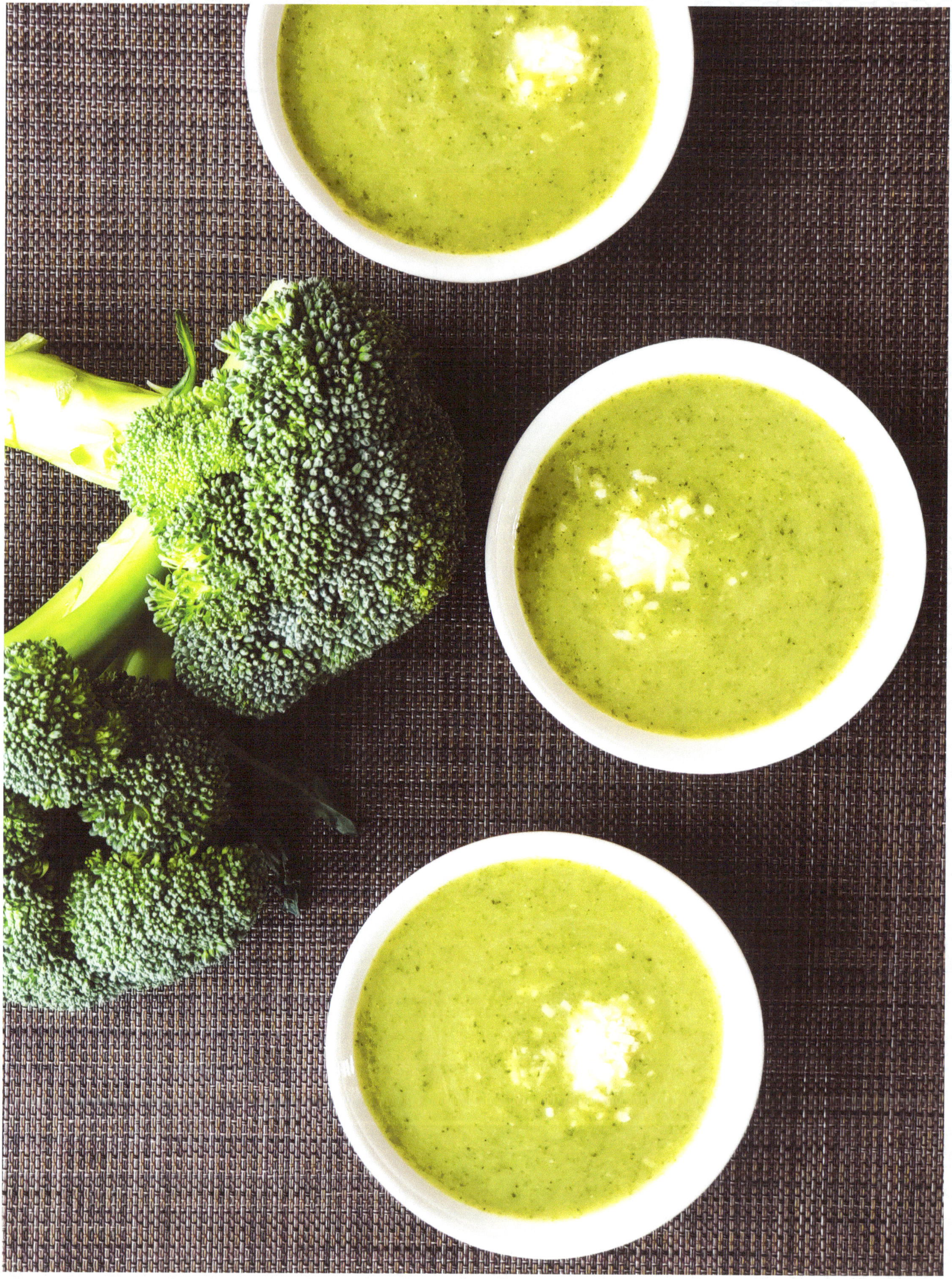

BROCCOLI SOUP

Rich in vitamin K, folate, and calcium, this soup is a healthier version of the traditional broccoli soup made with cream. One can make it completely with broccoli, but I added some zucchini and kale to add an extra variety of nutritional benefits.

RECIPE YIELD 14 cups

GF EF Vt FF

INGREDIENTS

4 medium broccoli heads (with stalks), broken/chopped into pieces (1 kg)
4 medium zucchini, sliced into circles (450 g)
4 small curly kale stalks (leaves only), chopped (100 g)
1 medium yellow onion, diced (160 g)
1 tsp garlic, crushed
1 tbsp olive oil
7 cups water
1 cup liquid skim milk
½ cup finely grated parmesan cheese (50 g)
¼ tsp allspice
½ tsp cumin
1 ½ tsp salt
black pepper, to taste

INSTRUCTIONS

1. In a large pot, covered, cook the onions with the olive oil on low heat for 20 minutes, stirring occasionally.
2. Add the water, broccoli, zucchinis, kale, garlic, and spices, then stir to mix (volume of vegetables will look like a lot, but the vegetables start "melting" as they cook up).
3. Bring to a boil, then cook, covered, on low for 20 minutes, stirring occasionally.
4. Blend in 3 or 4 batches until smooth. Return the soup to the pot.
5. On medium-high heat, slowly stir in the milk, then add the parmesan cheese little by little, stirring well until melted.
6. Keep stirring until the soup just comes to a boil.
7. Garnish with extra grated parmesan cheese if desired.

NUTRITION FACTS PER CUP

66 Kcal	4.6 g Protein	2.4 g Fat	8 g Carbs	2.7 g Fiber	3.6 g Sugar

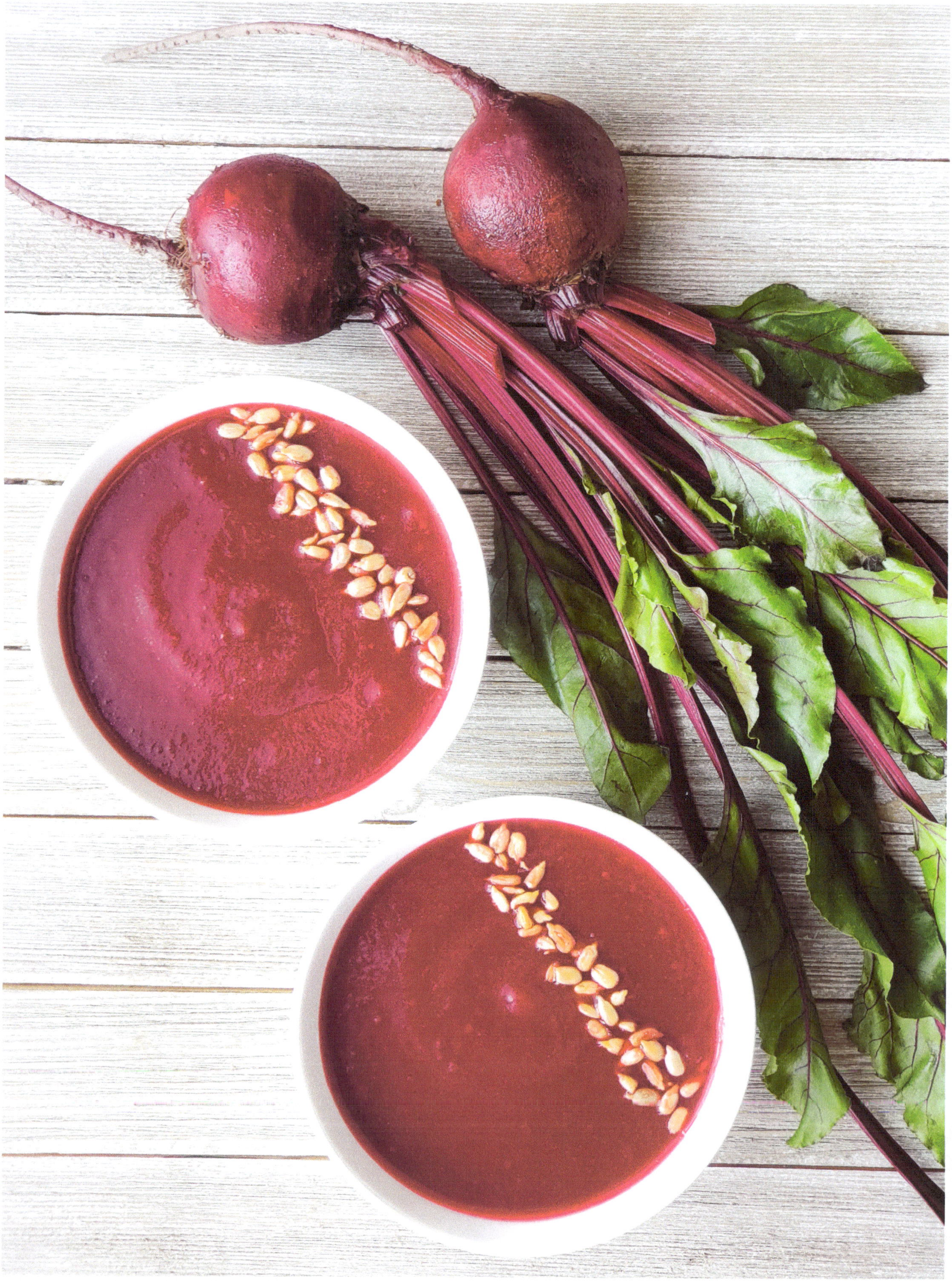

BEET SOUP

This beautiful ruby-red colored soup is super easy to make and is rich in a multitude of nutrients, namely fiber, folate, and vitamin C, not to mention unlimited antioxidant power.

RECIPE YIELD 13 cups

DF GF EF V FF

INGREDIENTS

5 small beets (no skin), chopped (375 g)
10 small red potatoes (with skin), chopped (675 g)
¼ small purple (red) cabbage, chopped (250 g)
1 large red onion, diced (375 g)
1 tsp garlic, crushed
1 tbsp olive oil
8 cups water
½ tsp ginger
1 ½ tsp salt
black pepper, to taste

NOTE

One can keep the beet skins on if they are not too dry or blemished, but make sure to scrub the beets well just as one would scrub potatoes.

INSTRUCTIONS

1. In a large pot, covered, cook the onions with the olive oil on low heat for 20 minutes, stirring occasionally.
2. Add the water, beets, potatoes, cabbage, garlic, and spices, then stir to mix. Bring to a boil, then cook, covered, on low for 25 minutes, stirring occasionally.
3. Blend in 3 or 4 batches until smooth. Return the soup to the pot, and mix.
4. Garnish with raw sunflower seeds if desired.

NUTRITION FACTS PER CUP

77 Kcal	2 g Protein	1 g Fat	15.4 g Carbs	3 g Fiber	5 g Sugar

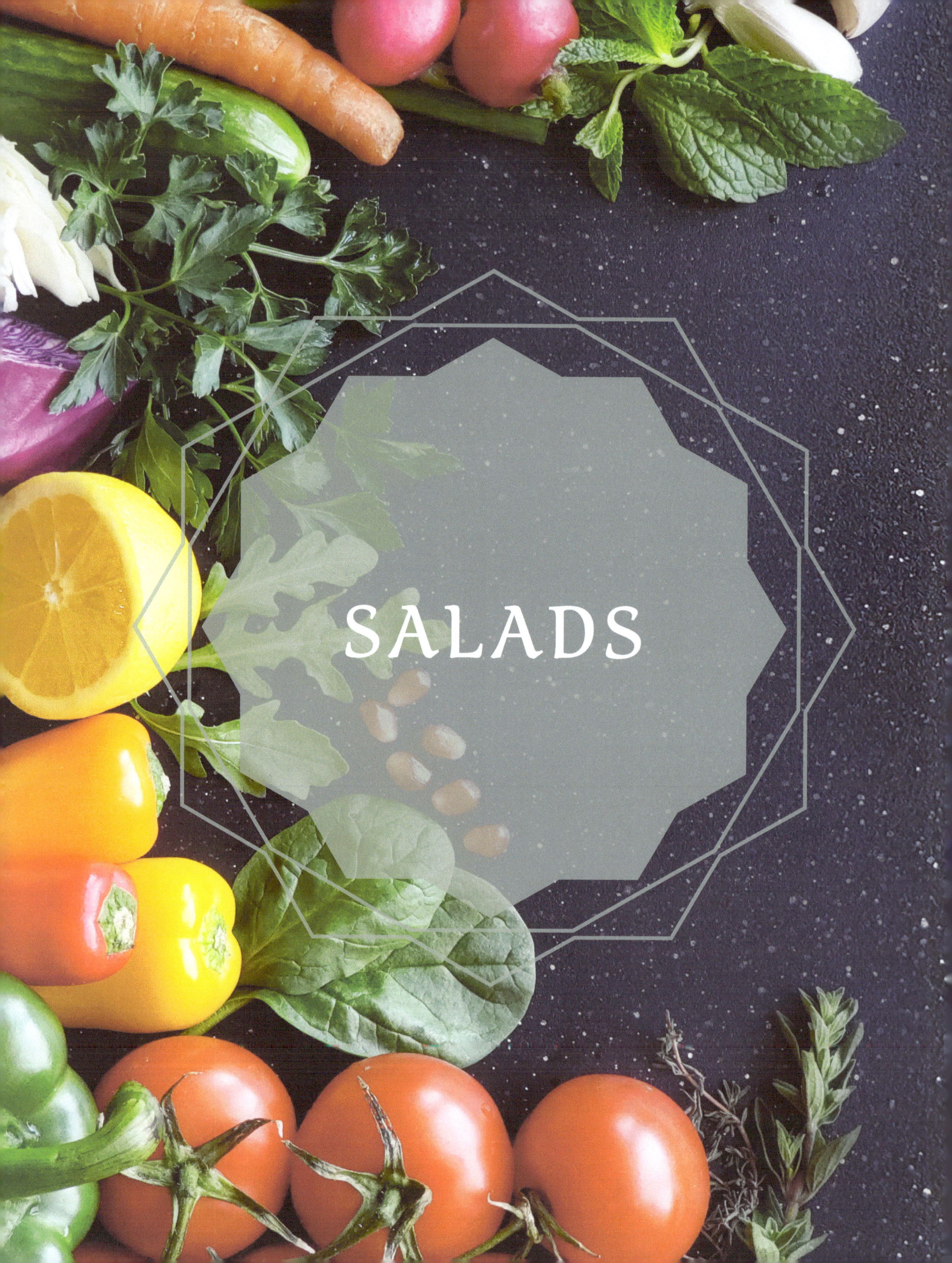

SALADS

Salads hold a special place in the Lebanese cuisine, acting as a starter to most lunch or dinner meals, especially in hot seasons. With a multitude of different vegetables, herbs, and dressings, salads are a great way to get a boost of micronutrients, phytochemicals, and fiber, while satisfying one's taste for pungent flavors and a fresh crunch. Lebanese and/or Middle Eastern salads presented in this section are named with the traditional Arabic name of the salad, along with an English transliteration of the Arabic. Salads without an Arabic name are not Lebanese/Middle Eastern. They are either recipes of my own creation or are ones adapted from recipes handed down to me by my mother.

SOME GENERAL REMARKS AND RECOMMENDATIONS

- It is extremely important in salad making to properly wash the vegetables, as salads are consumed raw. Vegetables can harbor soil particles from having been grown in the field, and soil in turn can be the source of many harmful bacteria. Properly washing vegetables under cold running water, with scrubbing and/or quick soaking, then rinsing as many times as needed, is important in preparing safe salads.

- Another key element in salad making is letting your vegetables dry completely prior to cutting, slicing, dicing or chopping, as this is vital in maintaining freshness and slowing down the wilting of vegetables, especially green-leafy vegetables, once the salt and dressing ingredients have been added. For maximum freshness and crispness, mix salad vegetables with the dressing right before serving.

- Proper refrigeration plays a role in maintaining freshness of the vegetables before being prepared for the salad, but also for the salad itself once mixed. Storing left-over salads in an airtight container will make day-old salads taste better.

- The weights presented to the right-hand side of a vegetable ingredient relate to the final net weight of the vegetable added to the salad (i.e. the net weight after peeling, removing the inedible ends or core, and chopping off bad parts of the vegetable).

- Since fresh produce can vary widely in size, shape, and weight, it is recommended to go by the presented weights of called for ingredients, in order to obtain more accurate recipe outcomes and yields.

- All spices called for in a recipe are in their ground (powdered) form, unless otherwise specified (such as for oregano, dry oregano leaves will be indicated if the non-powdered dry oregano is called for. Same goes for mint).

- I am a big fan of spices and herbs, but not a fan of salt. Thus, the salt amounts called for in my salads tend to be on the lower end, so always taste the salad once prepared, and accordingly adjust the salt to your taste.

- The addition of salt as an ingredient is included with the spices in the instruction steps of the recipes, unless otherwise specified.

- When it comes to common dressing ingredients used such as garlic, lemon juice, or cider vinegar, let your food preferences guide how much you add to your salads. If you like the above ingredients, then follow my recipes exactly, as I like them, too (or even go ahead and bump up the quantities if need be)! If you like your salads weak in terms of these flavors, cut back a bit, have a taste, and then adjust according to your taste.

- I like to prepare my salads without too much oil, especially since I am not fond of oily/greasy food in general. However, I make sure that the lower amount of oil doesn't negatively affect the flavor of the salad. One can definitely add more oil if desired, but this will increase the caloric and fat content of the salad.

- A serving of 1 cup of salad is a good serving size if the salad is to be followed by a main dish. Otherwise, a serving of 2 to 2.5 cups is a good serving size if the salad is to be enjoyed as a light meal.

- The 'sugar' value in the nutrition facts of recipes refers to the total amount of sugar (both simple and complex) that is naturally occurring in the various ingredients.

- Food items suggested as garnish are NOT included in the nutrition facts.

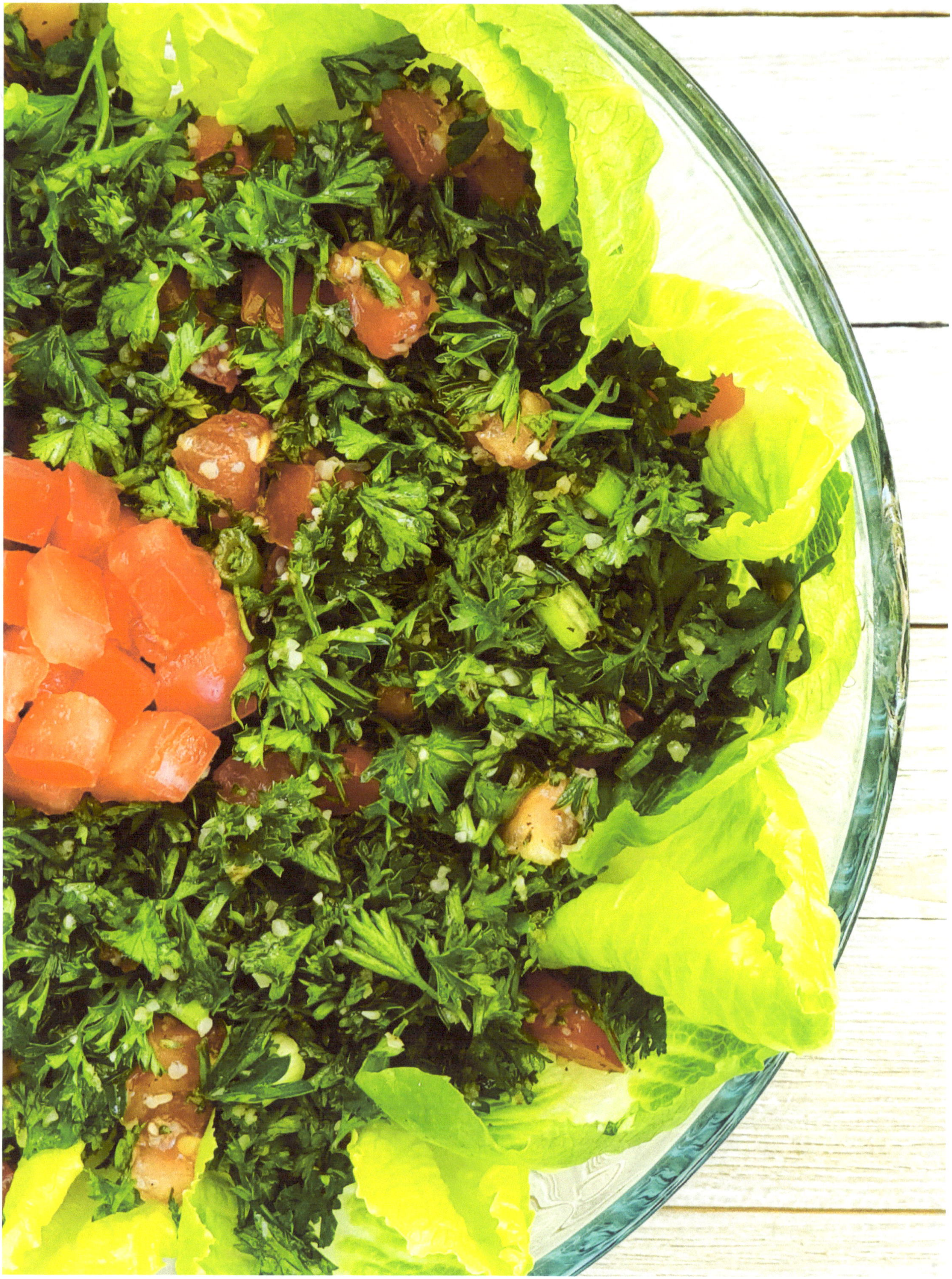

TABBOOLI SALAD

Salatit Tabbooli سلطة تبّولة

Tabbooli is the most world-wide famous Lebanese salad, loved for its fresh rich flavors and beautiful colors of green parsley, red tomatoes, and beige speckles of bulgur. Despite it being a very healthy salad, it is notorious for being a bit too rich in olive oil. Though the oil gives it a great flavor and moistness, it tends to increase the calories of the salad a bit more than desired. To decrease the need for so much olive oil while maintaining the juiciness of the salad, I use a lot of fresh lemon juice and many red ripe tomatoes. *Tabbooli* is traditionally made with flat leaf Italian parsley, but I love using curly parsley instead. While both impart somewhat similar flavor and nutritional benefits, the latter gives *tabbooli* a crunchier texture, allowing it to keep fresher and crisper for longer.

RECIPE YIELD 14 cups

DF EF V

INGREDIENTS

6 bunches curly parsley, finely chopped (450 g)
6 medium red tomatoes, diced (800 g)
6 medium green onion stalks, diced (95 g)
⅓ cup dry dark fine bulgur (grade 1) (47 g)
1 cup lemon juice
5 tbsp olive oil
2 tsp dry mint leaves
½ tsp 7-spices
½ tsp cinnamon
⅔ tsp salt
⅛ tsp black pepper

NOTE

- If Italian parsley is to be used in the making of *tabbooli*, the yield may be slightly less given that Italian parsley shrinks more when mixed in with the salad dressing, and thus will pack more than curly parsley.

INSTRUCTIONS

1. Rinse the bulgur a couple times. Drain and press away all water by hand. Set aside.
2. In a small bowl, mix the dressing ingredients. Add the bulgur and mix well. Cover, then let sit for at least an hour or two for the bulgur to soften.
3. In a large bowl, toss the chopped onions and tomatoes over the chopped parsley.
4. Add the bulgur and dressing mixture to the chopped salad vegetables, tossing together until well mixed.
5. Serve with fresh romaine lettuce leaves.

RECIPE ALTERNATIVES

- For a gluten-free tabbooli recipe, use cooked quinoa (~ 1 cup) instead of bulgur.
- An equally delicious but quite different version of tabbooli was commonly made by my paternal grandmother using significantly more bulgur and no parsley. To prepare this salad version, eliminate the parsley and green onions, substituting with a ½ large white onion (minced). Increase the bulgur to 1 cup, add the lemon juice, oil, and diced tomatoes, and let sit for about an hour. Substitute the 7-spices and cinnamon with 1 tsp of cumin and increase the mint to 1 tbsp (can also use fresh mint if desired). Add more olive oil as desired and serve with lettuce.

NUTRITION FACTS PER CUP

83 Kcal	2 g Protein	5 g Fat	8.6 g Carbs	2.5 g Fiber	2 g Sugar

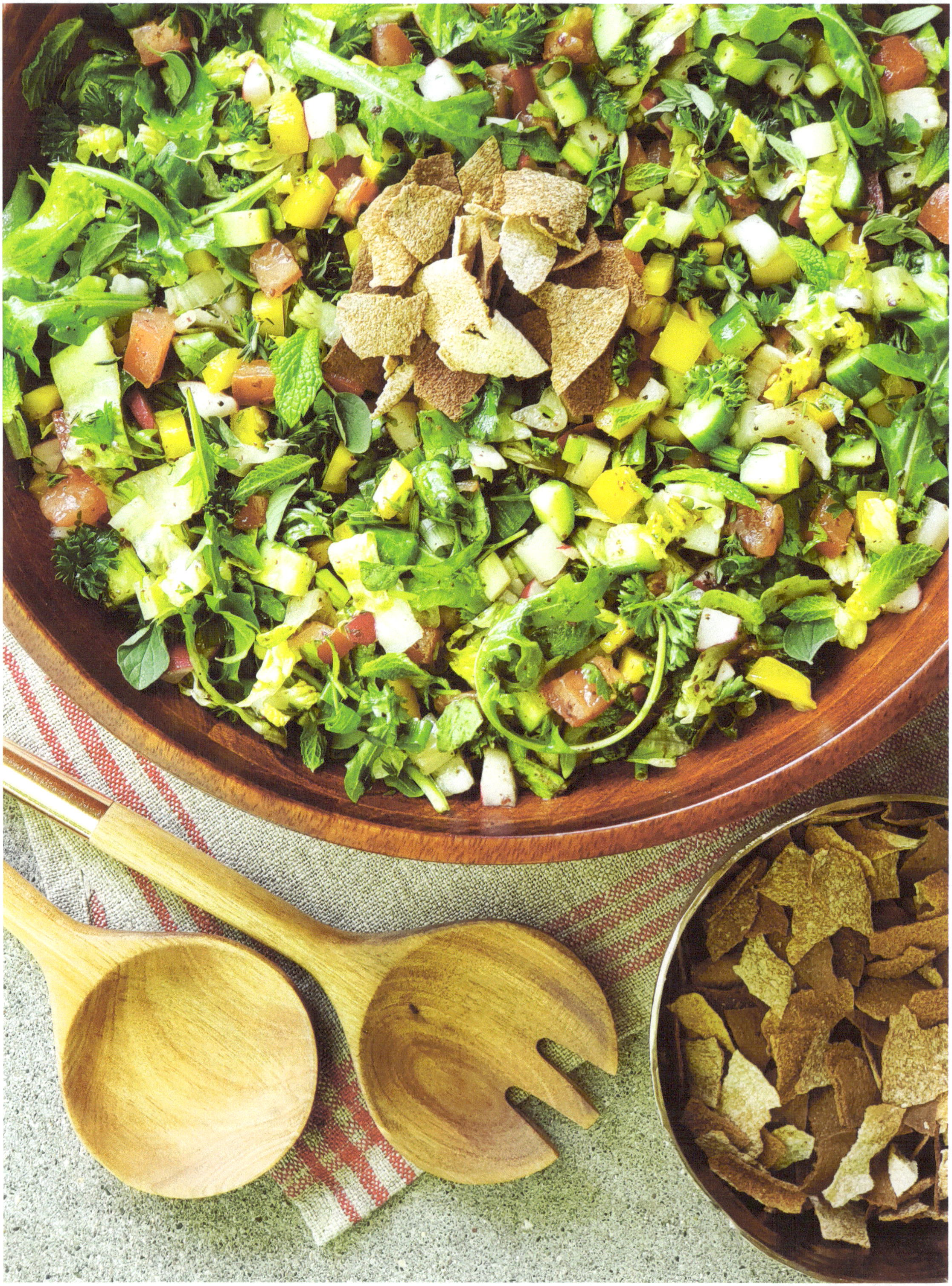

FATTOUSH SALAD

Salatit Fattoush سلطة فتّوش

This salad is the second most famous among Lebanese salads after *tabbooli*, commonly eaten during the month of Ramadan. Made with over eight kinds of vegetables, I like to describe this salad as a 'multivitamin with fiber'. Some will throw in additional vegetables such as cabbage, fresh mint, thyme, oregano, and/or purslane leaves, further adding to its nutritional power. Vegetables for this salad are meant to be chopped finely so that one gets a full combination with every bite. As with most traditional salads, however, Fattoush is notorious for being high in fat - fat from too much added olive oil, and also from fried pita bread that is meant to be mixed in with the salad vegetables. This salad can taste as delicious adding much less olive oil and using toasted pita bread.

RECIPE YIELD 16 cups

DF EF V

INGREDIENTS

1 medium romaine lettuce heart, finely chopped (375 g)
1 bunch curly parsley, coarsely chopped (75 g)
3 cups (packed) baby arugula, whole (60 g)
4 medium red tomatoes, diced (540 g)
2 small cucumbers, diced (176 g)
1 medium yellow bell pepper, diced (165 g)
6 medium green onion stalks, diced (95 g)
10 medium radishes, diced (175 g)
1 ½ loaves whole wheat Arabic bread (medium size) (110 g)
2 tbsp apple cider vinegar (or red grape vinegar)
1 tbsp pomegranate molasses
6 tbsp olive oil
2 tbsp sumac
2 tsp dry mint leaves
⅔ tsp salt

INSTRUCTIONS

1. Separate the pita bread loaves into 3 individual halves. Brush each half with 1 tsp of olive oil then place in a preheated oven at 350 °F and toast for 7 to 10 minutes (until lightly browned and completely toasted). Let cool, then break up (by hand) into small pieces.
2. In a small bowl, mix the remaining 5 tbsp oil with the vinegar, molasses, sumac, mint, and salt.
3. In a large bowl, toss the chopped vegetables, then mix in the dressing.
4. Fold in the pita bread right before serving.
5. Add more pomegranate molasses and sumac if desired.

NUTRITION FACTS PER CUP

89 Kcal	2 g Protein	5.6 g Fat	9 g Carbs	2.5 g Fiber	3 g Sugar

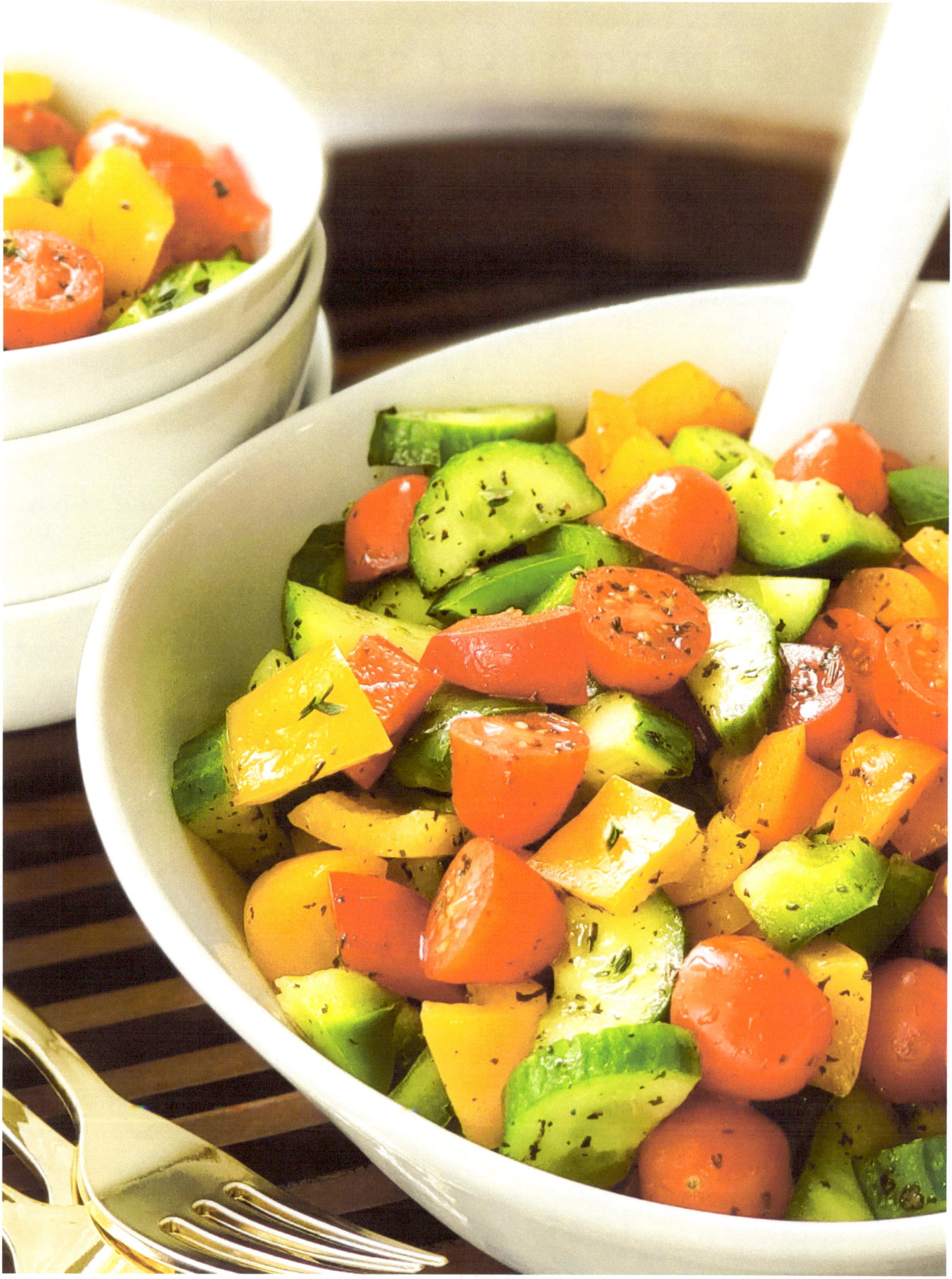

MIXED VEGGIE SALAD

Salatit Khudra Mshakkaleh سلطة خضرة مشكّلة

This salad is one of the simplest to prepare, yet is full of flavor and nutrients, including loads of vitamin C and phytochemicals. Variations of this salad between households exists, with some adding more cucumbers and less bell peppers, while others adding onions.

RECIPE YIELD 10 cups

DF GF EF V

INGREDIENTS

40 large grape tomatoes, sliced (400 g)
4 medium bell peppers (1 green, 1 red, 1 orange, 1 yellow), chopped (660 g)
4 small cucumbers, chopped (352 g)
2 tsp garlic, crushed
⅓ cup lemon juice
2 tbsp olive oil
2 tsp dry mint leaves
⅓ tsp salt

INSTRUCTIONS

1. In a small bowl, mix the garlic and salt (until a paste is formed), then add the lemon juice.
2. Place the chopped vegetables in a medium bowl, then add the olive oil and mint.
3. Pour in the garlic and lemon mixture, then stir to mix.
4. Add fresh thyme leaves if desired before serving.

NUTRITION FACTS PER CUP

56 Kcal	1 g Protein	3 g Fat	7.4 g Carbs	2 g Fiber	4 g Sugar

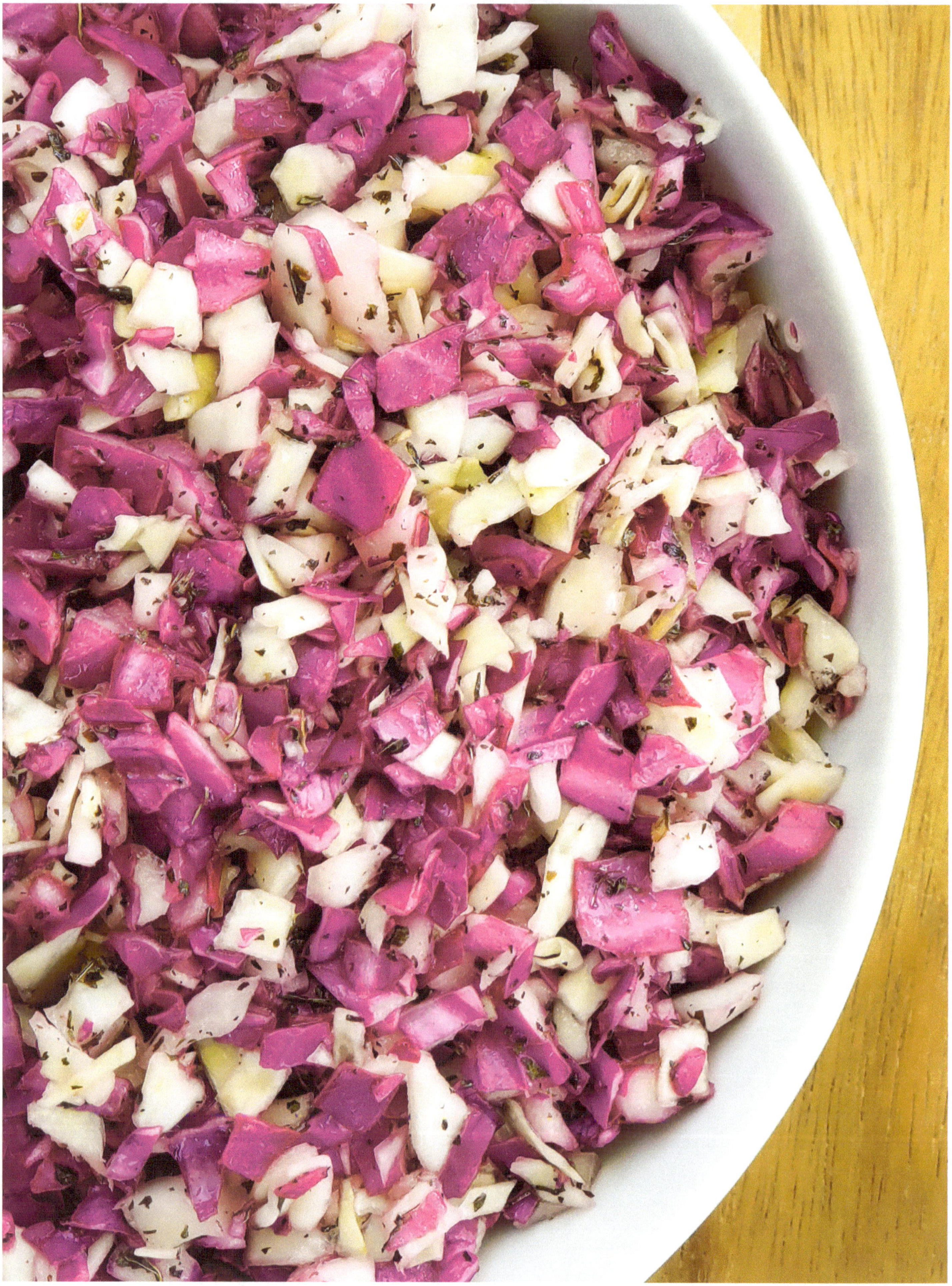

CABBAGE SALAD

Salatit Malfoof سلطة ملفوف

This is a garlicy and lemony salad traditionally made with green (white) cabbage or with romaine lettuce. As with most traditional salads, people often add too much olive oil, whereas I like to add extra lemon juice to moisten the salad and add flavor.

RECIPE YIELD 9 cups

DF GF EF V

INGREDIENTS

½ small red (purple) cabbage, finely chopped (500 g)
¼ medium green (white) cabbage, finely chopped (375 g)
1 tbsp garlic, crushed
⅓ cup lemon juice
2 tbsp olive oil
2 tbsp dry mint leaves
¼ tsp salt

INSTRUCTIONS

1. In a small bowl, mix the garlic and salt (until a paste is formed), then add the lemon juice.
2. Place the chopped cabbage in a medium bowl, then add the olive oil and mint.
3. Pour in the garlic and lemon mixture, then stir to mix.

NUTRITION FACTS PER CUP

59 Kcal	1.5 g Protein	3 g Fat	7.6 g Carbs	2.4 g Fiber	4 g Sugar

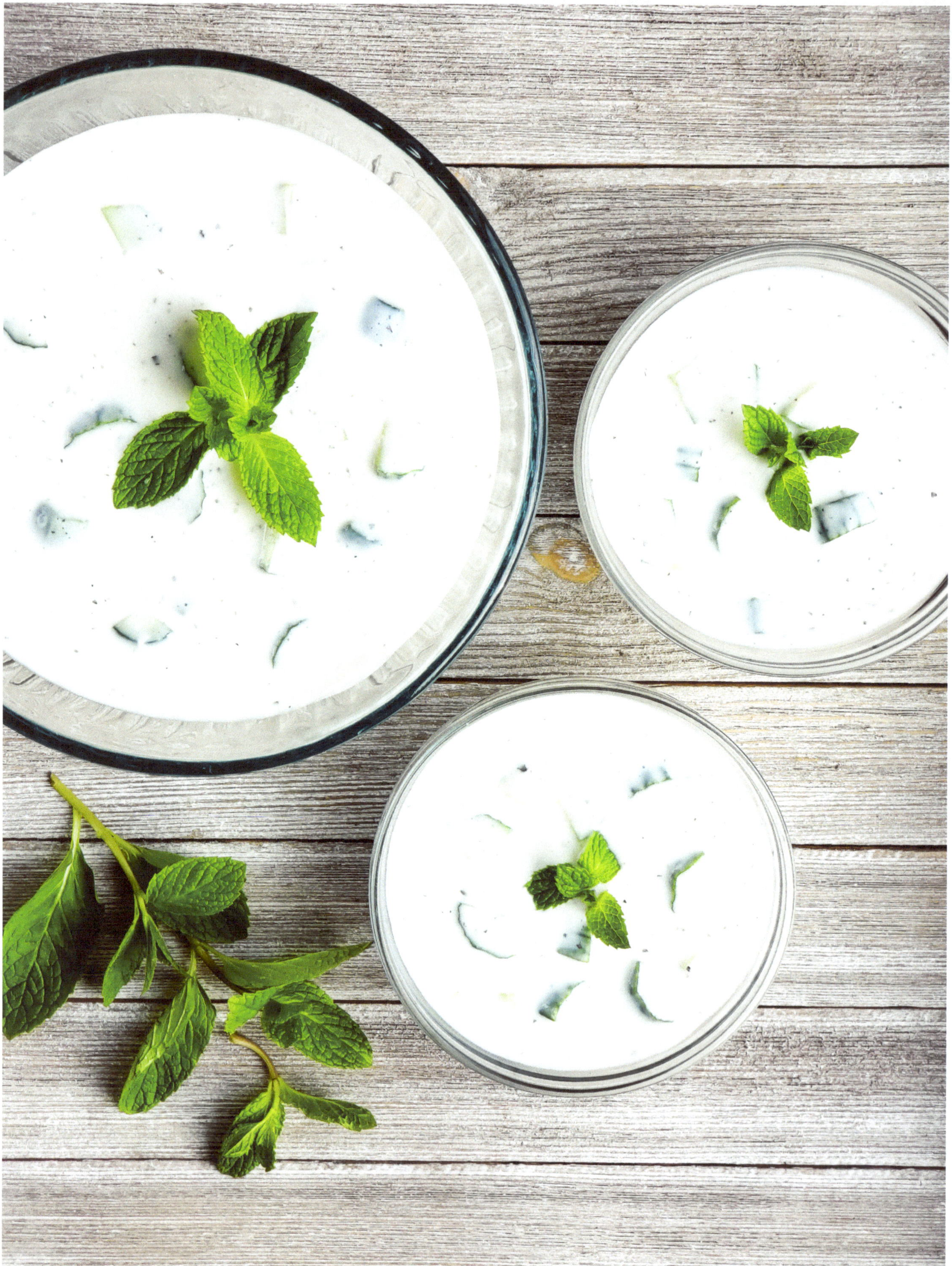

CUCUMBER YOGURT SALAD

Salatit Khyar bi Laban سلطة خيار بلبن

This salad is quite the unconventional salad. Traditionally eaten as a side to rice or *freekeh* dishes, this cooling yogurt-based salad is delicious and super flavorful. My healthier version is made with homemade skim yogurt and is light on the olive oil. Some prefer keeping the oil out of the salad, and then drizzling some on top of individual servings.

RECIPE YIELD 7 cups

GF EF Vt

INGREDIENTS

5 cups skim yogurt (1,175 g)
6 small cucumbers (528 g)
2 tsp garlic, crushed
2 tsp olive oil
1 ½ tsp dry mint leaves
½ tsp salt

INSTRUCTIONS

1. In a small bowl, mix the garlic and salt (until a paste is formed).
2. In a medium bowl, add the olive oil and mint to the yogurt, then stir to mix.
3. Stir in the garlic, then fold in the cucumbers.
4. Garnish with fresh mint leaves and add some lemon juice if desired before serving.

NUTRITION FACTS PER CUP

122 Kcal	10.6 g Protein	2 g Fat	16.5 g Carbs	0.5 g Fiber	15 g Sugar

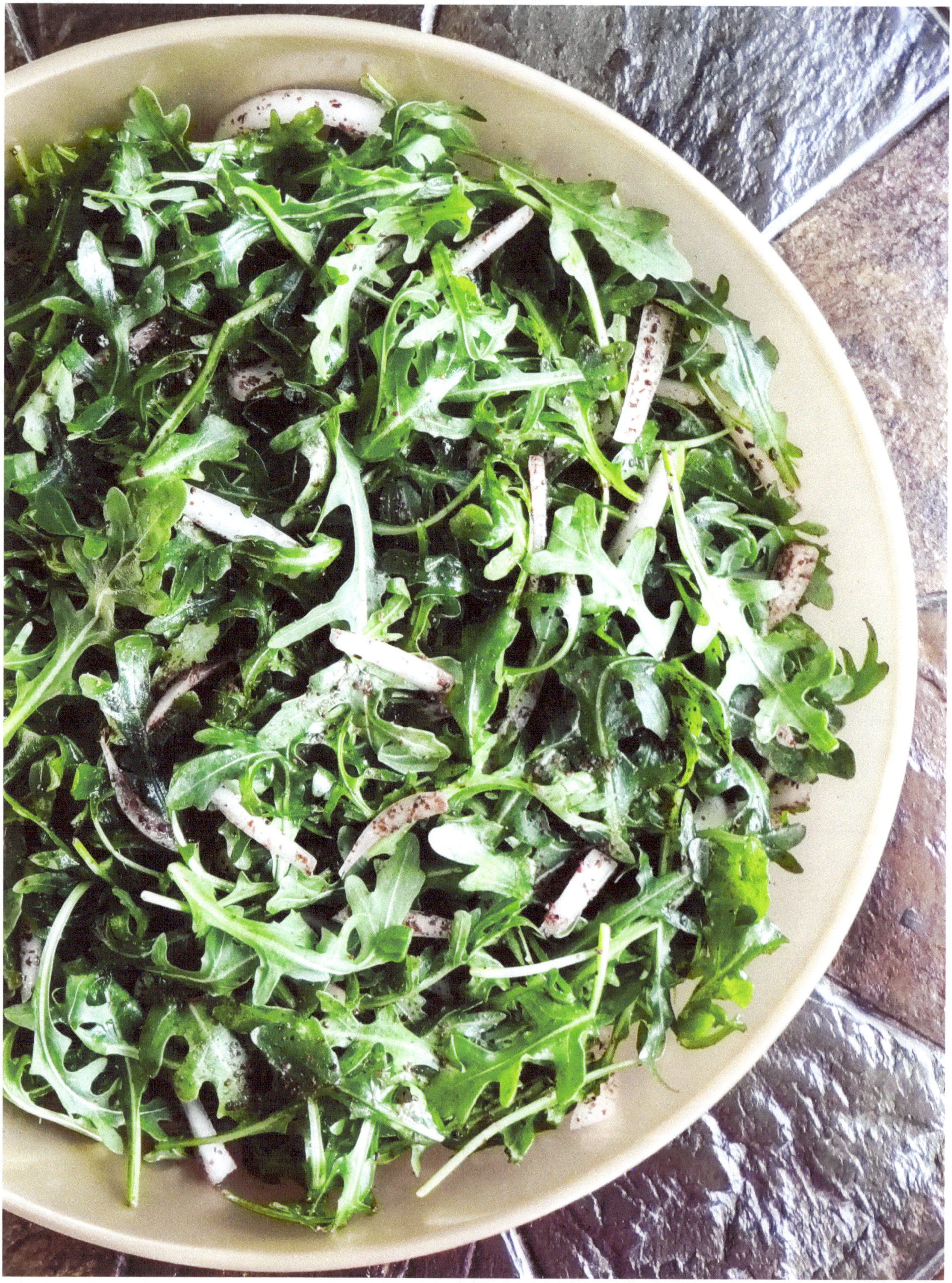

CLASSIC ARUGULA SALAD

Salatit Jarjeer سلطة جرجير

This simple two-vegetable salad is one of the most pungent salads one may taste. Traditionally, this salad is not eaten alone, but is instead served as a side to main dishes such as beef *kibbeh* (recipe on page 201) or Arabian rice with beef (recipe on page 165).

RECIPE YIELD 12 cups

DF GF EF V

INGREDIENTS

14 cups (packed) baby arugula, whole (280 g)
½ large white onion, sliced into slivers (160 g)
⅓ cup lemon juice
4 tbsp olive oil
2 tbsp sumac
⅓ tsp salt

RECIPE ALTERNATIVES

- A traditional sister recipe of the above salad calls for fresh wild thyme leaves instead of arugula.
- An equally delicious and strong-flavored two-vegetable salad I enjoy making includes diced steamed beets (2 large; 675 g) with diced fresh red or white onions (⅓ large; 125 g), dressed with crumbled fetta cheese (200 g), olive oil (2 tbsp), balsamic vinegar (2 tbsp), and salt (¼ tsp). Add more balsamic vinegar as desired.

INSTRUCTIONS

1. In a small bowl, rub the onions with 1 tbsp sumac.
2. In a separate bowl, mix the lemon juice, olive oil, salt, and the remaining sumac.
3. Toss the arugula into a medium bowl, add the onions, then pour the dressing over the vegetables and fold.
4. Garnish with sliced grape tomatoes if desired.

NUTRITION FACTS PER CUP

56.5 Kcal	1 g Protein	5 g Fat	3 g Carbs	1 g Fiber	1 g Sugar

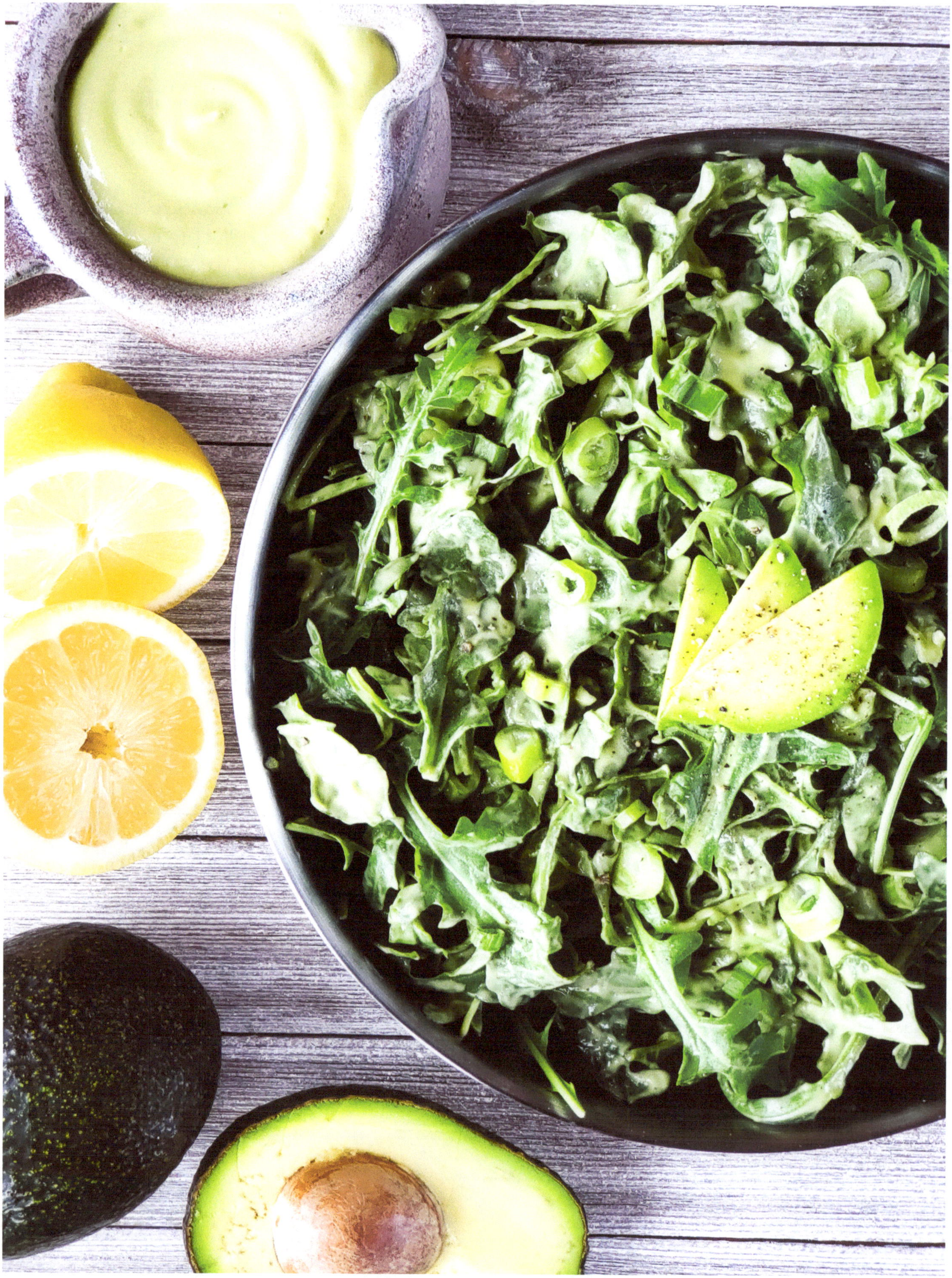

AVOCADO ARUGULA SALAD

Inspired by the classic arugula salad (on the previous page) and my love for avocados, this rich yet super healthy salad is a great variation to be enjoyed as a side salad, or on top of toast or in sandwiches.

RECIPE YIELD 10 cups

DF GF EF V

INGREDIENTS

14 cups (packed) baby arugula, whole (280 g)
6 medium green onion stalks, diced (95 g)
2 medium ripe pitted Hass avocados (no skin) (310 g)
1 cup lemon juice
1 tsp olive oil
⅓ tsp salt
⅛ tsp black pepper

NOTE

- The dressing of this salad is thick (dense) and thus will weigh the vegetables down a bit. If desired, one can dice the avocados instead of having them mashed up as part of the dressing.

RECIPE ALTERNATIVES

- Instead of using only arugula, one can toss in some chopped lettuce and cucumbers.
- For a Middle Eastern flavor, one can omit the avocados and olive oil, and add ½ cup *tahini* and 1½ tsp crushed garlic instead (process the *tahini* and garlic in the food processor with the lemon juice and spices).

INSTRUCTIONS

1. In a medium bowl, toss the arugula and onions.
2. In a small food processor, add the avocados, lemon juice, olive oil, and spices, then process well, scraping down the sides, until smooth and well blended.
3. Pour the dressing over the vegetables and fold.

NUTRITION FACTS PER CUP

71.4 Kcal	1.6 g Protein	5.5 g Fat	6 g Carbs	3 g Fiber	1.5 g Sugar

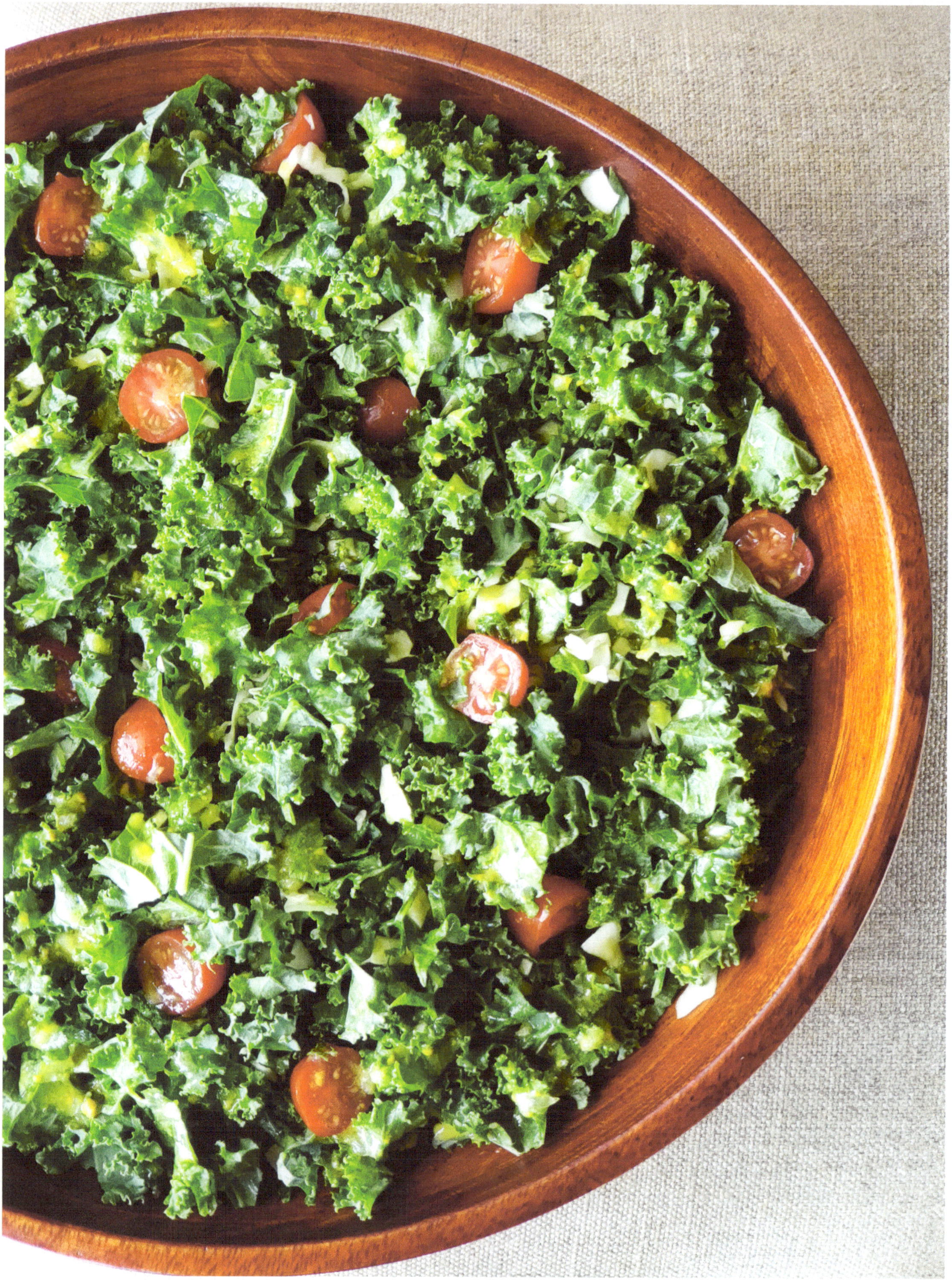

KALE SALAD

Inspired by my love for kale and sour salad flavors, this simple salad is very nutritious and goes well with many Middle Eastern dishes.

RECIPE YIELD 12 cups

DF GF EF V

INGREDIENTS

9 small curly kale stalks (leaves only), finely chopped (225 g)
1/6 medium green (white) cabbage, finely chopped (265 g)
25 large grape tomatoes, sliced (250 g)
2 tbsp mustard
¼ cup lemon juice
3 tbsp olive oil
1/3 tsp salt
black pepper, to taste

NOTE

Some may find kale to be too tough to chew or too hard to digest. A technique often followed to soften kale is to massage it by hand with oil and salt, pressing and working it hard with one's fingers for a few minutes. I simply prefer finely chopping kale for my salad, and that works just fine for me, but one can massage the kale if a softer kale texture is desired.

INSTRUCTIONS

1. In a medium bowl, toss the kale, cabbage, and tomatoes.
2. Mix the mustard, lemon juice, olive oil, and spices in a separate small bowl.
3. Pour the dressing over the vegetables and fold.
4. Add more lemon juice if desired.

NUTRITION FACTS PER CUP

48.5 Kcal	1 g Protein	4 g Fat	3.4 g Carbs	2 g Fiber	1.6 g Sugar

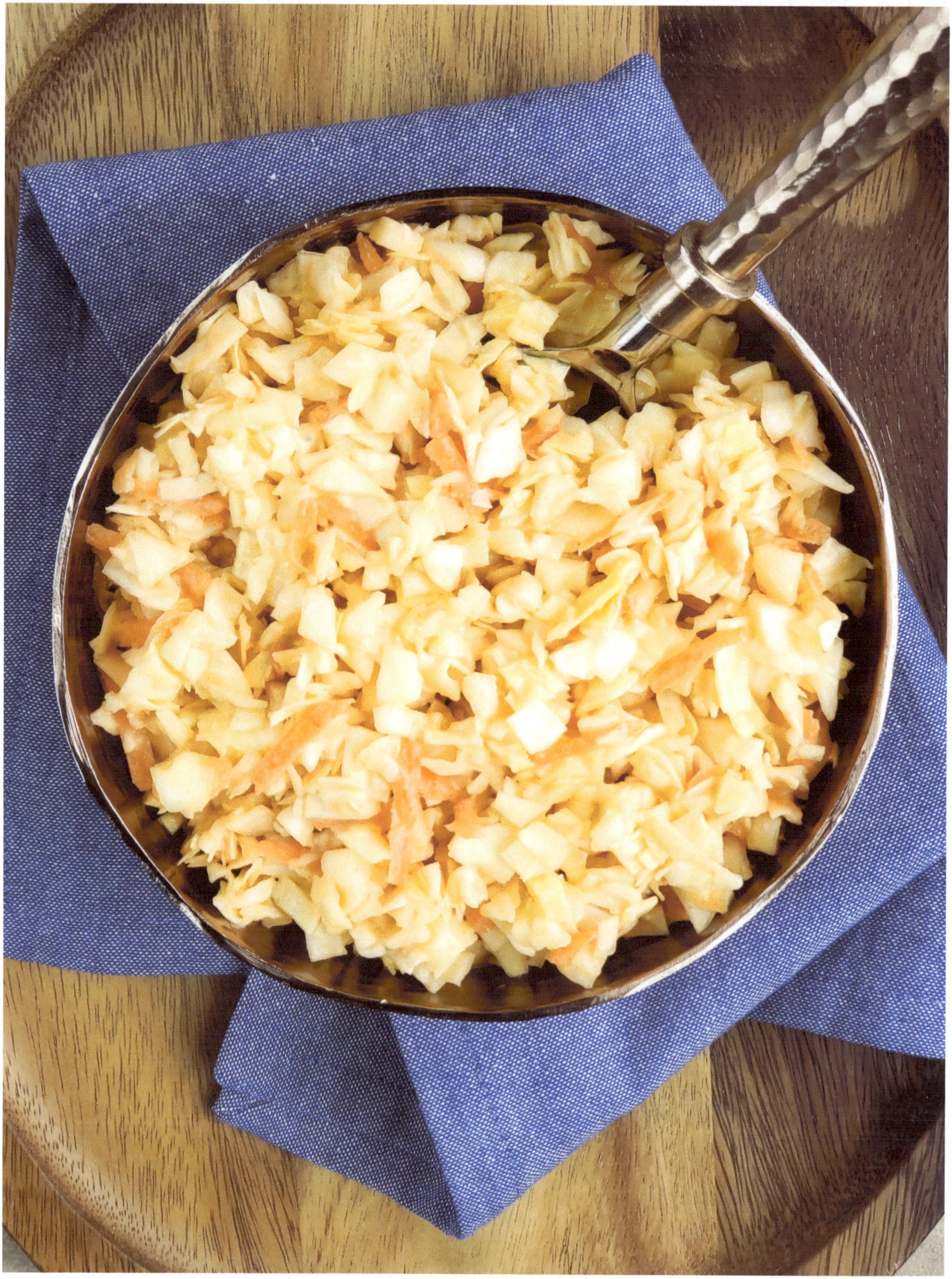

COCKTAIL COLESLAW SALAD

Growing up, my mom would always make us a quickie salad of chopped cabbage mixed with ketchup and mayonnaise - which I loved. To me that was the 'coleslaw salad' I got used to eating, but later, I came to learn that coleslaw salad is quite different. Since I quit using mayonnaise in my cooking years ago, I decided to recreate the flavors of a coleslaw salad but with ketchup and skim *labneh* for the dressing - giving it a Middle Eastern touch.

RECIPE YIELD 9 cups

GF EF Vt

INGREDIENTS

⅔ medium green (white) cabbage, finely chopped (1 kg)
1 medium carrot (no skin), coarsely shredded (60 g)
½ cup skim labneh (110 g)
4 tbsp ketchup
1 tbsp honey
1 tbsp white vinegar
2 tbsp olive oil
⅓ tsp salt
black pepper, to taste

NOTE

- If more juiciness in the salad is desired, one can add extra vinegar, ketchup, or a couple tablespoons of skim yogurt.

INSTRUCTIONS

1. In a medium bowl, toss the cabbage and carrot.
2. Put the dressing ingredients all together in a small bowl, then whisk to mix.
3. Pour the dressing over the vegetables and fold.

NUTRITION FACTS PER CUP

91 Kcal	3 g Protein	3 g Fat	14 g Carbs	3 g Fiber	10.4 g Sugar

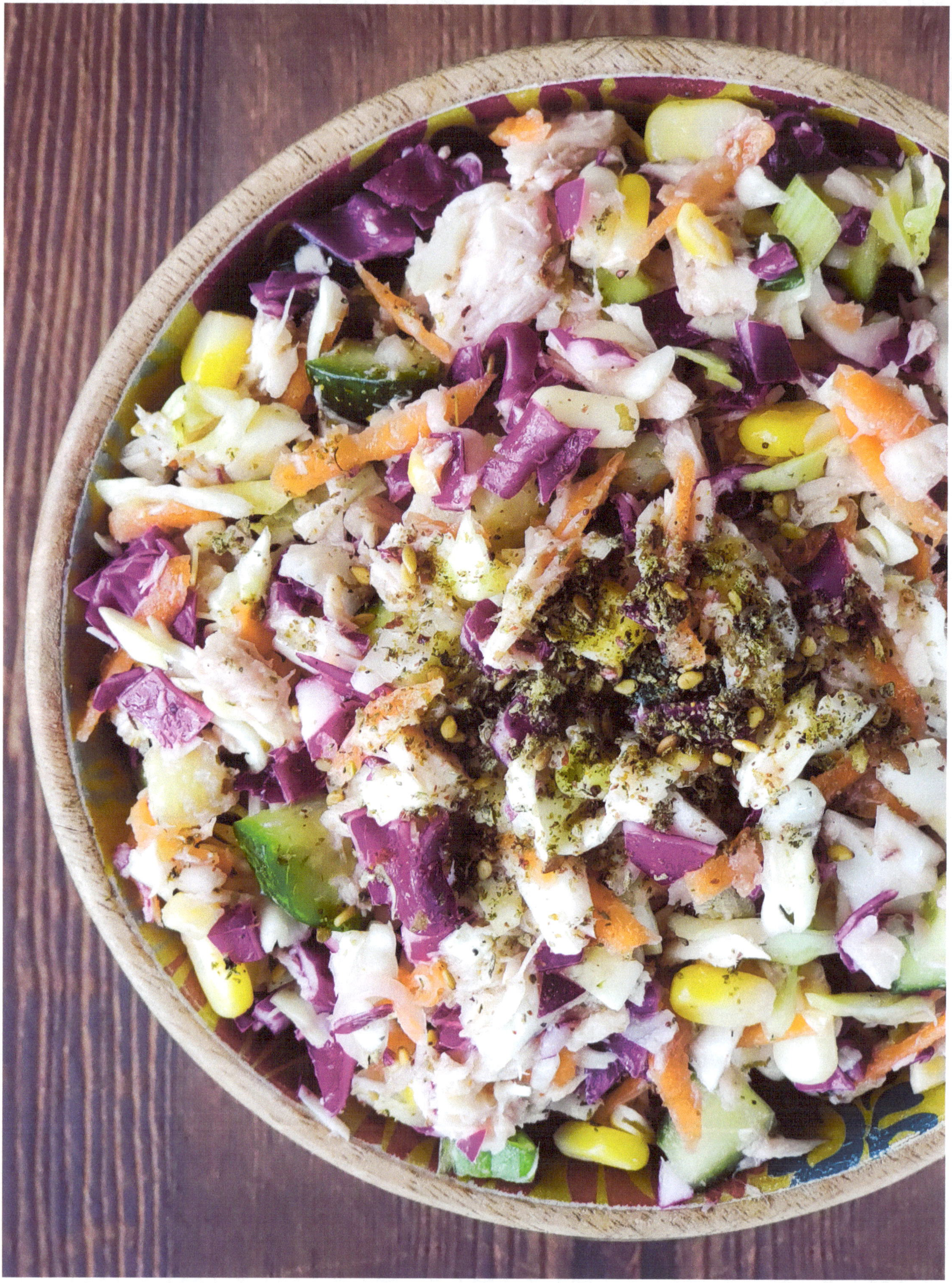

TUNA SALAD

Tuna salads are commonly made in households everywhere. My healthy version is light but flavorful, seasoned with lots of fresh lemon juice, some olive oil, and dry wild thyme (*zaatar*) for a Middle Eastern touch!

RECIPE YIELD 13 cups

DF GF EF

INGREDIENTS

2 (7 oz) cans light tuna fish (water-based), drained (350 g)
⅓ medium green (white) cabbage, finely chopped (500 g)
¼ small red (purple) cabbage, finely chopped (250 g)
2 small cucumbers, diced (176 g)
2 medium carrots (no skin), coarsely shredded (120 g)
1 cup sweet corn kernels (160 g)
3 medium green onion stalks, diced (48 g)
2 tbsp zaatar
½ cup lemon juice
4 tbsp olive oil
⅓ tsp salt
black pepper, to taste

NOTE

Zaatar can vary in saltiness between households and brands. As such, I kept the salt quantity for this salad at a minimum, in order for one to increase the salt as needed, depending on the saltiness of the added *zaatar*.

RECIPE ALTERNATIVE

An equally delicious but simpler tuna salad can be prepared with 1 can tuna (175 g), 1 chopped medium lettuce heart (375 g), and 1 ½ cups sweet corn (240 g), dressed with lemon juice (¼ cup), olive oil (2 tbsp), mustard (2 tbsp), ground ginger (⅛ tsp), salt (¼ tsp), and black pepper (⅛ tsp). For a vegan twist of this version, substitute the tuna with cooked quinoa (~ ¾ cup).

INSTRUCTIONS

1. After draining the tuna, lightly squeeze out any excess water.
2. In a small bowl, add the dressing ingredients to the tuna and mix well, breaking up the large tuna pieces into smaller ones.
3. Toss the vegetables together in a large bowl.
4. Add the tuna in the dressing to the vegetable bowl and mix.
5. Sprinkle more *zaatar* if desired before serving.

NUTRITION FACTS PER CUP

105 Kcal	8.4 g Protein	5 g Fat	8 g Carbs	2.5 g Fiber	3 g Sugar

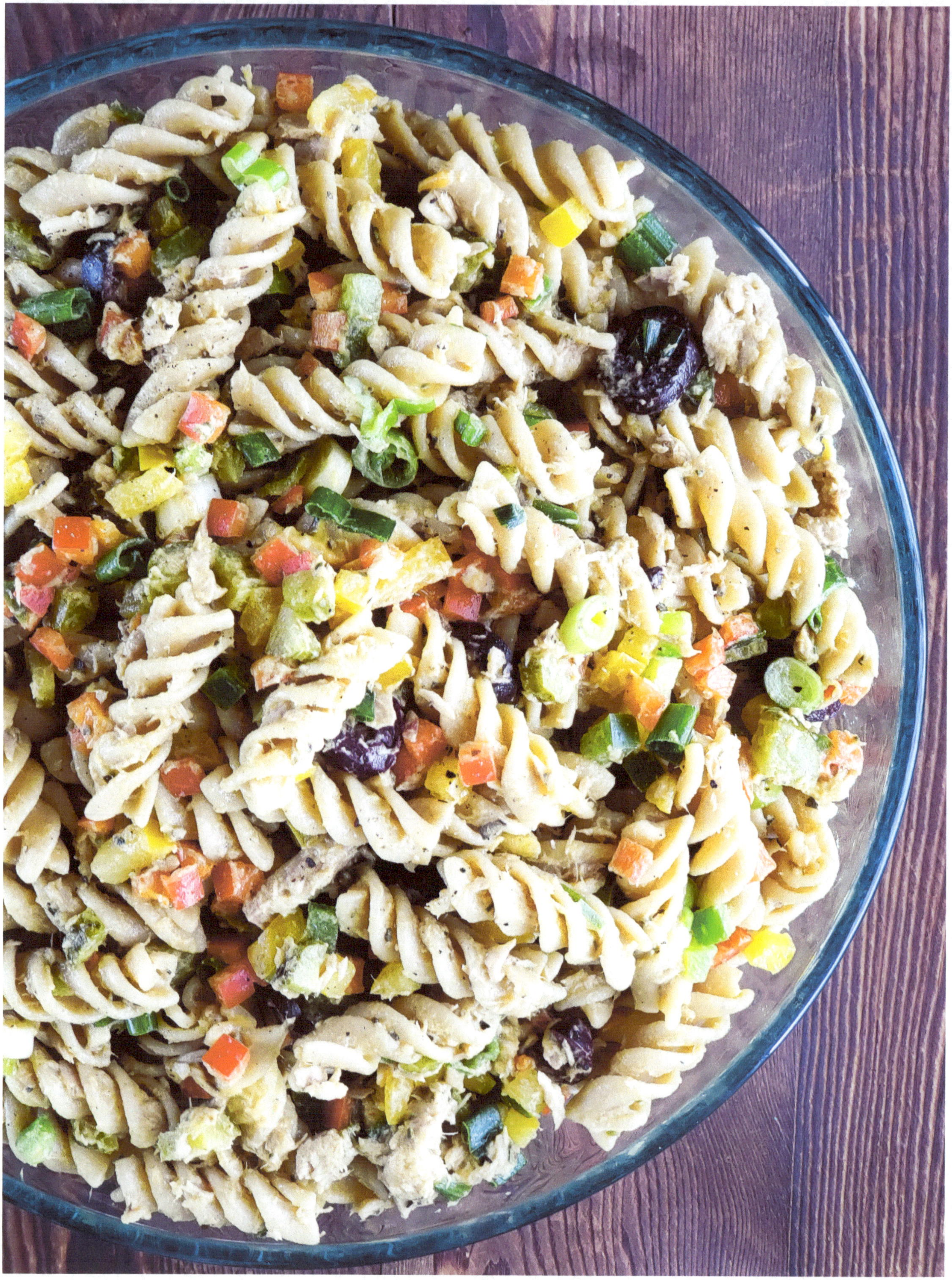

TUNA PASTA SALAD

As with tuna salad, almost every household has their own creation of a tuna past salad, tossing in various ingredients alongside canned tuna and boiled pasta. My version is light yet flavorful, serving as a hearty salad that can be eaten as a light meal.

RECIPE YIELD 13 cups

EF

INGREDIENTS

Dry whole wheat rotini pasta (350 g)
2 (7 oz) cans light tuna fish (water-based), drained (350 g)
1 ½ medium bell peppers (½ yellow, ½ red, ½ green), diced (248 g)
6 medium green onion stalks, diced (95 g)
15 large black olives (pitted), sliced (65 g)
7 baby dill cucumber pickles, diced (70 g)
5 tbsp mustard
3 tbsp skim yogurt
3 tbsp lemon juice
3 tbsp olive oil
1 tbsp dry oregano leaves
⅓ tsp salt
black pepper, to taste

NOTE

Olives and pickles can vary in saltiness between households and brands. As such, I kept the salt quantity for this salad at a minimum, in order for one to increase the salt as needed, depending on the saltiness of the used olives and pickles.

INSTRUCTIONS

1. After draining the tuna, lightly squeeze out any excess water.
2. In a small bowl, add the dressing ingredients to the tuna and mix well, breaking up the large tuna pieces into smaller ones.
3. Toss the vegetables together in a large bowl.
4. Add the tuna in the dressing to the vegetable bowl and mix.
5. Boil the pasta until cooked to al dente. Drain, then rinse well with cold water. Let sit to drain.
6. Gently fold in the pasta to the salad bowl.
7. Add more lemon juice and oregano if desired before serving.

NUTRITION FACTS PER CUP

165.5 Kcal	11.6 g Protein	5 g Fat	22 g Carbs	4.5 g Fiber	2 g Sugar

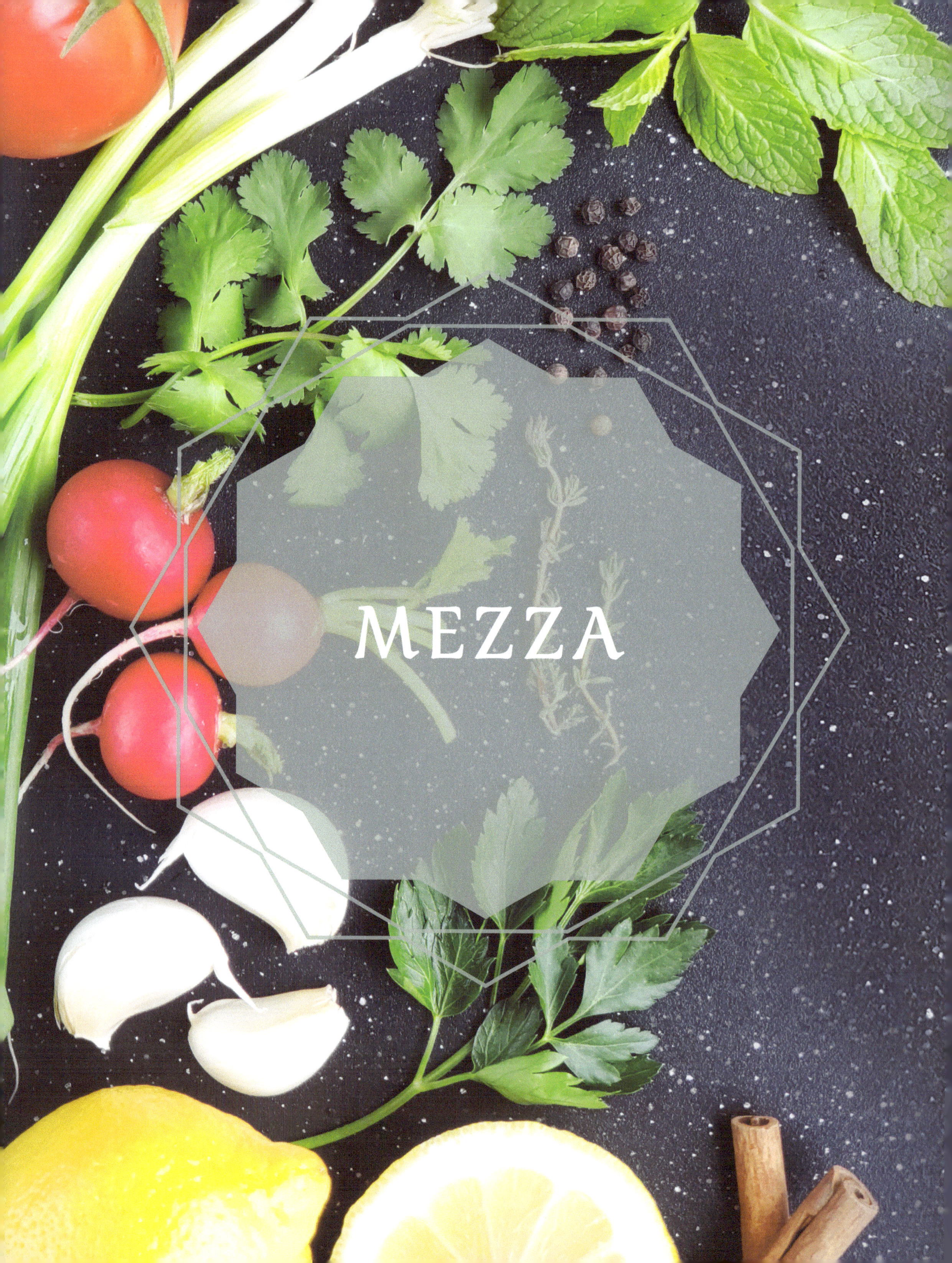

MEZZA

Pronounced as Mai-zah, this course is uniquely Middle Eastern, resembling somewhat the course of appetizers in other cultures, but including a wide selection of delicious small plates of very different and distinct dishes. Mezza dishes are most commonly served at restaurants or at large gatherings at homes as starters to a meal, but any mezza dish can be eaten as a separate meal, making up a healthy and light brunch or dinner. The mezza dishes I have shared are my favorites among the many Lebanese mezza dishes available. Lebanese and/or Middle Eastern mezza dishes presented in this section are named with the traditional Arabic name of the dish, along with an English transliteration of the Arabic.

SOME GENERAL REMARKS AND RECOMMENDATIONS

- It is very important to wash all vegetables called for in a recipe prior to starting. Vegetables can harbor soil particles from having been out in the field, and soil in turn can be the source of many harmful bacteria. Properly washing vegetables under cold running water, with scrubbing and/or quick soaking, then rinsing as many times as needed, is important. Since I do not peel my potatoes, make sure to rub the skins very well with a clean brush during washing.

- The weights presented to the right-hand side of a vegetable ingredient relate to the final net weight of the vegetable added to the mezza dish (i.e. the net weight after peeling, removing the inedible ends or core, and chopping off bad parts of the vegetable), unless otherwise specified.

- Since fresh produce can vary widely in size, shape, and weight, it is recommended to go by the presented weights of called for ingredients, in order to obtain more accurate recipe outcomes and yields.

- Bake an ingredient/dish on the middle rack of the oven, unless otherwise specified.

- All spices called for in a recipe are in their ground (powdered) form, unless otherwise specified (such as for oregano, dry oregano leaves will be indicated if the non-powdered dry oregano is called for. Same goes for mint).

- I am a big fan of spices and herbs, but not a fan of salt. Thus, the salt amounts called for in my mezza dishes tend to be on the lower end, so always taste the dish once prepared, and accordingly adjust the salt to your taste.

- The addition of salt as an ingredient is included with the spices in the instruction steps of the recipes, unless otherwise specified.

- When it comes to ingredients used such as garlic and lemon juice, let your food preferences guide how much you add to your mezza dishes. If you like them, then follow my recipes exactly, as I like them, too (or even go ahead and bump up the quantities if need be)! Otherwise, cut back a bit, have a taste, and then adjust accordingly.

- I like to prepare my mezza dishes without too much oil, especially since I am not fond of oily/greasy food in general. However, I make sure that the lower amount of oil doesn't negatively affect the flavor of the dish. One can definitely add more oil if desired, but this will increase the caloric and fat content of the dish.

- A serving of 1 cup of a mezza dish is a good serving size if it is to be followed by a main dish. Otherwise, a serving of 2 to 2.5 cups is a good serving size if the mezza dish is to be enjoyed as a light meal.

- The 'sugar' value in the nutrition facts of recipes refers to the total amount of sugar (both simple and complex) that is naturally occurring in the various ingredients.

- Food items suggested as garnish are NOT included in the nutrition facts.

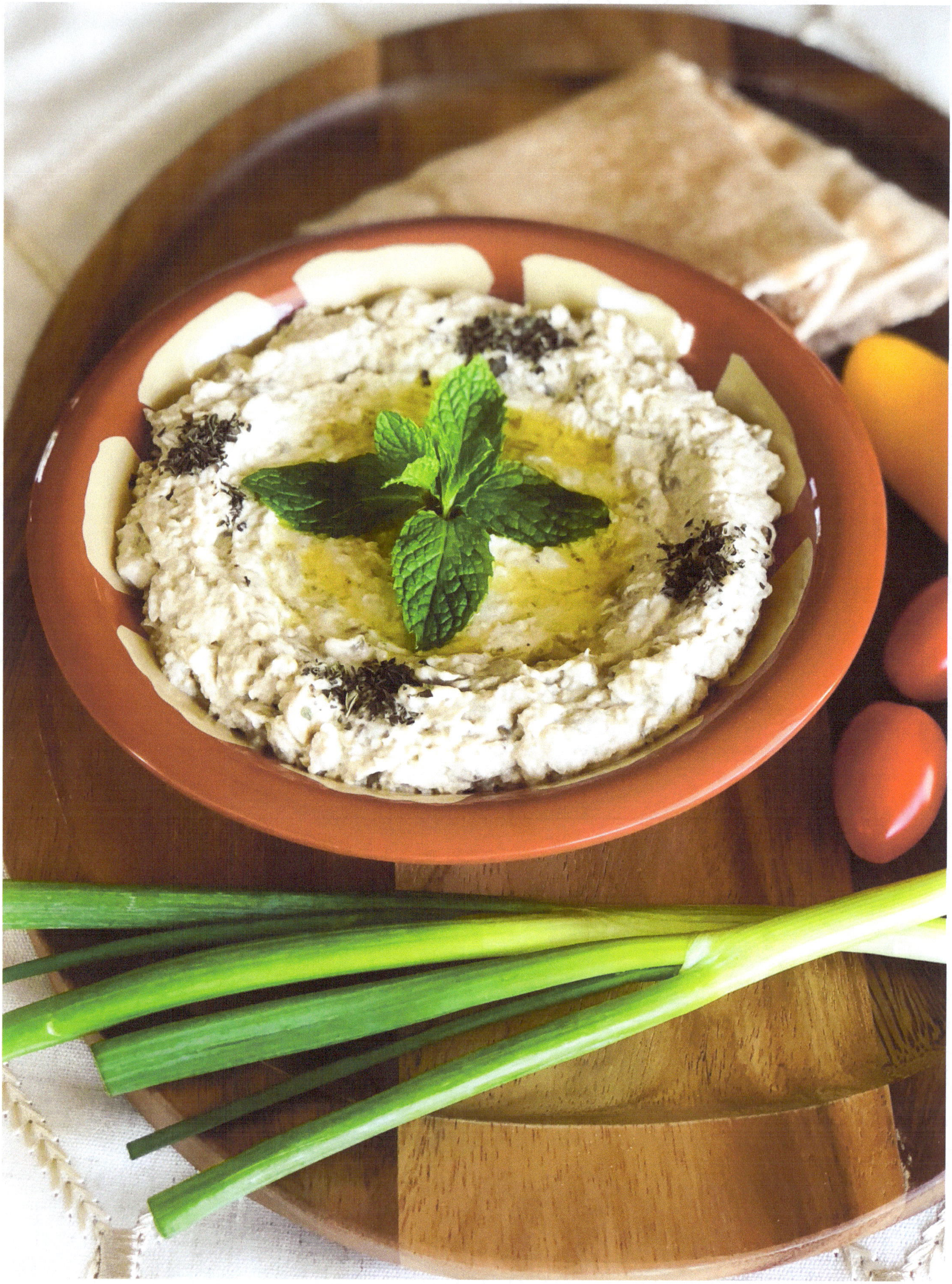

EGGPLANT DIP

Baba Ghanouj (Mtabbal Bathinjan) بابا غنوج (متبّل باذنجان)

This famous and nutritious mezza dip has similar ingredients to the all-famous *hummus* dip (on the next page), except that instead of boiled chickpeas, this recipe calls for cooked eggplant (aubergines). Whereas some traditional *baba ghanouj* recipes call for the eggplants to be 'roasted' on the stove-top wrapped in foil or as is, a method that gives them a very tasty smoked flavor, I opt for the healthier and faster method of cooking, which is baking them in the oven. Many will also add yogurt in place of some *tahini* to brighten up the color of the dip and decrease the fat content, but I prefer the full flavor of *tahini* only. My family and I will often enjoy this dip for a light lunch or dinner, wrapped up as a pita bread sandwich or eaten on a plate with bread to the side.

RECIPE YIELD 5 ½ cups (11 servings)

DF GF EF OF V FF

INGREDIENTS

4 medium Italian eggplants (with skin and ends) (1.5 kg)
1 ¼ cups tahini (300 g)
1 tbsp garlic, crushed
½ cup lemon juice
⅓ tsp salt

NOTES

- The *baba ghanouj* dip will firm up further once refrigerated.
- Each serving includes ½ cup of the dip.

INSTRUCTIONS

1. Keep the eggplants whole, then cut into each one with a knife, creating an inch-long slit, running vertically along the body of the eggplant (this will prevent the build-up of pressure inside the eggplant during the baking process, thus preventing it from bursting open).
2. Place the eggplants, slit facing up, in a preheated oven at 450 °F, then bake for 50 to 60 minutes, or until the eggplants are soft and look quite wrinkly and deflated (inserting a knife into the center of a done eggplant will go in and out with ease) (line the bottom of the oven with aluminum foil since the eggplants may ooze during baking).
3. Remove the eggplants from the oven and place on a tray to let cool just enough to be able to handle with one's hands. Slice open and scoop out the insides with a spoon into a large bowl, discarding the skins.
4. With a whisk, mash up the warm eggplant until all big chunks are gone and the texture is quite smooth (should yield 4 cups mashed eggplant; 860 g). If the baked eggplant has a lot of liquid, drain some of it away to reach the required weight.
5. In a small bowl, mix the garlic and salt (until a paste is formed), then add the lemon juice.
6. Add the tahini to the mashed eggplant and whisk well, until well mixed.
7. Add the garlic and lemon mixture, then whisk well to mix (all ingredients could be placed in a food processor for a very smooth texture, but using a whisk adds air and fluffiness to the dip).
8. Serve at room temperature or chilled from the refrigerator, and garnish with dry mint leaves and olive oil if desired. Serve with fresh or toasted pita bread, as well a variety of vegetables such as green onions, tomatoes, and/or sweet peppers.

NUTRITION FACTS PER SERVING

185.4 Kcal	6 g Protein	15 g Fat	11 g Carbs	4 g Fiber	3 g Sugar

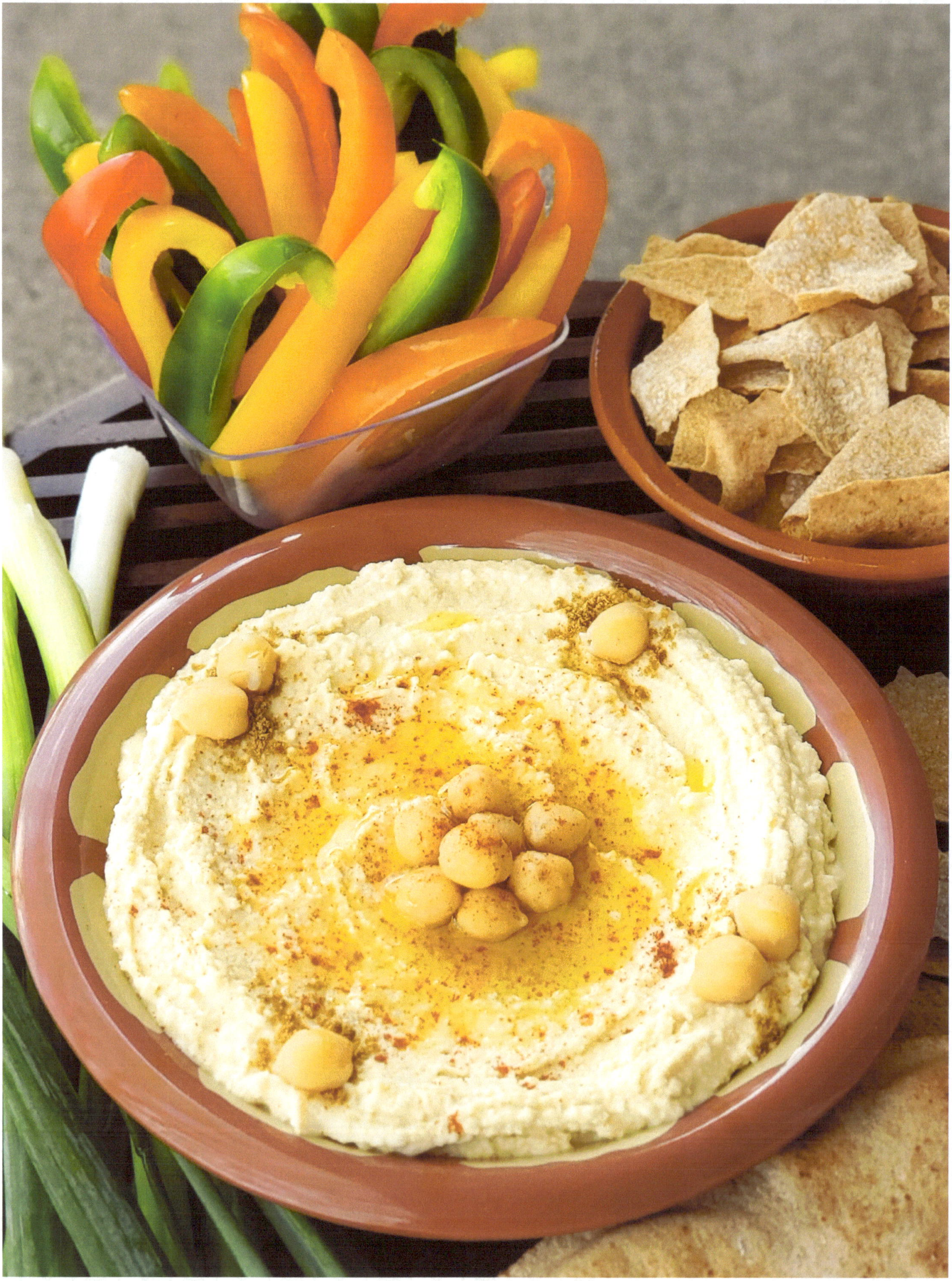

CHICKPEA DIP

Hummus bi Tahini حمّص بطحينة

This world-renowned creamy chickpea mezza dish has become popular in almost every part of the world. Made with simple ingredients, this hearty dish is full of flavor and nutrients. Making creamy and very smooth hummus at home, however, is not that easy, and many will revert to ready-made hummus dips, but the homemade version is indeed totally worth the time and effort it takes to make. My hummus is smooth but definitely not the smoothest, however, I prefer putting flavor and nutrition first over simply texture (read more below in the notes). As with the eggplant dip mezza dish (on the previous page), yogurt is often added in place of some tahini to brighten up the color of the dip, while decreasing the fat content a bit, but I prefer the flavor with only tahini. Enjoy this dip as a brunch or light dinner, wrapped up as a pita bread sandwich or eaten on a plate with bread to the side.

RECIPE YIELD 8 cups (16 servings)

DF GF EF OF V FF

INGREDIENTS

2 ½ cups dry chickpeas (463 g)
1 ¼ cups tahini (300 g)
2 tbsp garlic, crushed
1 ¼ cups lemon juice
¼ cup chickpea water
2 medium ice cubes (40 g)
2 tsp salt
2 ½ tsp baking soda

INSTRUCTIONS

1. Soak the chickpeas and 1 ½ tsp baking soda in water for 12 hours. Drain and rinse, discarding any bad pieces.

2. Transfer the chickpeas to a pot, cover with water and add the remaining 1 tsp of baking soda, then bring to a boil. Skim off the white foam that floats to the surface, then cook, covered, on low heat for 50 to 60 minutes (or until overcooked but not mushy).

3. Drain the chickpeas, saving ¼ cup of the chickpea water (set in the refrigerator until ready to use), then remove ¼ cup chickpeas to add whole later on when serving the dip. Lightly cover the drained chickpeas to keep from drying out. Let cool to room temperature.

4. In a small bowl, mix the garlic and salt (until a paste is formed), then add the lemon juice.

5. Pour into a large food processor, then add in the tahini and blend well until mixed, scraping down the sides as needed. Remove half and set aside in a bowl.

6. Add half of the chickpeas and half of the water to the food processor, blending well and scraping down the sides as needed.

7. Once all mixed, add an ice cube, then continue blending for a few until the hummus is smooth. Scrape out into a bowl.

Instructions continued on the next page »

NUTRITION FACTS PER SERVING

236 Kcal	10 g Protein	12 g Fat	25.4 g Carbs	7 g Fiber	4 g Sugar

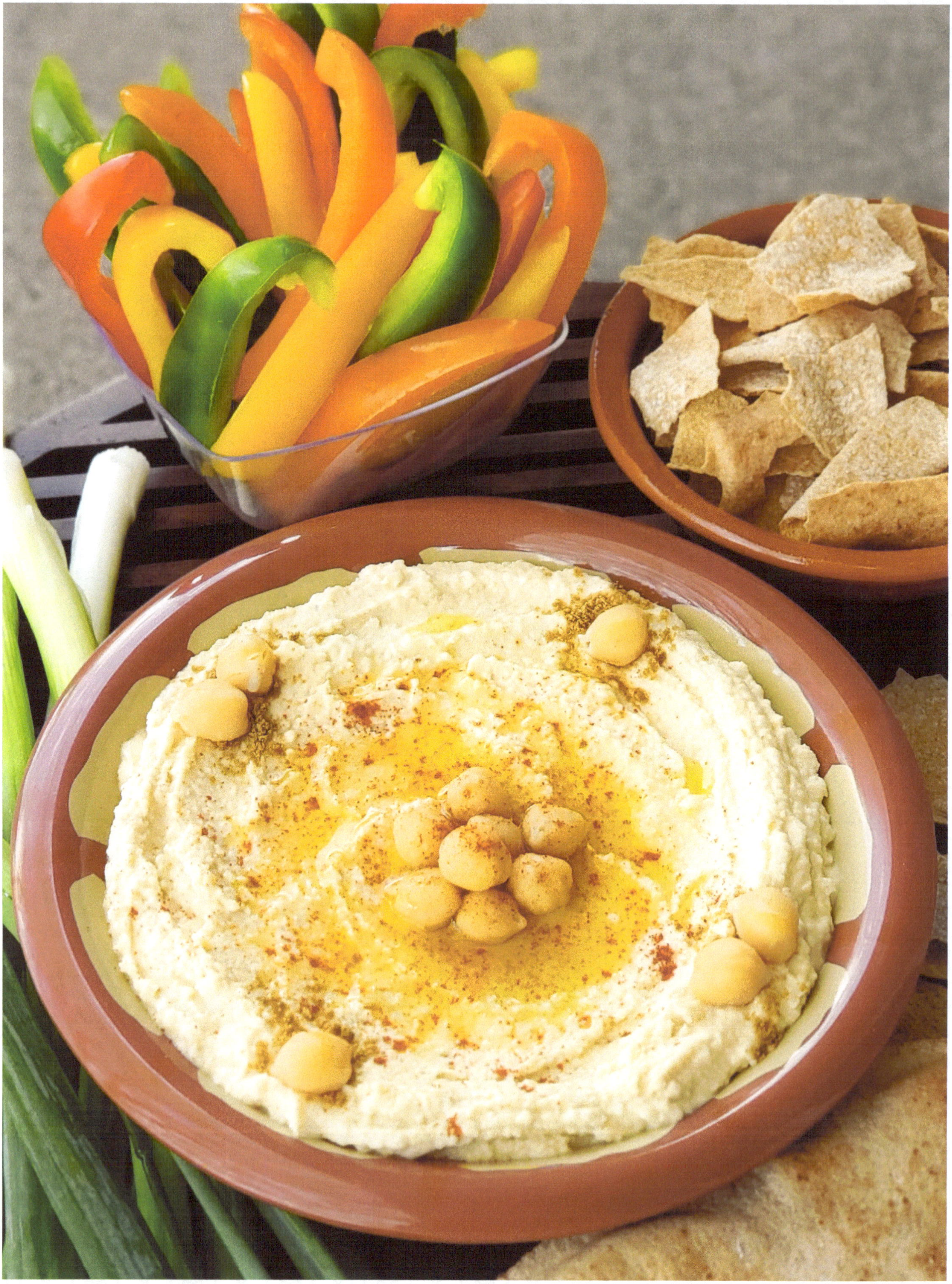

INGREDIENTS

2 ½ cups dry chickpeas (463 g)
1 ¼ cups tahini (300 g)
2 tbsp garlic, crushed
1 ¼ cups lemon juice
¼ cup chickpea water
2 medium ice cubes (40 g)
2 tsp salt
2 ½ tsp baking soda

NOTES

- The *hummus* dip will firm up further once refrigerated.
- Patience is key when making *hummus*, and the longer one allows the food processor to blend the ingredients at every step in the making of *hummus*, the smoother the final outcome will be.
- When I make this recipe, I normally set aside 3 cups of the plain *hummus* (freezing part of it if desired), and then I use the remaining 5 cups of *hummus* to make a variety of veggie chickpea dips (on the next page), the next day after the *hummus* has set and thickened up a bit in the refrigerator.
- My *hummus* is on the lemony side. For those who prefer a less lemony flavor, cut down the amount of lemon juice to 1 cup and bump up the chickpea water to ½ cup.
- For super smooth hummus, canned chickpeas are often used (but I definitely prefer the flavor of hummus when dry chickpeas are used), and many will often peel each individual chickpea (a step that is time consuming and ends up discarding the fiber-rich chickpea skin).
- The water obtained from the boiling of chickpeas is known as aquafaba, which becomes viscous upon cooling. This liquid is often saved and used as a replacement for egg whites.
- Each serving includes ½ cup of the dip.

INSTRUCTIONS

1. Soak the chickpeas and 1 ½ tsp baking soda in water for 12 hours. Drain and rinse, discarding any bad pieces.

2. Transfer the chickpeas to a pot, cover with water and add the remaining 1 tsp of baking soda, then bring to a boil. Skim off the white foam that floats to the surface, then cook, covered, on low heat for 50 to 60 minutes (or until overcooked but not mushy).

3. Drain the chickpeas, saving ¼ cup of the chickpea water (set in the refrigerator until ready to use), then remove ¼ cup chickpeas to add whole later on when serving the dip. Lightly cover the drained chickpeas to keep from drying out. Let cool to room temperature.

4. In a small bowl, mix the garlic and salt (until a paste is formed), then add the lemon juice.

5. Pour into a large food processor, then add in the tahini and blend well until mixed, scraping down the sides as needed. Remove half and set aside in a bowl.

6. Add half of the chickpeas and half of the water to the food processor, blending well and scraping down the sides as needed.

7. Once all mixed, add an ice cube, then continue blending for a few until the hummus is smooth. Scrape out into a bowl.

8. Process the remaining chickpeas in the same way, with the remaining water, *tahini*/garlic mix, and ice cube.

9. Add back the initial batch of prepared hummus to the processor and blend the two batches together until well mixed.

10. Serve at room temperature or chilled from the refrigerator, and garnish with whole chickpeas, sprinkle some cumin or paprika, and drizzle with some olive oil if desired. Serve with fresh or toasted pita bread, as well a variety of vegetables such as green onions, tomatoes, and/or sweet peppers.

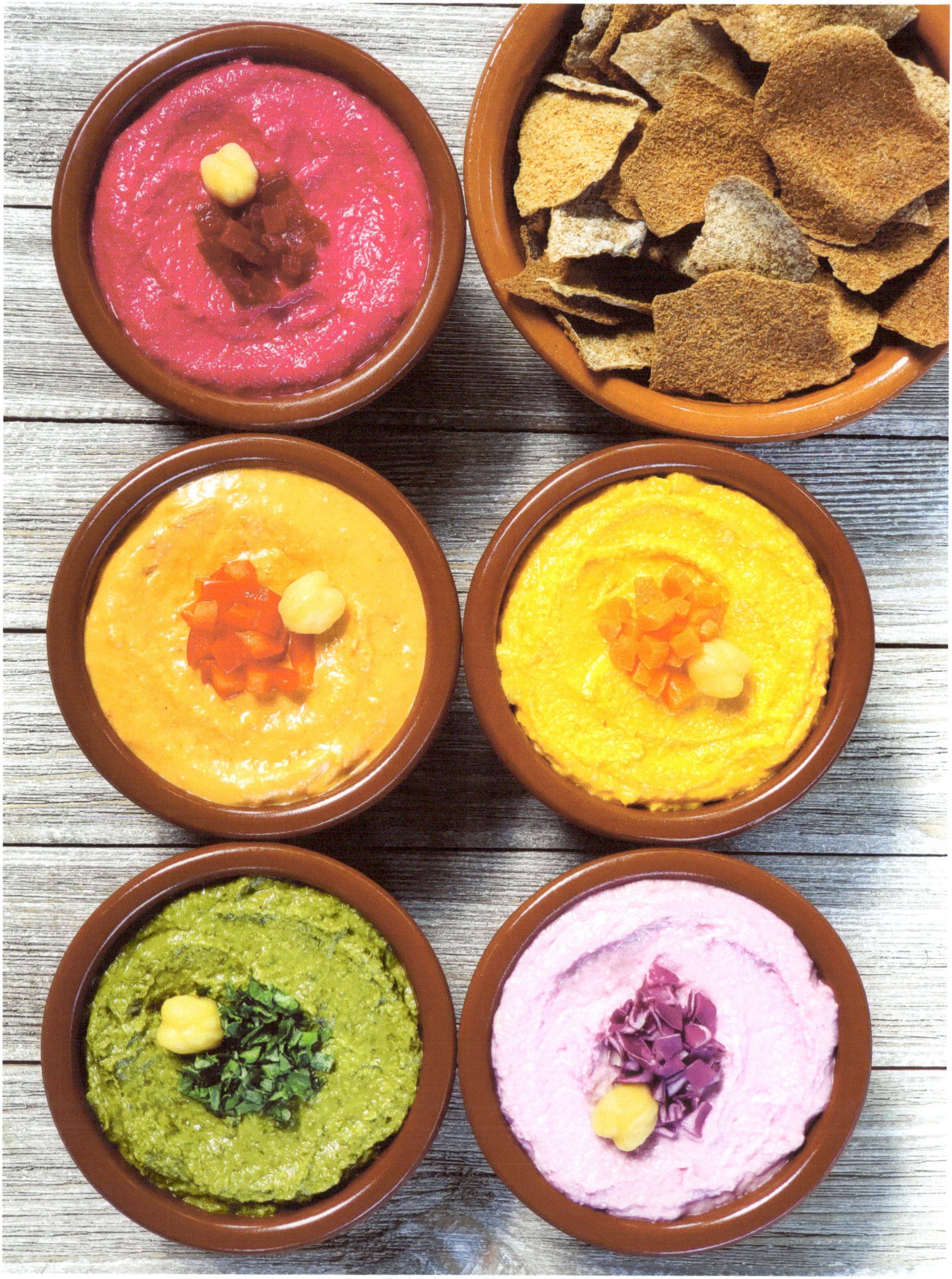

VEGGIE CHICKPEA DIP

This is my healthy rainbow-inspired take on the classic world-renowned *hummus* mezza dish (on the previous page). Mixing vegetables into creamy *hummus* not only adds a multitude of nutrients, but also enhances the rich flavors, while giving the dip beautiful and vibrant colors. This delicious and pretty dish is great for parties and makes for a great finger-food dish when hosting guests.

RECIPE YIELD 1 2/3 cups* 1 ½ cups** 1 1/3 cups***

DF GF EF OF V FF

INGREDIENTS

5 cups plain chickpea dip (1,150 g)
2 ½ small beets (no skin), sliced into circles (188 g)
1 ½ medium red bell peppers, quartered (248 g)
3 medium carrots (no skin), halved lengthwise (180 g)
4 small curly kale stalks (leaves only), torn by hand (100 g)
⅛ small red (purple) cabbage, separated into slices (125 g)
⅓ tsp paprika
⅓ tsp turmeric

INSTRUCTIONS

1. Because bell peppers are so moist, it is best to roast them in the oven. Spread the bell peppers (skin side down) on a large sheet pan (recommended dimensions: 30 cm x 40 cm) lined with parchment paper, then bake in a preheated oven at 400 °F for 40 minutes. Peel off any charred parts of the skin then set the peppers aside to cool slightly.

2. For all other vegetables, steam separately for 20 minutes in a steamer basket placed inside a closed large pot with boiling water covering the bottom (don't let the water touch the basket.) Make sure to check the water level in the pot after steaming each vegetable, adding more as needed (sometimes changing the water is recommended if the water starts changing color).

3. Set each type of steamed vegetable aside on a paper towel and dab to dry. Let cool for at least 5 minutes.

4. With the help of a small food processor, process 1 cup of *hummus* dip with each type of vegetable, separately. Blend well until smooth, scraping down the sides as needed (the paprika should be added when making the bell pepper *hummus*, while the turmeric should be added when making the carrot *hummus*).

5. One can work on blending one type of veggie *hummus* dip while another vegetable is being cooked. After blending each type of veggie *hummus*, make sure to scrape clean the food processor cup with a spatula or rinse under hot water then dry, to prevent the colors of the different veggie *hummus* dips from blending into one another. Store each veggie *hummus* dip in a separate air-tight container.

6. Garnish with boiled chickpeas and/or matching vegetables, and drizzle with olive oil, if desired. Serve with fresh or toasted pita bread.

See next page for notes »

NUTRITION FACTS PER SERVING

116 Kcal	5 g Protein	5.4 g Fat	13.6 g Carbs	4 g Fiber	3 g Sugar

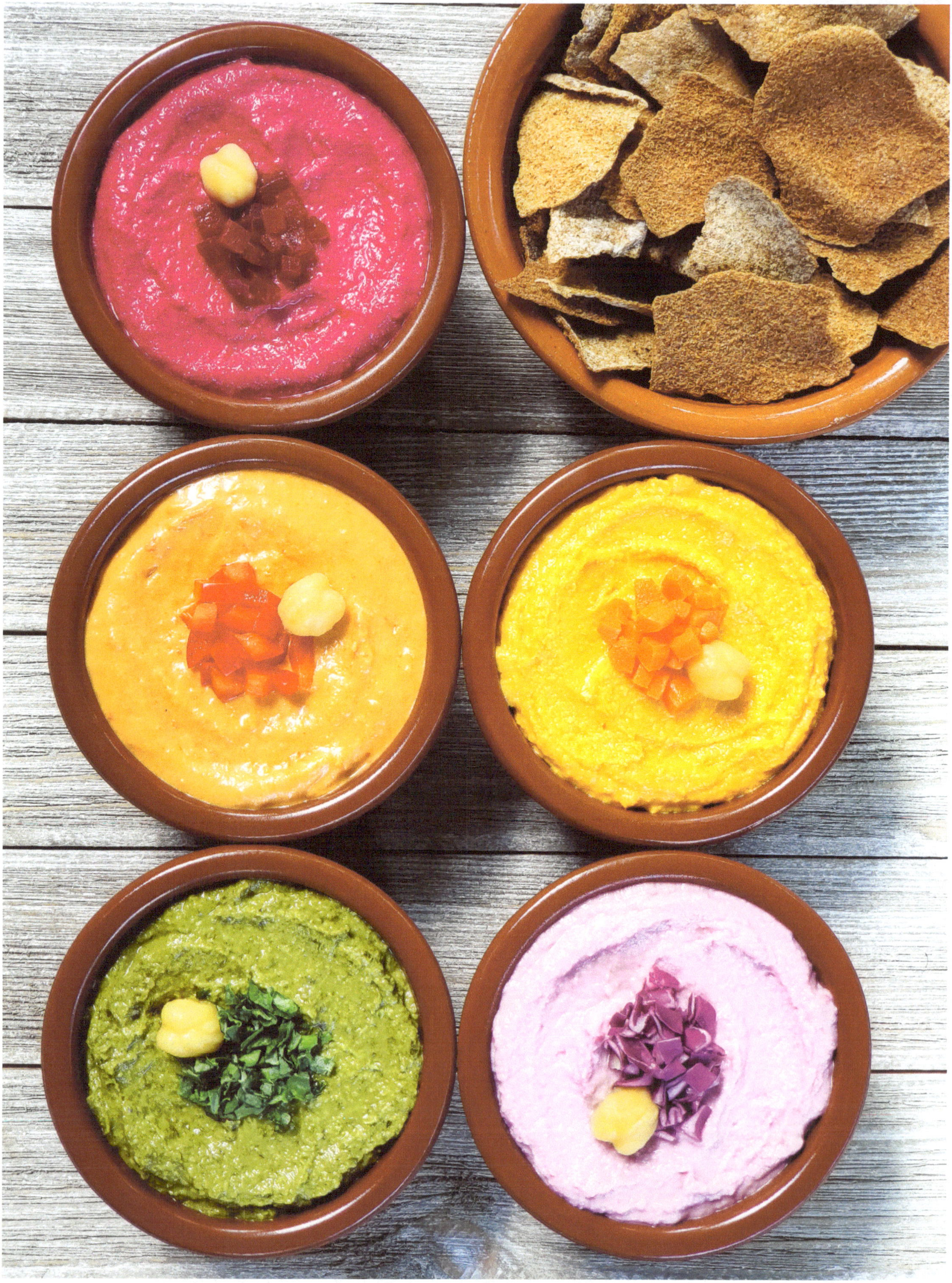

INGREDIENTS

5 cups plain chickpea dip (1,150 g)
2 ½ small beets (no skin), sliced into circles (188 g)
1 ½ medium red bell peppers, quartered (248 g)
3 medium carrots (no skin), halved lengthwise (180 g)
4 small curly kale stalks (leaves only), torn by hand (100 g)
⅛ small red (purple) cabbage, separated into slices (125 g)
⅓ tsp paprika
⅓ tsp turmeric

NOTES

- For steaming, I let the water reach a rapid boil on high heat, then I put the vegetables in the steamer basket, cover the pot, then turn down the heat to medium, while making sure a rapid boil is maintained.
- The veggie *hummus* dips will firm up further once refrigerated.
- The purple veggie *hummus* could be made with purple sweet potatoes instead, if desired, while the green veggie *hummus* could be made with spinach instead, if desired.
- Since the different veggie *hummus* dips have only slight differences in nutritional value, the numbers were averaged between them.
- Each serving includes ⅓ cup of the dip.

* Recipe yield for the beet *hummus* and the carrot *hummus*
** Recipe yield for the bell pepper *hummus* and the cabbage *hummus*
*** Recipe yield for the kale *hummus*

INSTRUCTIONS

1. Because bell peppers are so moist, it is best to roast them in the oven. Spread the bell peppers (skin side down) on a large sheet pan (recommended dimensions = 30 cm x 40 cm) lined with parchment paper, then bake in a preheated oven at 400 °F for 40 minutes. Peel off any charred parts of the skin then set the peppers aside to cool slightly.

2. For all other vegetables, steam separately for 20 minutes in a steamer basket placed inside a closed large pot with boiling water covering the bottom (don't let the water touch the basket.) Make sure to check the water level in the pot after steaming each vegetable, adding more as needed (sometimes changing the water is recommended if the water starts changing color).

3. Set each type of steamed vegetable aside on a paper towel and dab to dry. Let cool for at least 5 minutes.

4. With the help of a small food processor, process 1 cup of *hummus* dip with each type of vegetable, separately. Blend well until smooth, scraping down the sides as needed (the paprika should be added when making the bell pepper *hummus*, while the turmeric should be added when making the carrot *hummus*).

5. One can work on blending one type of veggie *hummus* dip while another vegetable is being cooked. After blending each type of veggie *hummus*, make sure to scrape clean the food processor cup with a spatula or rinse under hot water then dry, to prevent the colors of the different veggie *hummus* dips from blending into one another. Store each veggie *hummus* dip in a separate air-tight container.

6. Garnish with boiled chickpeas and/or matching vegetables, and drizzle with olive oil, if desired. Serve with fresh or toasted pita bread.

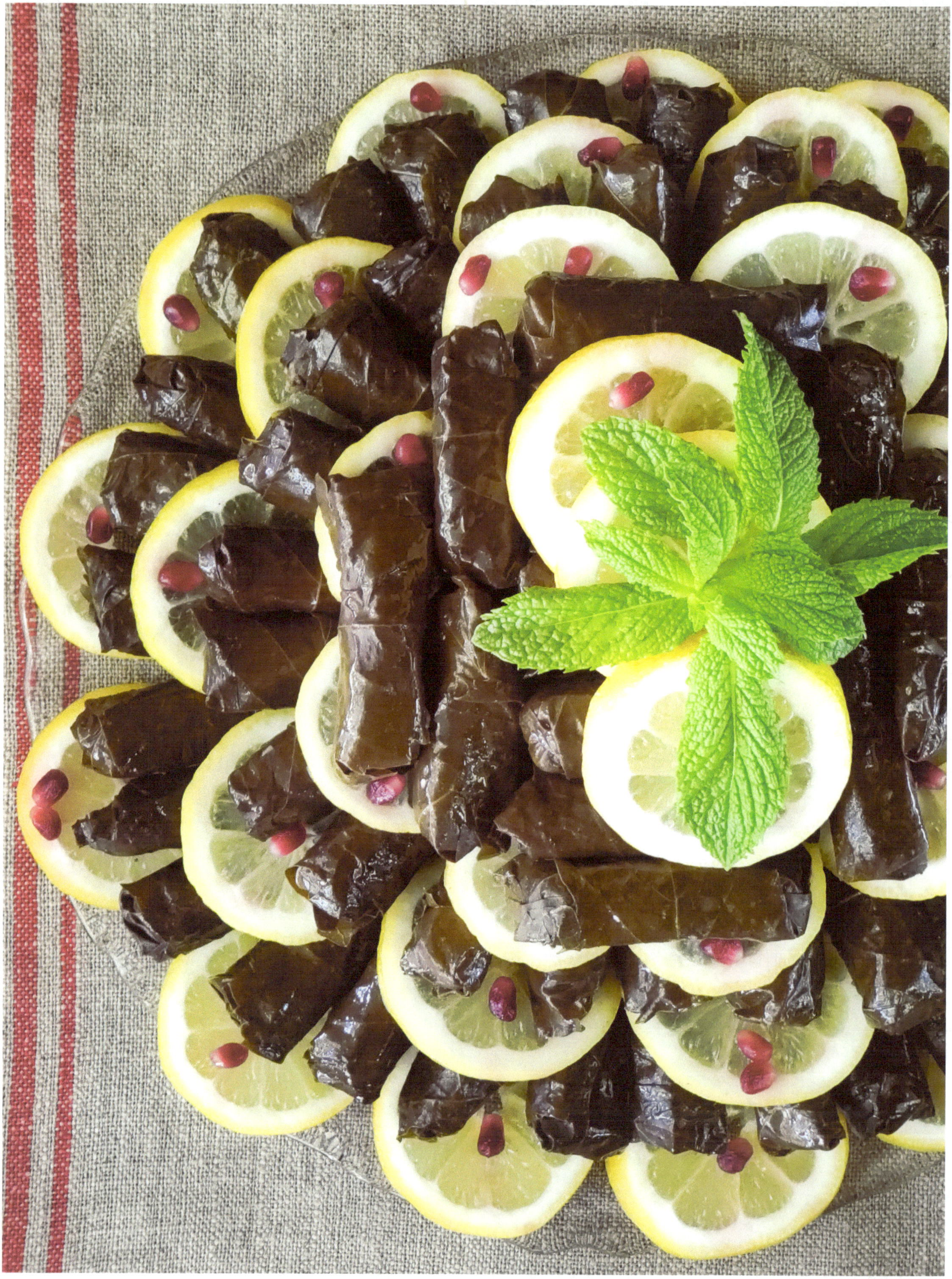

STUFFED GRAPE LEAVES IN OIL

Warak Enab bi Zait   ورق عنب بزيت

Vegan grape leaf dolma is one of my favorite Middle Eastern mezza dishes. While this dish is tedious to prepare, especially the part that involves rolling the grape leaves around the prepared rice and vegetable stuffing, the end result is totally worth the time and effort. Gathering up some friends or family members to help in the making of a pot of stuffed grape leaves is definitely a deal breaker when it comes to preparing this dish. There are a few variations to this classic, with some being non-vegan and containing a source of red meat and made alongside stuffed zucchinis. My take on the vegan version of this dish is very close to the Lebanese traditional way of making it, with the main difference being that I use brown rice and less olive oil.

RECIPE YIELD 90 pieces (18 servings)

DF GF EF V FF

INGREDIENTS

1 jar (454 g) grape leaves in brine
2 cups dry parboiled brown rice (364 g)
1 medium yellow onion, minced (160 g)
4 medium red tomatoes, diced (540 g)
1 medium carrot, finely grated (60 g)
2 bunches Italian parsley, finely chopped (210 g)
2 bunches mint (leaves only), finely chopped (40 g)
4 cups boiling water
⅔ cup lemon juice
6 tbsp olive oil
1 tbsp pomegranate molasses
1 tbsp dry mint leaves
1 tbsp sumac
2 ¼ tsp salt
⅓ tsp black pepper
1 medium russet potato (sliced into circles)

INSTRUCTIONS

1. Drain away the brine, then soak the leaves in warm water for 10 minutes. Soak again in a new bowl of clean warm water for another 10 minutes (this helps decrease the taste/smell of the brine solution), then rinse well. Lay out on a towel to dry and cover with another towel to keep from drying out (net weight of the leaves is 370 g).
2. Pick over the rice, removing any bad pieces. Rinse well, then drain.
3. Place the rice in a large bowl, toss in all the prepared vegetables (except for the potato), and mix in the herbs, spices, 2 tsp salt, 5 tbsp olive oil, pomegranate molasses, and 1/3 cup lemon juice. Stir well to mix.
4. Using a scissors, cut away the thick end of the middle vein of each grape leaf. Lay out on the counter (veiny side up), then scoop out a level tablespoon of stuffing onto the center of the leaf and spread out horizontally. Fold in the side of the leaf (starting from the wider side) over the stuffing, then fold the edges, then roll up tightly.
5. Repeat steps 4 and 5 until all the stuffing has been used up (save any remaining juices). Set aside any torn leaves that cannot be stuffed and rolled.
6. Line the bottom of a big pot with one row of potato slices to prevent any sticking/burning of the grape leaves while cooking.

Instructions continued on the next page »

NUTRITION FACTS PER SERVING

151.6 Kcal	3.5 g Protein	6 g Fat	22 g Carbs	4 g Fiber	3 g Sugar

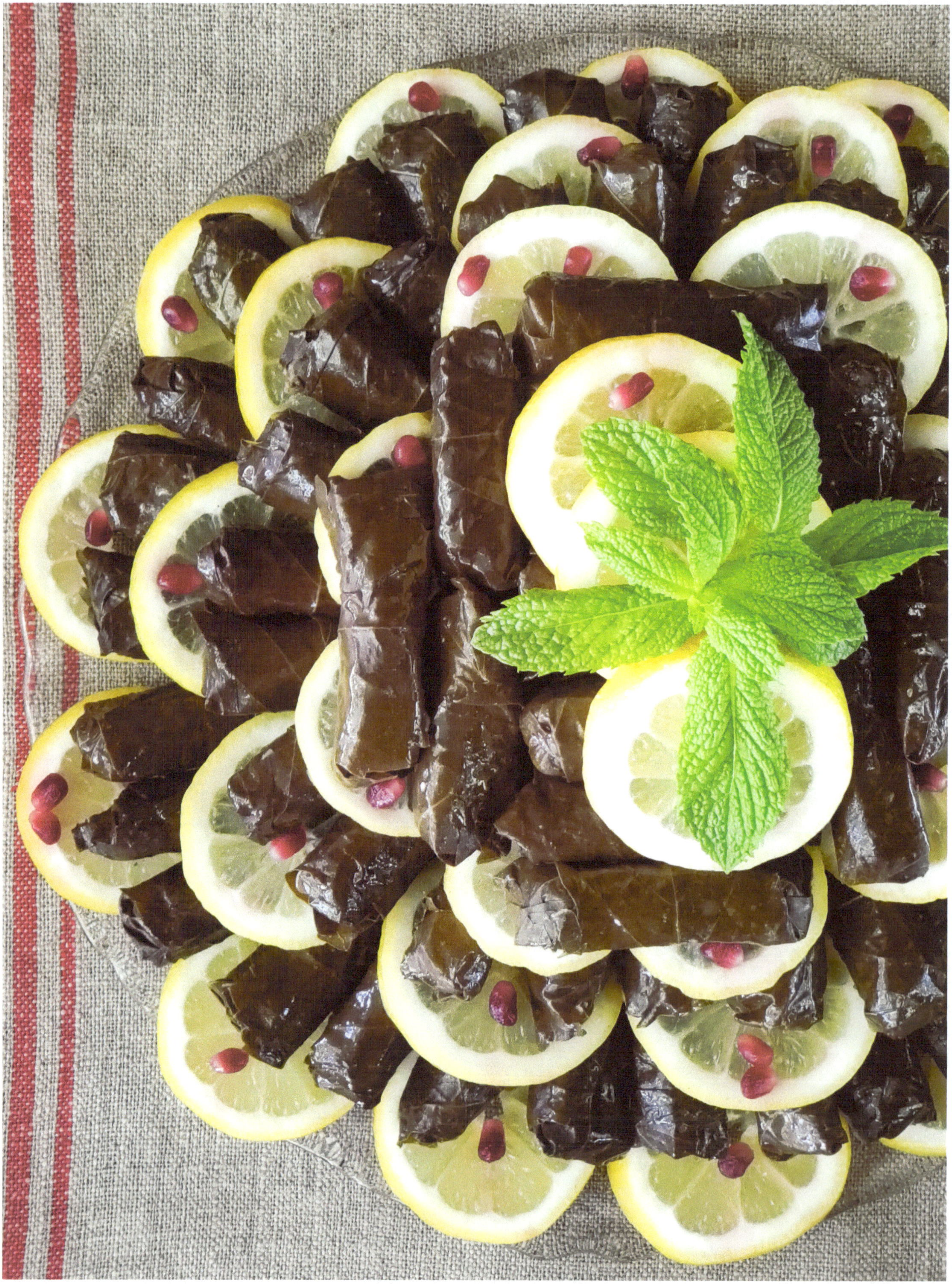

INGREDIENTS

1 jar (454 g) grape leaves in brine
2 cups dry parboiled rice (364 g)
1 medium yellow onion, minced (160 g)
4 medium red tomatoes, diced (540 g)
1 medium carrot, finely grated (60 g)
2 bunches Italian parsley, finely chopped (210 g)
2 bunches mint (leaves only), finely chopped (40 g)
4 cups boiling water
⅔ cup lemon juice
6 tbsp olive oil
1 tbsp pomegranate molasses
1 tbsp dry mint leaves
1 tbsp sumac
2 ¼ tsp salt
⅓ tsp black pepper
1 medium russet potato (sliced into circles)

NOTES

- If freshly picked grape leaves are to be used, aim for 90 mostly large leaves washed well with ends removed. Soaking in very hot water for 15 minutes after washing helps soften the leaves enough to roll up better. A fun fact: many states in the US have wild grape vines growing in the woods and around parks and neighborhoods. Minnesota is full of wild grape vines and that is where I mostly harvest my grape leaves. Fresh grape leaves normally take less time to cook (2 hours or less) than those pre-packed in brine.
- Since grape leaves often come in large, medium, and small sizes, one can use two small leaves to create a medium sized grape leaf. Similarly, one can use a small leaf as well as a medium one to create a large grape leaf. Place the two leaves next to each other vertically, slightly overlapping, before stuffing and rolling.
- The yield of this dish may vary slightly depending on the size of the grape leaves used. A yield of 90 rolled grape leaves is obtained if leaves are mostly the large size (thus able to accommodate a 1 tbsp of stuffing). If leaves are mostly medium and small, more leaves will be needed to use up the whole stuffing.
- Each serving includes 5 stuffed grape leaves.
- The potato slices are not included in the nutrition facts (carrot slices can also be used alongside the potato).

INSTRUCTIONS

1. Drain away the brine, then soak the leaves in warm water for 10 minutes. Soak again in a new bowl of clean warm water for another 10 minutes (this helps decrease the taste/smell of the brine solution), then rinse well. Lay out on a towel to dry and cover with another towel to keep from drying out (net weight of the leaves is 370 g).

2. Pick over the rice, removing any bad pieces. Rinse well, then drain.

3. Place the rice in a large bowl, toss in all the prepared vegetables (except for the potato), and mix in the herbs, spices, 2 tsp salt, 5 tbsp olive oil, pomegranate molasses, and 1/3 cup lemon juice. Stir well to mix.

4. Using a scissors, cut away the thick end of the middle vein of each grape leaf. Lay out on the counter (veiny side up), then scoop out a level tablespoon of stuffing onto the center of the leaf and spread out horizontally. Fold in the side of the leaf (starting from the wider side) over the stuffing, then fold the edges, then roll up tightly.

5. Repeat steps 4 and 5 until all the stuffing has been used up (save any remaining juices). Set aside any torn leaves that cannot be stuffed and rolled.

6. Line the bottom of a big pot with one row of potato slices to prevent any sticking/burning of the grape leaves while cooking.

7. Start arranging the rolled grape leaves over the layer of potatoes placing them snug together. Once one layer is formed, brush the grape leaves with some of the remaining 1 tbsp of olive oil, sprinkle some salt (from the remaining ¼ tsp), and continue on to form another layer of rolled grape leaves (alternating the directions of the placed leaves). Again, brush the layer with olive oil then sprinkle some salt. Continue in this manner until all the grape leaves have been neatly arranged inside the pot.

8. Place an inverted heat-resistant plate to cover the surface and to weigh down the grape leaves in order to keep them in place, then pour in the boiling water (and any remaining juices from the stuffing), and assess if more is needed (the water level should be just covering the bottom of the inverted plate).

9. Cover the pot, bring to a boil, then cook, covered, on low heat for about 2 to 3 hours (do a taste test to make sure the grape leaf itself, especially the center vein, is well cooked and soft).

10. Uncover then carefully remove the plate. Pour the remaining 1/3 cup lemon juice over the top, then loosely place a piece of foil over the surface, and let cool for at least two hours before placing in the refrigerator (too fast of a cooling process will cause excess darkening in color of the surface of the grape leaves).

11. Serve at room temperature or cold out of the refrigerator. Squeeze extra lemon juice if desired.

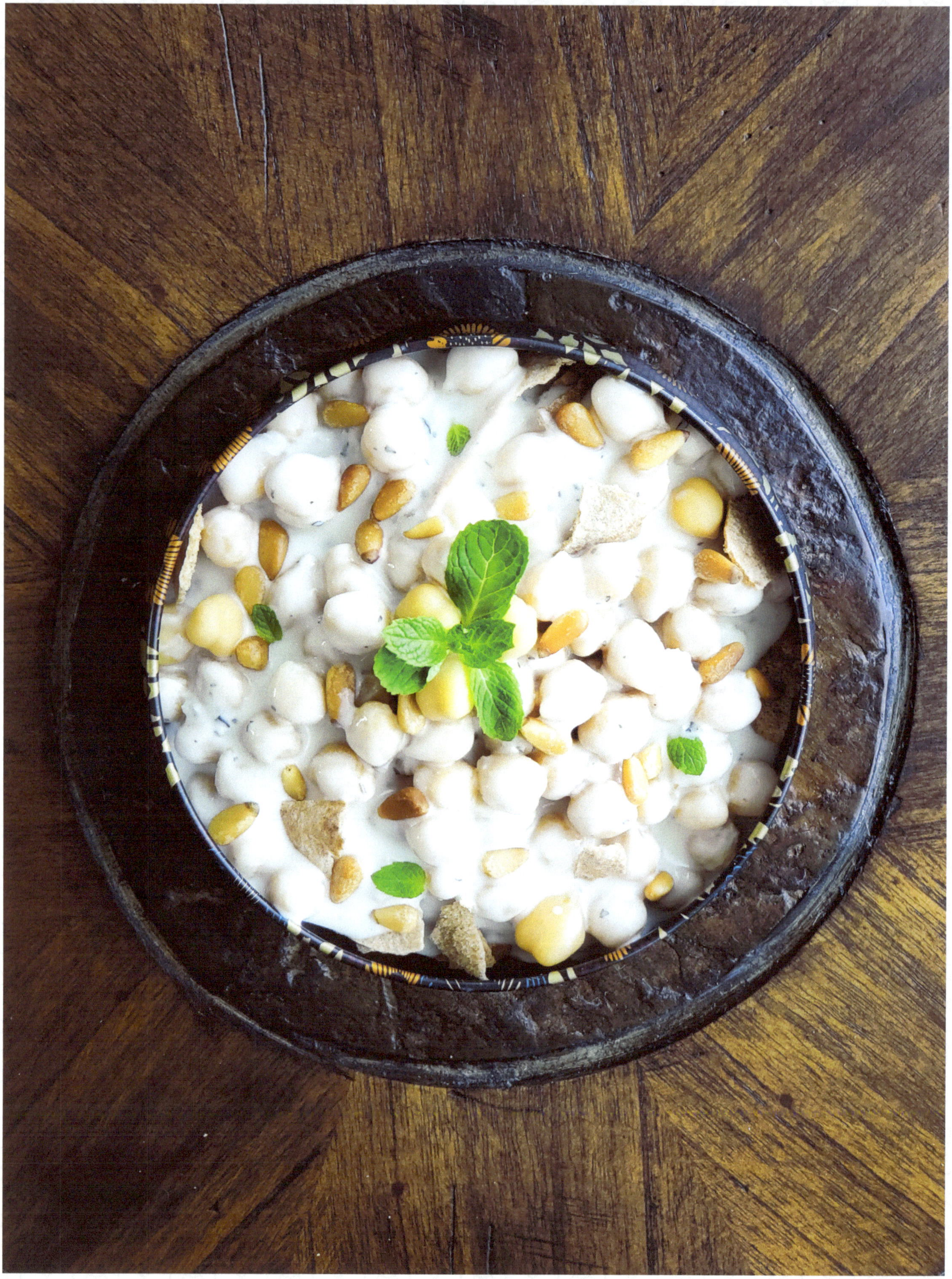

CHICKPEAS WITH PITA IN YOGURT

Fatteh bi Hummus فتّة بحمّص

This garlicy warm yogurt mezza dish is a signature of the Middle Eastern cuisine. Commonly consumed as part of a hearty breakfast or brunch, it is traditionally made with fried pita bread, a garlicky full-fat yogurt sauce with *tahini*, and sometimes a meat source (usually beef or chicken). My healthy and light take on this dish is vegetarian and made with toasted pita bread and skim yogurt.

RECIPE YIELD 12 servings

EF Vt

INGREDIENTS

2 cups dry chickpeas (370 g)
2 ½ loaves whole wheat Arabic bread (medium size) (183 g)
5 ½ cups skim yogurt (1,293 g)
4 tbsp skim labneh
4 tbsp tahini
1 tbsp garlic, crushed
5 tsp olive oil
2 tsp dry mint leaves
1 tsp salt
1 tsp baking soda

NOTES

- I like placing the serving dish in a hot (but turned off) oven for around 10 to 15 minutes before layering in the ingredients, as this helps keep the ingredients warmer.
- Each serving roughly includes ½ cup yogurt mixture, a little under ½ cup boiled chickpeas, and ⅓ cup (12 g) toasted pita bread pieces.

INSTRUCTIONS

1. Soak the chickpeas and baking soda in water for 12 hours. Drain and rinse, discarding any bad pieces.
2. Transfer the chickpeas to a pot, cover with water, then bring to a boil. Skim off the white foam that floats to the surface, then cook, covered, on low heat for 30 minutes (or until tender). Uncover and place the lid ajar.
3. Separate the pita bread loaves into 5 individual halves. Brush each half with 1 tsp of olive oil then place in a preheated oven at 350 °F and toast for 7 to 10 minutes (until lightly browned and completely toasted). Let cool slightly, then break up (by hand) into small pieces.
4. In a small bowl, mix the garlic and salt (until a paste is formed), then add the *labneh* and mix.
5. Transfer to a bigger bowl, then add the yogurt, *tahini*, and mint. Stir to mix.
6. Drain the hot chickpeas well, then spread evenly over the bottom of a deep serving dish (glass or stoneware of recommended dimensions: 23.5 cm x 33.5 cm or similar).
7. Sprinkle the warm pita bread pieces over the chickpeas, then pour the yogurt mixture over the pita bread, covering it well.
8. Garnish with fresh mint leaves as well as dry roasted pine nuts if desired. Serve immediately while warm and before the bread becomes soggy.

NUTRITION FACTS PER SERVING

281 Kcal	16 g Protein	7 g Fat	40.4 g Carbs	7 g Fiber	13.6 g Sugar

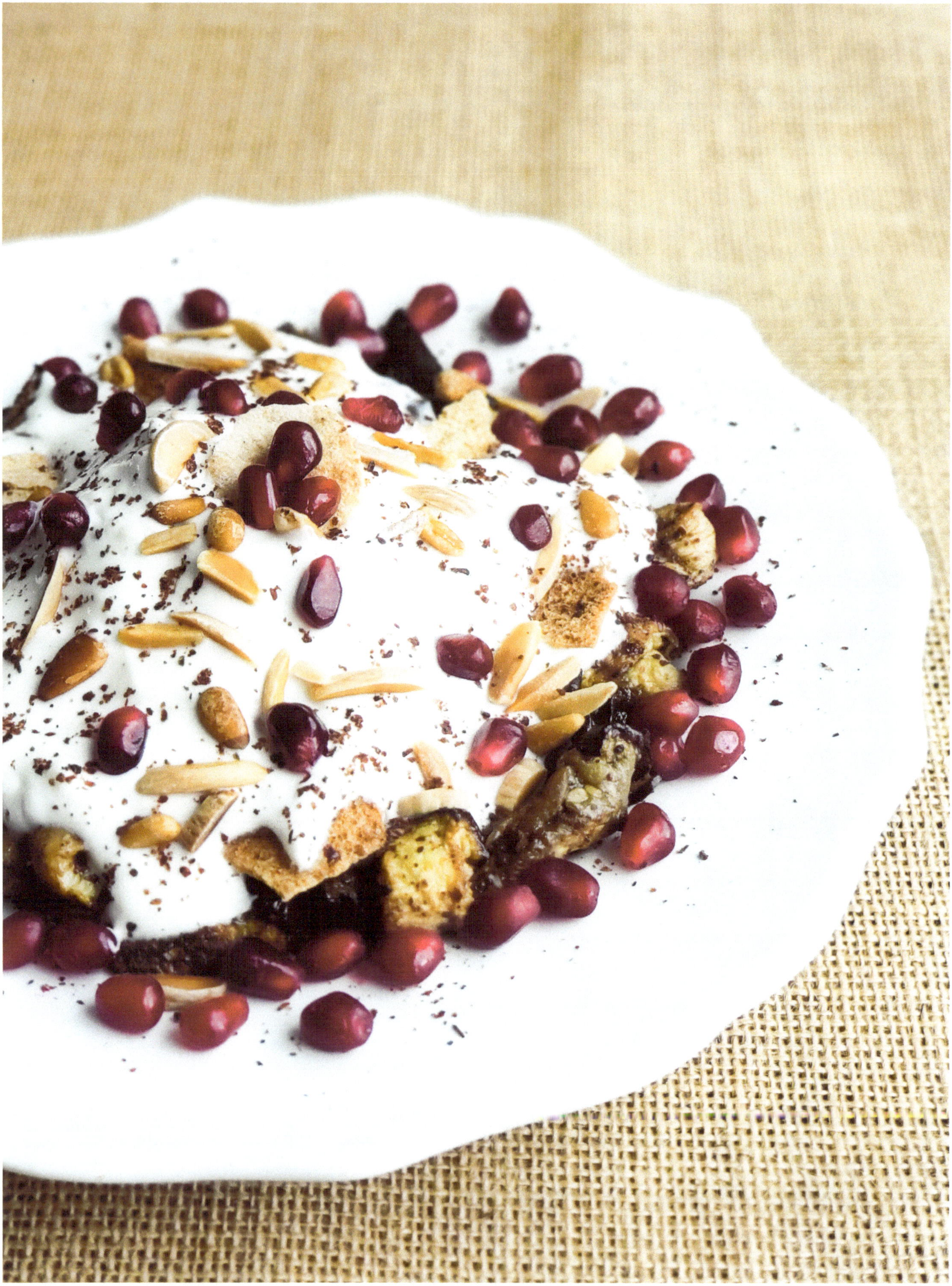

EGGPLANT WITH PITA IN YOGURT

Fatteh bi Bathinjan فتّة بباذنجان

This warm eggplant mezza dish is similar to the chickpea dish on the previous page, but is distinct in many ways. It is a layered dish composed of a garlicky yogurt sauce with tahini, eggplant seasoned with pomegranate molasses (and I also add sumac), pita bread, and nuts (other variations of the dish include adding red meat, usually lamb, as well as some tomato paste). While the traditional dish is quite heavy being made with full-fat yogurt and all other ingredients fried (fried eggplant, pita bread, as well as nuts), my healthy version calls for low-fat yogurt and oven roasting of the former 3 ingredients without any oil, then drizzling a little heart-healthy olive oil afterwards on top of the eggplant.

RECIPE YIELD 12 servings

EF Vt

INGREDIENTS

4 medium Italian eggplants (with skin, no ends), sliced (1,450 g)
2 ½ loaves whole wheat Arabic bread (medium size) (183 g)
5 ½ cups skim yogurt (1,293 g)
4 tbsp skim labneh
3 tbsp tahini
2 tbsp garlic, crushed
2 tsp pomegranate molasses
6 tsp olive oil
1 tbsp sumac
1 tsp salt

NOTES

- I like placing the serving dish in a hot (but turned off) oven for around 10 to 15 minutes before layering in the ingredients, as this helps keep the ingredients warmer.
- Each serving roughly includes ½ cup yogurt mixture, ⅓ cup baked eggplant, and ⅓ cup (12 g) toasted pita bread pieces.

INSTRUCTIONS

1. Separate the pita bread loaves into 5 individual halves. Brush each half with 1 tsp of olive oil then place in a preheated oven at 350 °F and toast for 7 to 10 minutes (until lightly browned and completely toasted). Let cool slightly, then break up (by hand) into small pieces.
2. Place the finger-sized eggplant slices on 2 large sheet pans (recommended dimensions: 30 cm x 40 cm or similar) lined with parchment paper (make sure the slices are spread out and not laying on top of one another), then bake in a preheated oven at 400 °F for 45 minutes (or until tender). There is no need to flip the eggplant slices halfway through.
3. In the meantime, mix the garlic and salt (until a paste is formed) in a small bowl, then add the *labneh* and mix.
4. Transfer to a bigger bowl, then add the yogurt and *tahini*. Stir to mix.
5. Spread the cooked eggplant evenly over the bottom of a deep serving dish (glass or stoneware of recommended dimensions: 23.5 cm x 33.5 cm or similar), then gently mix in the pomegranate molasses, the remaining 1 tsp of olive oil, and sumac.
6. Sprinkle the warm pita bread pieces over the eggplant, then pour the yogurt mixture over the pita bread, covering it well.
7. Garnish with extra sumac, pomegranate seeds, and dry roasted pine nuts and/or almond slivers if desired. Serve immediately while warm and before the bread becomes soggy.

NUTRITION FACTS PER SERVING

187 Kcal	10 g Protein	5 g Fat	27 g Carbs	5 g Fiber	15 g Sugar

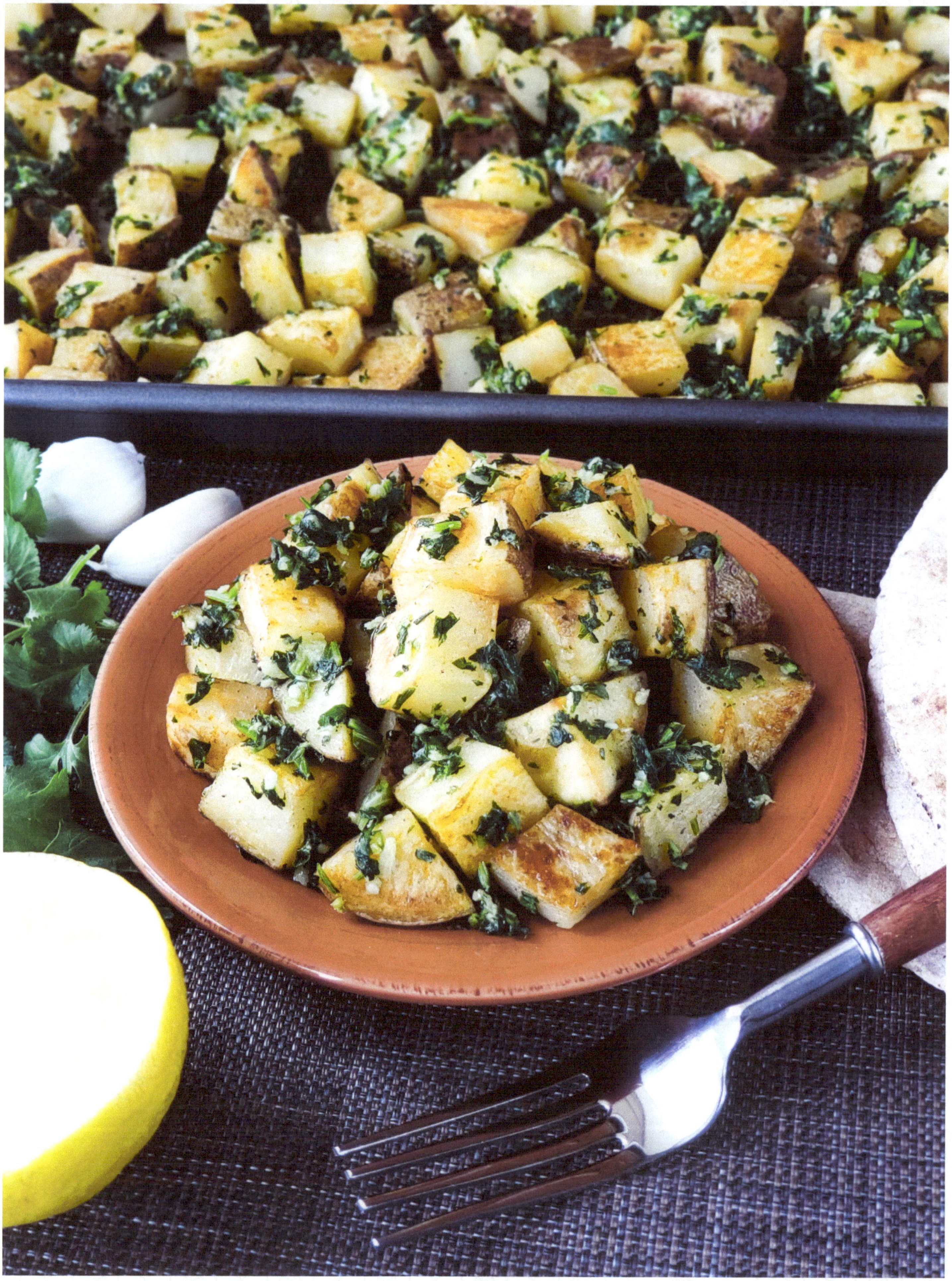

GARLICY POTATOES WITH CORIANDER

Batata bi Kizbara wa Toom بطاطا بكزبرة و توم

This is a simple but flavorful potato mezza dish. Traditionally, the potatoes are peeled then deep fried, and often the coriander and garlic are sautéed in oil as well before being mixed in with the fried potatoes. I prefer keeping potato skins on for added fiber, then roasting them in the oven with some heart-healthy extra-virgin olive oil. A hot spicy sister dish is commonly made as well, whereby red pepper is added. I personally prefer the dish without the spicy hot flavor, thus enjoying the sole strong flavors of garlic, coriander, and fresh lemon juice.

RECIPE YIELD 9 cups

DF GF EF V

INGREDIENTS

4 medium russet potatoes (with skin), cubed (1.7 kg)
3 bunches coriander, finely chopped (255 g)
3 tbsp garlic, crushed
2 tbsp lemon juice
1 tbsp olive oil
1 tsp dry oregano leaves
½ tsp paprika
1 tsp salt
⅛ tsp black pepper

RECIPE ALTERNATIVE

- For a spicy hot flavor, garnish with ground cayenne pepper or red pepper flakes.

INSTRUCTIONS

1. Wash the potatoes very well, then cut into cubes.
2. Add to a pot of hot water then let sit for 10 minutes.
3. Drain, then rinse with cold water. Drain well, then pat dry.
4. Transfer to a large bowl containing the olive oil, herbs, spices and ½ tsp salt, then rub the potatoes well until evenly covered.
5. Lay out on a large sheet pan (recommended dimensions: 30 cm x 40 cm or bigger) lined with parchment paper (make sure the potatoes are spread out and not on top of one another), then bake in a preheated oven at 375 °F for 50 minutes (if using refined olive oil, one can bake the potatoes in a hotter oven, such as at 400 °F or higher, and for a shorter time, about 40 minutes or less).
6. In a small bowl, mix the garlic and ½ tsp salt (until a paste is formed).
7. Transfer the garlic to a medium pan or skillet and mix in the coriander. Stir on medium/high heat for 5 minutes, or until the coriander has wilted a bit, then mix in the lemon juice.
8. Add the garlic/coriander mix over the pan of potatoes, then gently fold.
9. Squeeze extra lemon juice and add more paprika if desired before serving. Eat plain on a plate or with pita bread.

NUTRITION FACTS PER CUP

174.6 Kcal	5 g Protein	2 g Fat	36.5 g Carbs	3.4 g Fiber	1.5 g Sugar

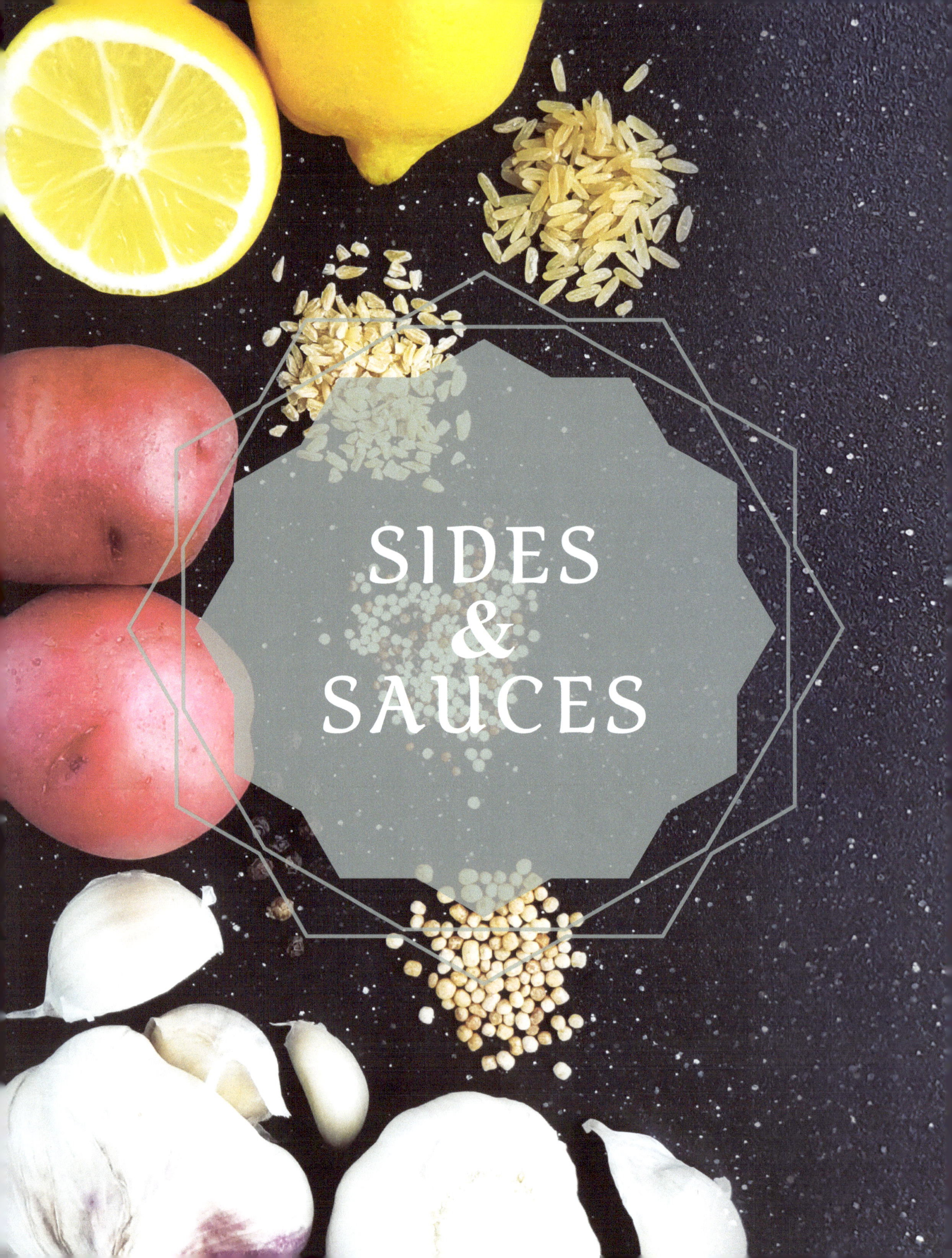

SIDES & SAUCES

The Lebanese cuisine combines a wide selection of main dishes that are either commonly served with a side dish, usually rice, such as beef-based stews, or eaten with a side of Arabic bread smothered in a flavorful and strong traditional sauce. Lebanese and/or Middle Eastern side dishes and sauces presented in this section are named with the traditional Arabic name, along with an English transliteration of the Arabic. Side dishes without an Arabic name are not Lebanese/Middle Eastern. They are either recipes of my own creation or are ones adapted from recipes handed down to me by my mother.

SOME GENERAL REMARKS AND RECOMMENDATIONS

- It is very important to wash all vegetables called for in a recipe prior to starting. Vegetables, such as potatoes, can harbor soil particles from having been out in the field, and soil in turn can be the source of many harmful bacteria. Properly washing vegetables under cold running water, with scrubbing and/or quick soaking, then rinsing as many times as needed, is important. Since I do not peel my potatoes, make sure to rub the skins very well with a clean brush during washing.

- The weights presented to the right-hand side of a vegetable ingredient relates to the final net weight of the vegetable added to the pot (i.e. the net weight after peeling, removing the inedible ends or core, and chopping off bad parts of the vegetable).

- Since fresh produce can vary widely in size, shape, and weight, it is recommended to go by the presented weights of called for ingredients, in order to obtain more accurate recipe outcomes and yields.

- Bake an ingredient/dish on the middle rack of the oven, unless otherwise specified.

- All spices such as cinnamon, turmeric, cumin, or ginger are called for in their ground (powdered) form, unless otherwise specified.

- I am a big fan of spices and herbs, but not a fan of salt. Thus, the salt amounts called for in my side dishes and sauces tend to be on the lower end, so always adjust the taste to your preference.

- The addition of salt as an ingredient is included with the spices in the instruction steps of the recipes, unless otherwise specified.

- I don't like to cook with too much oil, especially since I am not fond of oily/greasy food in general. However, I make sure that the lower amount of oil doesn't negatively affect the flavor of a dish. One can definitely add more oil if desired, but this will increase the caloric and fat content of the dish.

- A serving of 1 cup of a side dish is a good serving size to be consumed with around 1.5 to 2 cups of a main dish (such as a stew).

- The 'sugar' value in the nutrition facts of recipes refers to the total amount of sugar (both simple and complex) that is naturally occurring in the various ingredients.

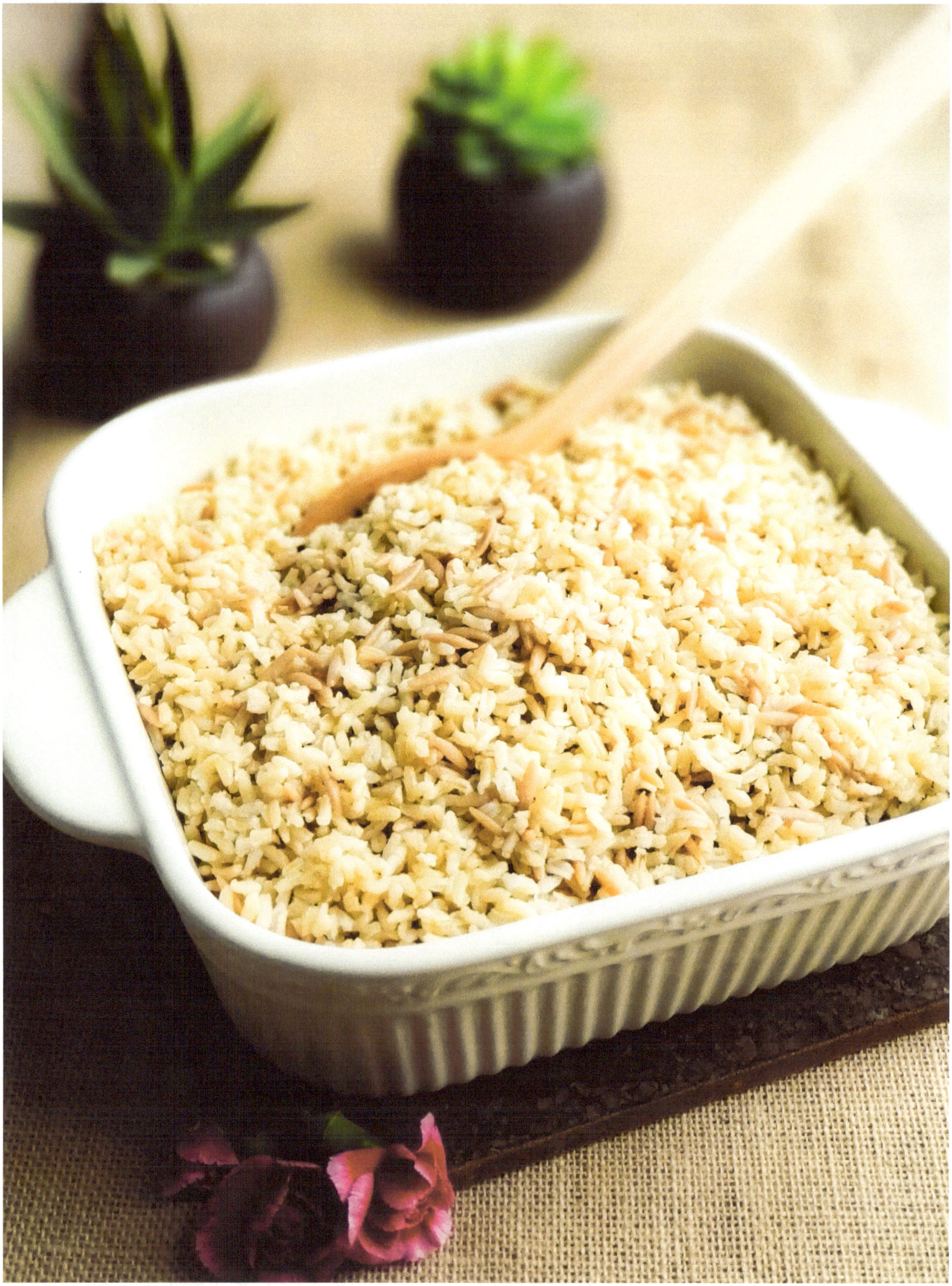

RICE WITH ORZO

Riz bi Shaeeriyyeh رز بشعيريّة

Plain white rice cooked with vermicelli is a common side dish eaten with traditional Lebanese stews. Vermicelli is normally browned by lightly sautéing it in vegetable oil or vegetable ghee, before adding the rice and water. My version of a healthier rice side dish calls for using parboiled brown rice which cooks up to be very close in tenderness to white rice. Since vermicelli is not widely available in the US, I turn to orzo as an alternative, only lightly browning it with some extra-virgin olive oil on medium heat.

RECIPE YIELD 12 cups

DF GF EF V FF

INGREDIENTS

3 cups dry parboiled brown rice (546 g)
4 tbsp orzo
3 tbsp olive oil
4 ½ cups water
2 ½ tsp salt

NOTES

- Each brand of parboiled brown rice may differ slightly in the amounts of water required for each cup of rice. The water quantity I use is slightly different than what is actually called for on the package's cooking instructions.
- I am not a big fan of freezing rice, as I believe the texture of freshly cooked rice is much better than thawed frozen rice. But if one wants to freeze rice, be sure to let it thaw completely in the refrigerator, before reheating it. I would suggest heating it in a baking dish covered with foil in the oven versus in a pot on the stove top.

INSTRUCTIONS

1. Pick over the rice, removing any bad pieces. Rinse well, then drain. Set aside.
2. In a large pot, sauté the orzo with the olive oil over medium heat, stirring frequently until lightly browned.
3. Pour in the water, then add the rice and salt. Stir to mix, then cover and bring to a boil.
4. Stir, then cover and cook on low heat for 25 minutes (do not stir during this time).
5. Turn off the heat, then fold the rice gently. Cover and let rest for 5 minutes.
6. Uncover, stir, then let rest, uncovered, for an additional 10 to 15 minutes (the rice will further fluff up as it cools). Stir again before serving.

NUTRITION FACTS PER CUP

215 Kcal	4 g Protein	5 g Fat	37 g Carbs	2 g Fiber	0.1 g Sugar

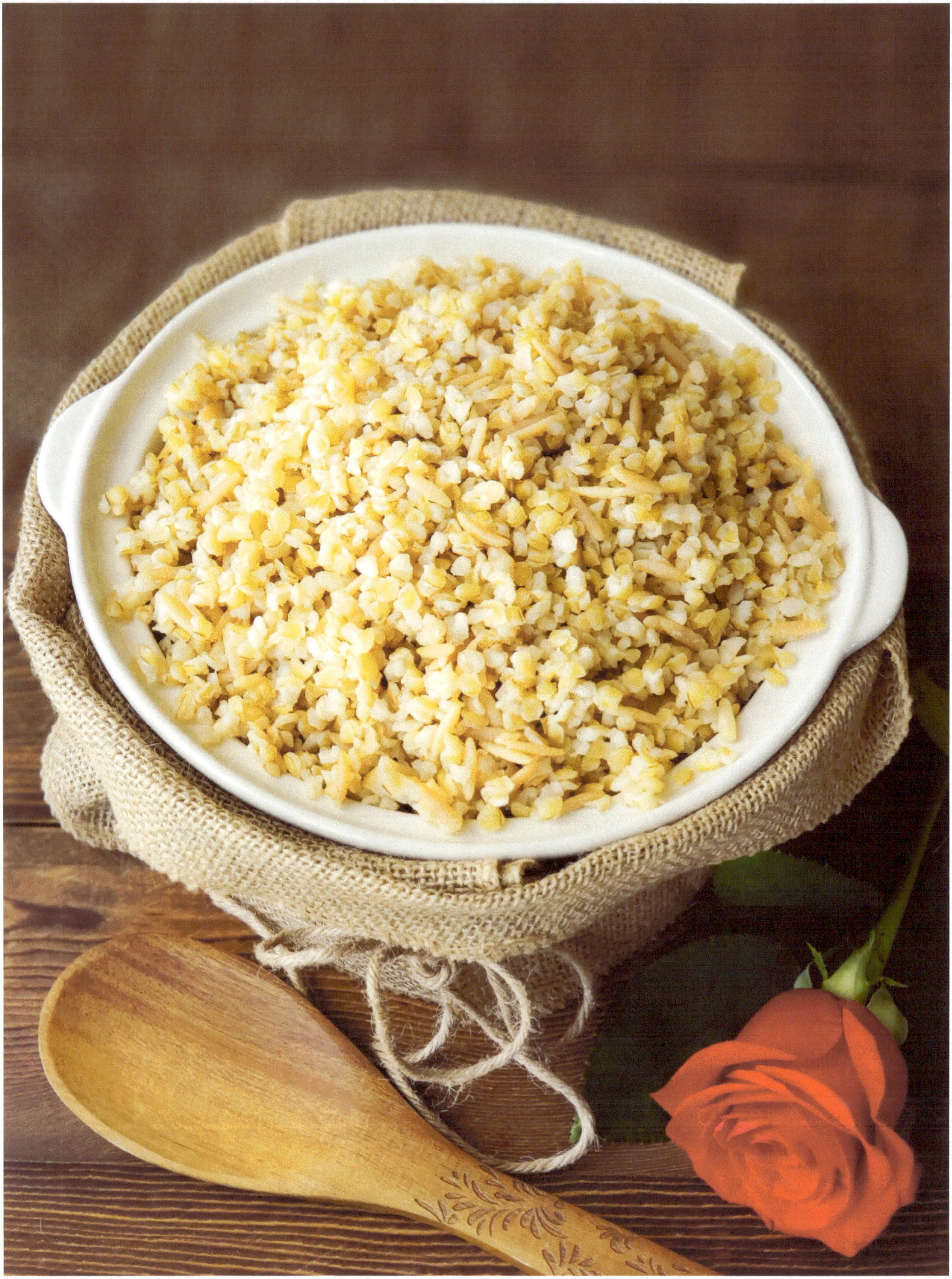

BULGUR WITH ORZO

Burghul bi Shaeeriyyeh بُرغل بشعيريّة

Plain bulgur cooked with vermicelli is also a common side dish eaten with traditional Lebanese stews, but tends to fall behind rice in popularity. As with my brown rice side dish, I use orzo as an alternative to vermicelli, lightly browning it on medium heat in some extra-virgin olive oil.

RECIPE YIELD 12 cups

DF EF V FF

INGREDIENTS

3 cups dry coarse bulgur (grade 4) (480 g)
4 tbsp orzo
3 tbsp olive oil
5 cups water
2 ½ tsp salt

NOTES

- Each brand of bulgur may differ slightly in the amounts of water required for each cup of bulgur. The water quantity I use is slightly different than what is actually called for on the package's cooking instructions.
- I am not a big fan of freezing bulgur, as I believe the texture of freshly cooked bulgur is much better than thawed frozen bulgur. But if one wants to freeze bulgur, be sure to let it thaw completely in the refrigerator, before reheating it. I would suggest heating it in a baking dish covered with foil in the oven versus in a pot on the stove top.

INSTRUCTIONS

1. Rinse the bulgur well, then drain. Set aside.
2. In a large pot, sauté the orzo with the olive oil over medium heat, stirring frequently until lightly browned.
3. Pour in the water, then add the bulgur and salt. Stir to mix, then cover and bring to a boil.
4. Stir, then cover and cook on low heat for 15 minutes (do not stir during this time).
5. Turn off the heat, then fold the bulgur gently. Cover and let rest for 5 minutes.
6. Uncover, stir, then let rest, uncovered, for an additional 10 to 15 minutes (the bulgur will further fluff up as it cools). Stir again before serving.

NUTRITION FACTS PER CUP

186.5 Kcal	4 g Protein	4 g Fat	34 g Carbs	4.6 g Fiber	0.1 g Sugar

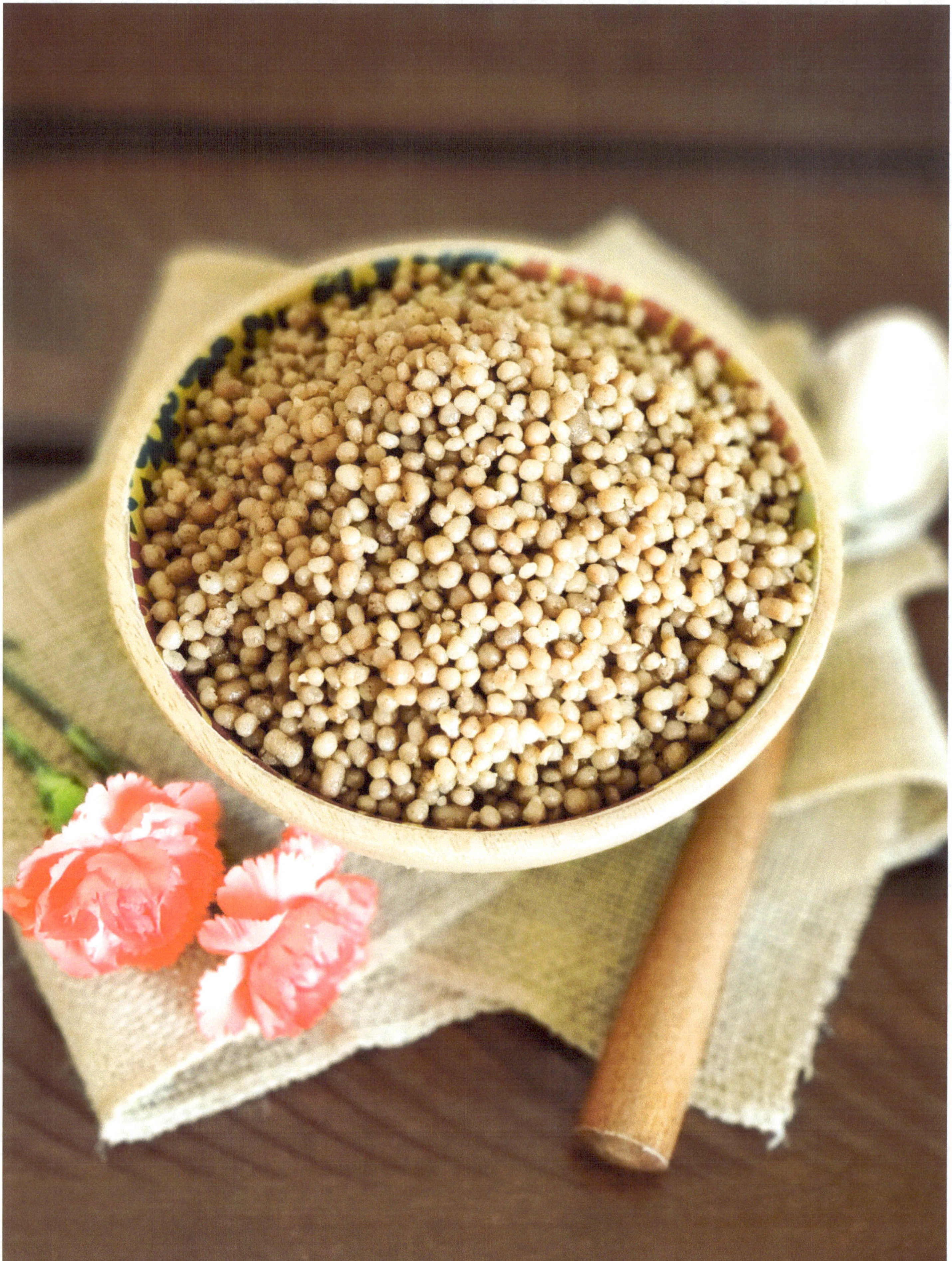

LEBANESE / PALESTINIAN COUSCOUS

Moghrabiyeh / Maftool مغربيّة / مفتول

This wheat-based product is traditionally served as a side dish with a chickpea stew (recipe on page 191) of the same name, and is called *moghrabiyeh* or Lebanese couscous in Lebanon and Syria, and *maftool* or Palestinian couscous in countries such as Palestine and Jordan. Growing up, I was accustomed to eating Lebanese couscous, but I have turned to making Palestinian couscous, since the latter contains more fiber and is thus, a heartier side dish. While Palestinian couscous is often cooked with vegetable ghee, I prefer using some extra-virgin olive oil for a healthier twist.

RECIPE YIELD 12 cups

DF EF V FF

INGREDIENTS

4 cups dry whole wheat Palestinian couscous (760 g)
2 tbsp olive oil
5 cups water
1 tsp cinnamon
1 tsp cumin
1 tsp caraway
2 tsp salt

NOTES

- Each brand of Palestinian couscous may differ slightly in the amounts of water required for each cup of couscous. The water quantity I use is slightly different than what is actually called for on the package's cooking instructions.
- I am not a big fan of freezing Palestinian couscous, as I believe the texture of freshly cooked Palestinian couscous is much better than thawed frozen Palestinian couscous. But if one wants to freeze Palestinian couscous, be sure to let it thaw completely in the refrigerator, before reheating it. I would suggest heating it in a baking dish covered with foil in the oven versus in a pot on the stove top.

INSTRUCTIONS

1. Pour the water into a large pot, then whisk in the oil and spices.
2. Add the couscous, then stir to mix. Cover and bring to a boil.
3. Stir, then cover and cook on low heat for 15 minutes. Stir lightly after 10 minutes to prevent any sticking to the bottom.
4. Turn off the heat, then fold the couscous gently. Cover and let rest for 5 minutes.
5. Uncover, stir, then let rest, uncovered, for an additional 10 to 15 minutes (the couscous will further fluff up as it cools). Stir again before serving.

NUTRITION FACTS PER CUP

250 Kcal	6.4 g Protein	3 g Fat	48.5 g Carbs	3 g Fiber	0.05 g Sugar

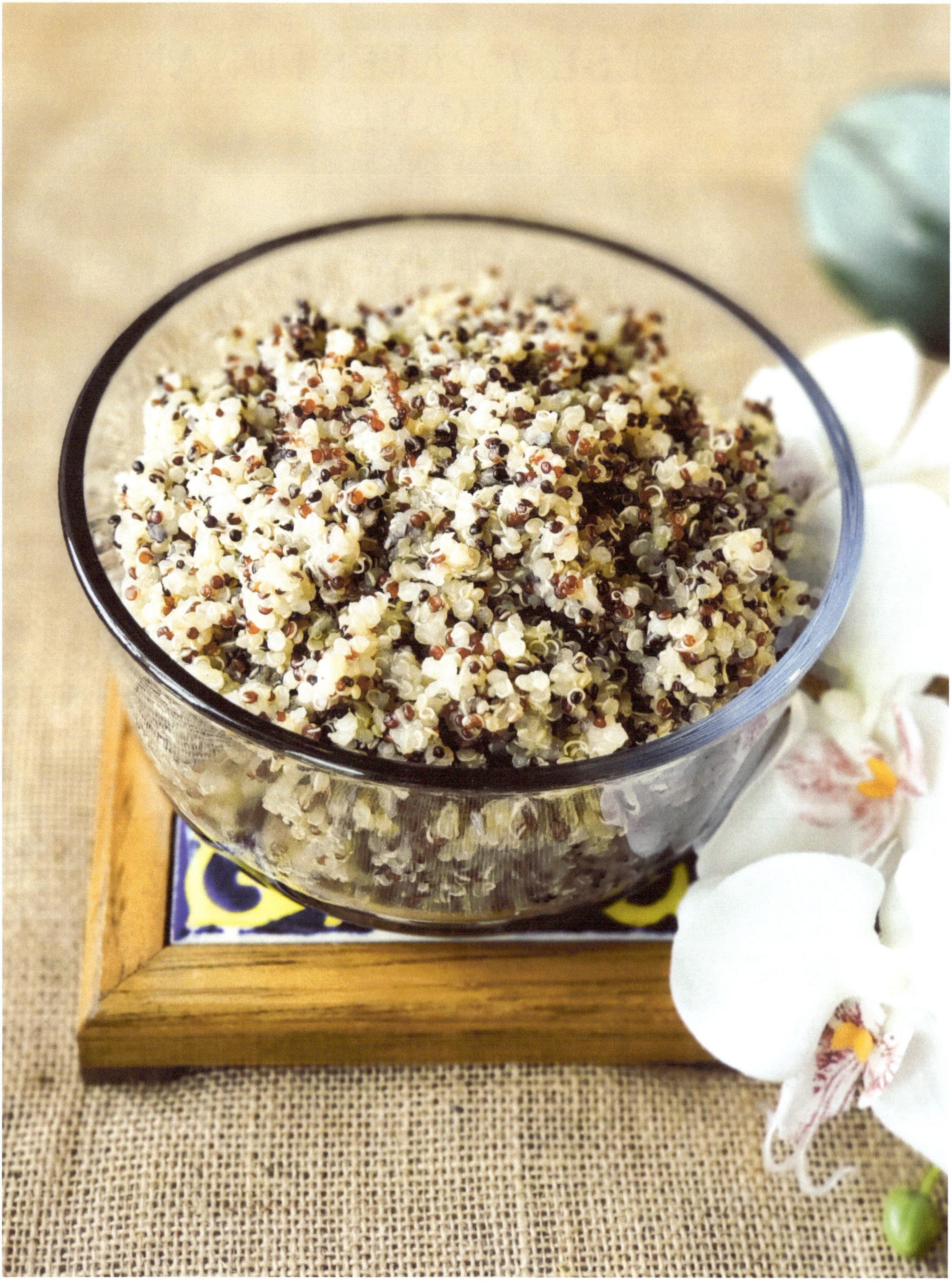

QUINOA

Quinoa is not native to the Middle East and is thus, not traditionally consumed in countries of the region. However, this nutritious protein-rich whole grain has recently become more available and is becoming more widely consumed. This plain quinoa side dish goes well with beef and chicken dishes otherwise served with rice.

RECIPE YIELD 11 cups

DF GF EF V FF

INGREDIENTS

3 cups dry quinoa (540 g)
5 cups water
2 tbsp olive oil
2 ¼ tsp salt

NOTES

- One can use either tri-colored or uni-colored quinoa.
- Each brand of quinoa may differ slightly in the amounts of water required for each cup of quinoa. The water quantity I use is slightly different than what is actually called for on the package's cooking instructions.
- I am not a big fan of freezing quinoa, as I believe the texture of freshly cooked quinoa is much better than thawed frozen quinoa. But if one wants to freeze quinoa, be sure to let it thaw completely in the refrigerator, before reheating it. I would suggest heating it in a baking dish covered with foil in the oven versus in a pot on the stove top.

INSTRUCTIONS

1. Rinse the quinoa well, then drain.
2. Transfer to a pot, pour in the water and oil, then mix in the salt.
3. Cover and bring to a boil.
4. Stir, then cover and cook on low heat for 15 minutes (do not stir during this time).
5. Turn off the heat, then fold the quinoa gently. Cover, and let rest for 5 minutes.
6. Uncover, stir, then let rest, uncovered, for an additional 10 to 15 minutes (the quinoa will further fluff up as it cools). Stir again before serving.

NUTRITION FACTS PER CUP

209 Kcal	7 g Protein	5.4 g Fat	35 g Carbs	3.5 g Fiber	3.5 g Sugar

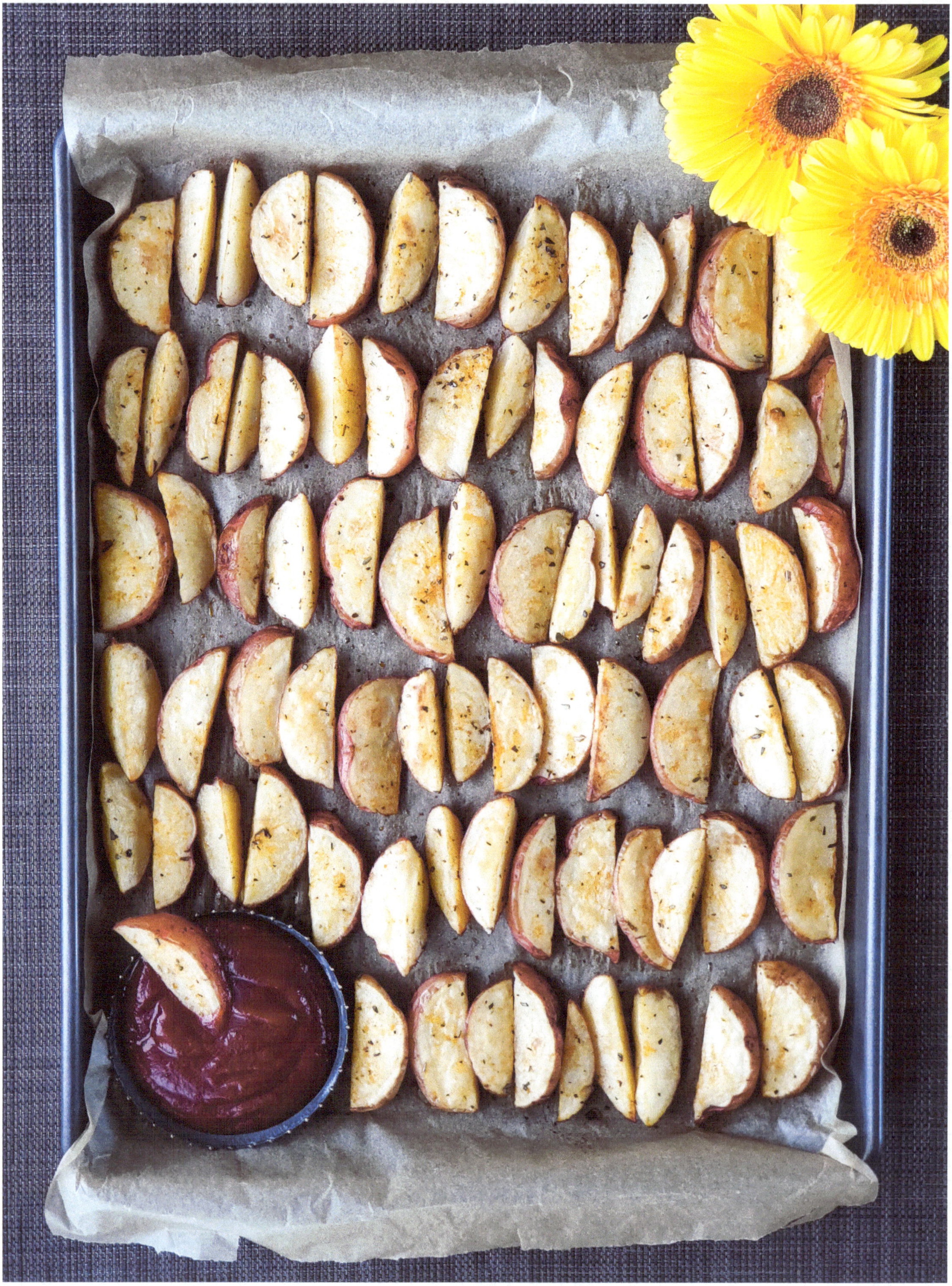

BAKED POTATO WEDGES

French fries are universally notorious, even in the Middle East. Baked potato wedges are my healthy homemade solution for when the craving for French fries strikes! They are not as calorically dense as their deep-fried counterparts, offering some heart-healthy extra-virgin olive oil that maintains a lot of its health benefits, being subjected to only moderate oven heat. I like using small red potatoes and keep their skins on for added fiber. While many will over roast their potatoes for extra outer crunchiness and crispness, I simply bake my wedges until the inside is soft and the outside is just starting to turn golden and lightly crisped.

RECIPE YIELD 96 wedges (12 servings)

DF GF EF V

INGREDIENTS

12 small red potatoes (with skin) (810 g)
2 tbsp olive oil
1 tsp dry oregano leaves
⅓ tsp paprika
¼ tsp cumin
½ tsp salt (or garlic salt)
⅛ tsp black pepper

NOTES

- One can add more of the called for herbs and spices as desired. The addition of onion powder is also nice.
- There is no need to flip the potatoes halfway through baking.
- Each serving includes 8 wedges.

INSTRUCTIONS

1. After washing the potatoes very well, slice each potato lengthwise into 8 slices.
2. Add to a pot of hot water then let sit for 10 minutes.
3. Drain, then rinse with cold water. Drain well, then pat dry.
4. Transfer to a large bowl containing the olive oil, spices, and herbs, then rub the potatoes well until evenly covered.
5. Lay out on a large sheet pan (recommended dimensions: 30 cm x 40 cm or bigger) lined with parchment paper (make sure the potatoes are spread out and not on top of one another), then bake in a preheated oven at 375 °F for 50 minutes (if using refined olive oil, one can bake the potatoes in a hotter oven, such as 400 °F or higher, and for a shorter time, about 40 minutes or less).
6. Serve the wedges warm out of the oven with a desired condiment such as ketchup or mustard.

NUTRITION FACTS PER SERVING

68 Kcal	1 g Protein	2.4 g Fat	11 g Carbs	1 g Fiber	1 g Sugar

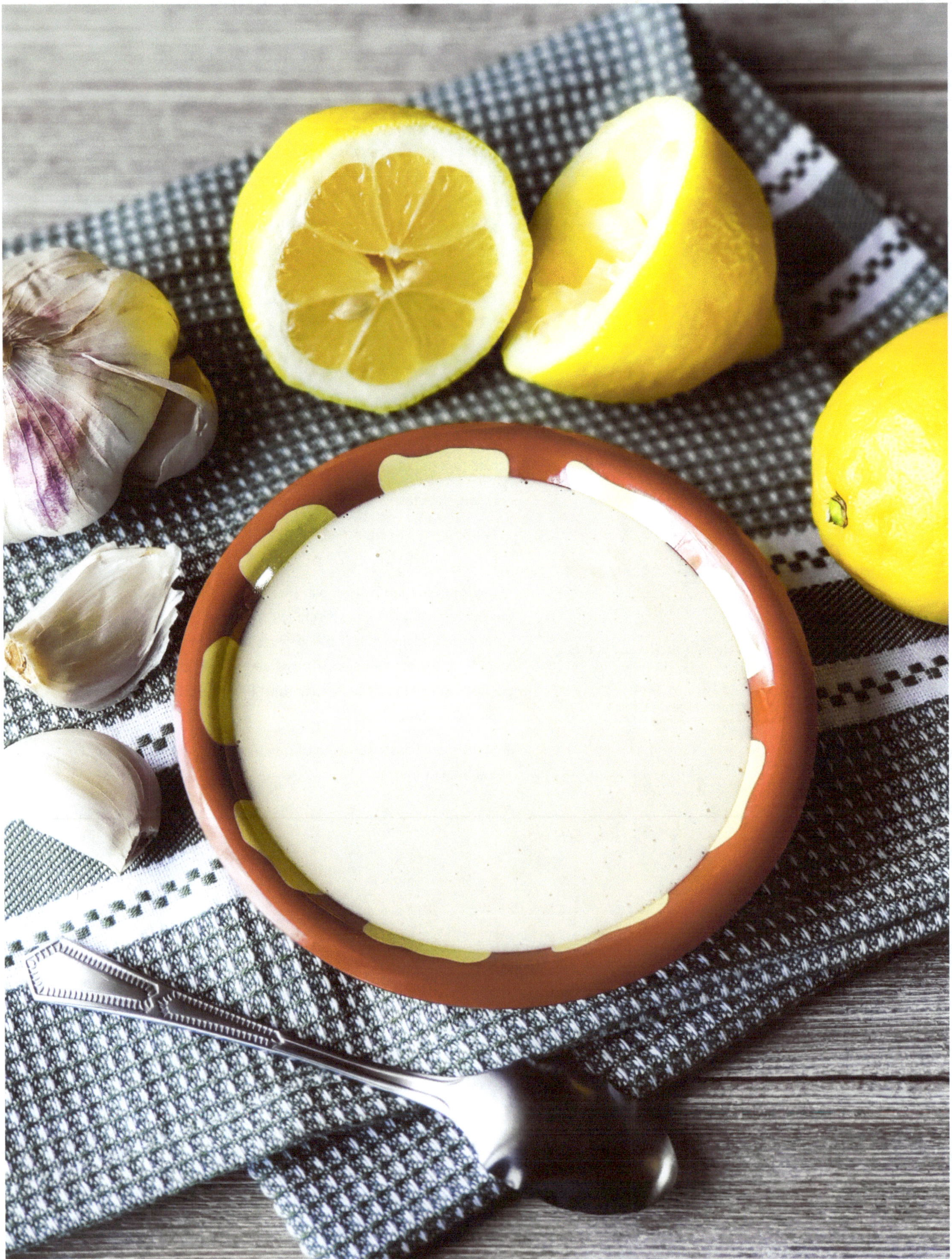

TAHINI SAUCE

Taratoor طرطور

This is a super simple garlicy and tangy *tahini* sauce that goes well with many Middle Eastern street foods such as *falafel* (recipe on page 199) and beef *shawarma* (recipe on page 221). While some may make their sauce with part *tahini* and part yogurt (for a lighter/whiter color), I like going all *tahini* for a richer flavor!

RECIPE YIELD 20 tbsp

DF GF EF OF V FF

INGREDIENTS

½ cup tahini (120 g)
½ cup water
¼ cup lemon juice
1 tbsp garlic, crushed
¼ tsp salt

NOTES

- It is normal for the *tahini* sauce to thicken with time as it sits in the refrigerator. One can whisk in some cold water if desired to thin it out slightly.
- The strength of the garlic flavor increases slightly as the *tahini* sauce sits in the refrigerator from day to day.

INSTRUCTIONS

1. In a small bowl, mix the garlic and salt (until a paste is formed), then add the lemon juice.
2. Add the *tahini* and water, then whisk well until a smooth homogenous sauce has been obtained (for a smoother effect, one can mix the ingredients in a blender. Let the garlic and salt melt together though before transferring to the blender).
3. Store in an airtight container and keep in the refrigerator. It is best consumed within a week (or send it off to the freezer).

NUTRITION FACTS PER TABLESPOON

37 Kcal	1 g Protein	3 g Fat	1.6 g Carbs	0.6 g Fiber	0 g Sugar

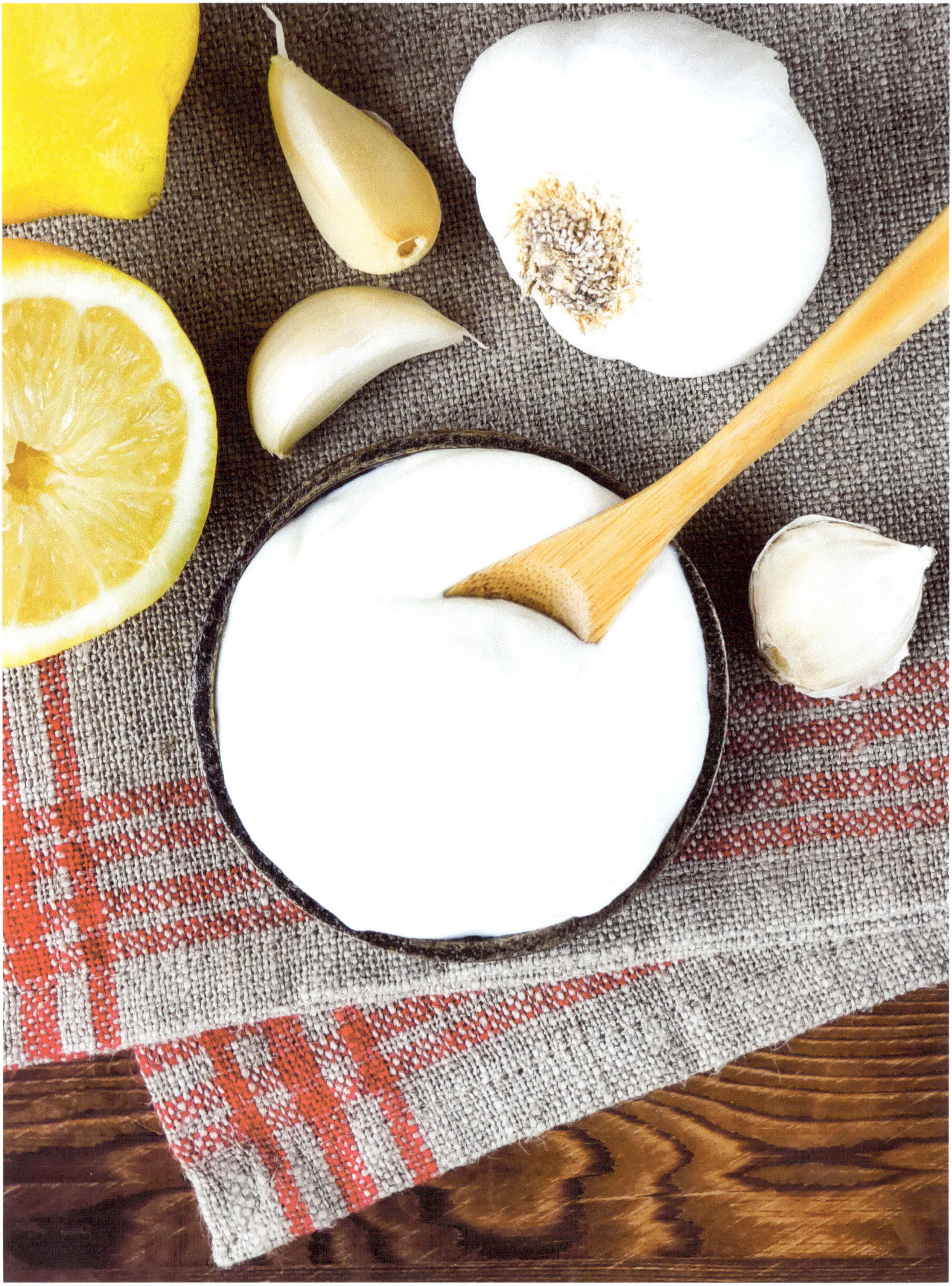

GARLIC SAUCE

Mtawwam متوّم

The traditional recipe of this garlic aioli or sauce calls for only two main ingredients, garlic and vegetable oil. Slowly trickling the oil over crushed garlic in a fast blender adds enough fluff to the garlic paste so that a thick white garlic sauce is formed. The end flavor is delicious, but it is so strong that only a slight amount is normally tolerated, even by the most ardent garlic lovers. However, this method is finicky and does not always succeed due to a few factors such as the speed of one's food processor and how fast one trickles the oil over the garlic. Thus, some will resort to adding whipped raw egg whites to add volume and thickness to the aioli, while others will add mayonnaise or even some baked potato. My simple, fast, and healthy take on this traditional sauce calls for using much less oil and includes skim *labneh* as an ingredient to thicken/firm up the sauce and increase the volume, thus also adding some protein to the sauce. This garlicy sauce goes well with many Middle Eastern street foods such as chicken *shish tawook* (recipe on page 227) as well as chicken *shawarma* (recipe on page 223).

RECIPE YIELD 15 tbsp

GF EF Vt FF

INGREDIENTS

5 tbsp avocado oil
⅔ cup skim labneh (146 g)
2 tsp garlic, crushed
¼ tsp salt

NOTES

- Mild tasting refined vegetable oils such as corn oil or safflower oil are traditionally used for making this garlic sauce. Olive oil is too strong in flavor to be used and may impart a slight bitterness, especially if extra-virgin olive oil is used. The color of the end product may also be impacted if olive oil is to be used instead of lighter-colored vegetable oils. For these reasons, it is recommended that lightly refined avocado oil is used for this sauce instead of virgin or extra-virgin oil.
- This garlic sauce will firm up a bit further as it sits in the refrigerator. For a thicker sauce, one can use *labneh* obtained from straining yogurt for 10 hours (instead of 8 hours).
- The strength of the garlic flavor increases slightly as the garlic sauce sits in the refrigerator from day to day.

INSTRUCTIONS

1. In a small bowl, mix the garlic and salt (until a paste is formed).
2. Transfer to a small food processor, then add the oil and *labneh*. Blend well, scraping down the sides as needed. Continue processing until a smooth, homogenous, and fluffy sauce has been obtained.
3. Store in an airtight container and keep in the refrigerator. It is best consumed within a week (or send it off to the freezer).

NUTRITION FACTS PER TABLESPOON

59 Kcal	1 g Protein	5 g Fat	2.5 g Carbs	0.1 g Fiber	2.4 g Sugar

MAIN DISHES

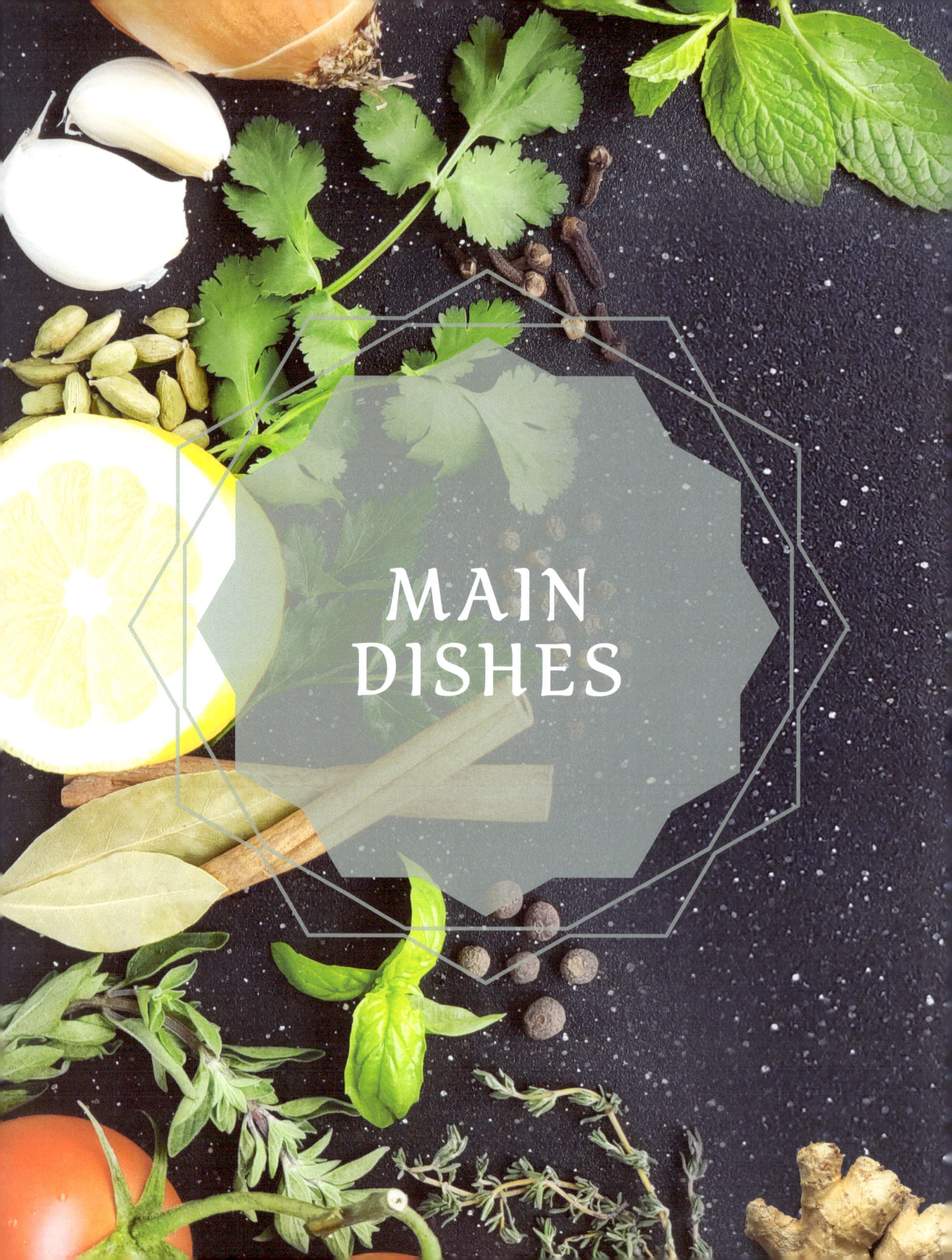

The Lebanese cuisine with its unique style of cooking combines a wide selection of main dishes. Varying from cold vegetarian dishes, to rice dishes with lentils, to rice dishes with meat, to vegetable stews, and to baked casserole-type dishes, each stands out from the other by differing ingredients and cooking methods, as well as in their multitude of distinct aromas, flavors, colors, and presentations. Lebanese and/or Middle Eastern main dishes presented in this section are named with the traditional Arabic name, along with an English transliteration of the Arabic. Main dishes without an Arabic name are not Lebanese/Middle Eastern. They are either recipes of my own creation or are ones adapted from recipes handed down to me by my mother.

SOME GENERAL REMARKS AND RECOMMENDATIONS

- Perhaps one of the trickiest aspects of cooking is stove-top heat variability. No stove is perfect, and no stove cooks and heats food in the same way as another stove. Get to know your stove, and use your personal experience in judging the heat level and length of time you cook your ingredients for.

- Along the same lines as the above remark, one of the trickiest aspects in baking is oven heat variability. No oven is perfect, and no oven bakes in the same way as another oven. Get to know your oven - how 'hot' it is and how it bakes your dishes. Using an inexpensive oven thermometer may be a good way to give you a sense of how your oven functions, allowing you to set your oven thermostat higher or lower depending on whether your oven tends to run cool or hot.

- Bake a dish on the middle rack of the oven, unless otherwise specified.

- For my baked main dishes, I prefer using metal stainless steel or ceramic baking pans, as these types of pans are better heat conductors than glass bakeware. If glassware is all one has, one may need to adjust the baking time.

- Whenever a cooking step calls for the addition of a main ingredient (such as water/broth, a meat source, vegetables, or rice) to a pot of ingredients cooking on low, follow the below steps. First turn up the heat to high, then add the ingredient(s) called for in that step, then cover. Wait until the dish returns to a rapid boil or a strong sizzle, then turn the heat back down to low. One can start timing the required cooking time from this point.

- It is very important to wash all vegetables called for in a recipe prior to starting. Vegetables can harbor soil particles from having been out in the field, and soil in turn can be the source of many harmful bacteria. Properly washing vegetables under cold running water, with scrubbing and/or quick soaking, then rinsing as many times as needed, is important. Since I do not peel my potatoes, make sure to rub the skins very well with a clean brush during washing.

- The weights presented to the right-hand side of a vegetable ingredient relate to the final net weight of the vegetable added to the pot (i.e. the net weight after peeling, removing the inedible ends or core, and chopping off bad parts of the vegetable), unless otherwise specified.

- Since fresh produce can vary widely in size, shape, and weight, it is recommended to go by the presented weights of called for ingredients, in order to obtain more accurate recipe outcomes and yields.

- When it comes to raw meats (especially for beef and chicken), always make sure to purchase a bit more than the amount called for in the recipe, to allow for some loss of weight during removal of the visible fat.

- All nuts and seeds called for in the main dishes recipes are shelled, raw, and unsalted (unless otherwise specified). Nuts and seeds not indicated as chopped or ground are intended to be added whole.

- All spices such as cinnamon, turmeric, cumin, or ginger are called for in their ground (powdered) form, unless otherwise specified.

- I am a big fan of spices and herbs, but not a fan of salt. Thus, the salt amounts called for in my main dishes tend to be on the lower end, so always taste the dish once made, and accordingly adjust the salt to your taste.

- The addition of salt as an ingredient is included with the spices in the instruction steps of the recipes, unless otherwise specified.

- I don't like to cook with too much oil, especially since I am not fond of oily/greasy food in general. However, I make sure that the lower amount of oil doesn't negatively affect the flavor of a dish. One can definitely add more oil if desired, but this will increase the caloric and fat content of the dish.

- Most main dishes can be made vegetarian simply by omitting the meat ingredient (red meat, chicken, or fish), as well as the substitution of meat broth with water or vegetable broth.

- A serving of 2 cups of a main dish is a good serving size to be consumed.

- The 'sugar' value in the nutrition facts of recipes refers to the total amount of sugar (both simple and complex) that is naturally occurring in the various ingredients.

- I grease my baking pans with olive oil, unless otherwise specified.

- The fat source called for greasing baking pans is NOT included in the nutrition facts. Reasons include the fact that different foods absorb the pan grease differently, and some people may opt to covering all their pans with parchment paper or foil before adding in the food item.

- Food items suggested as garnish are NOT included in the nutrition facts.

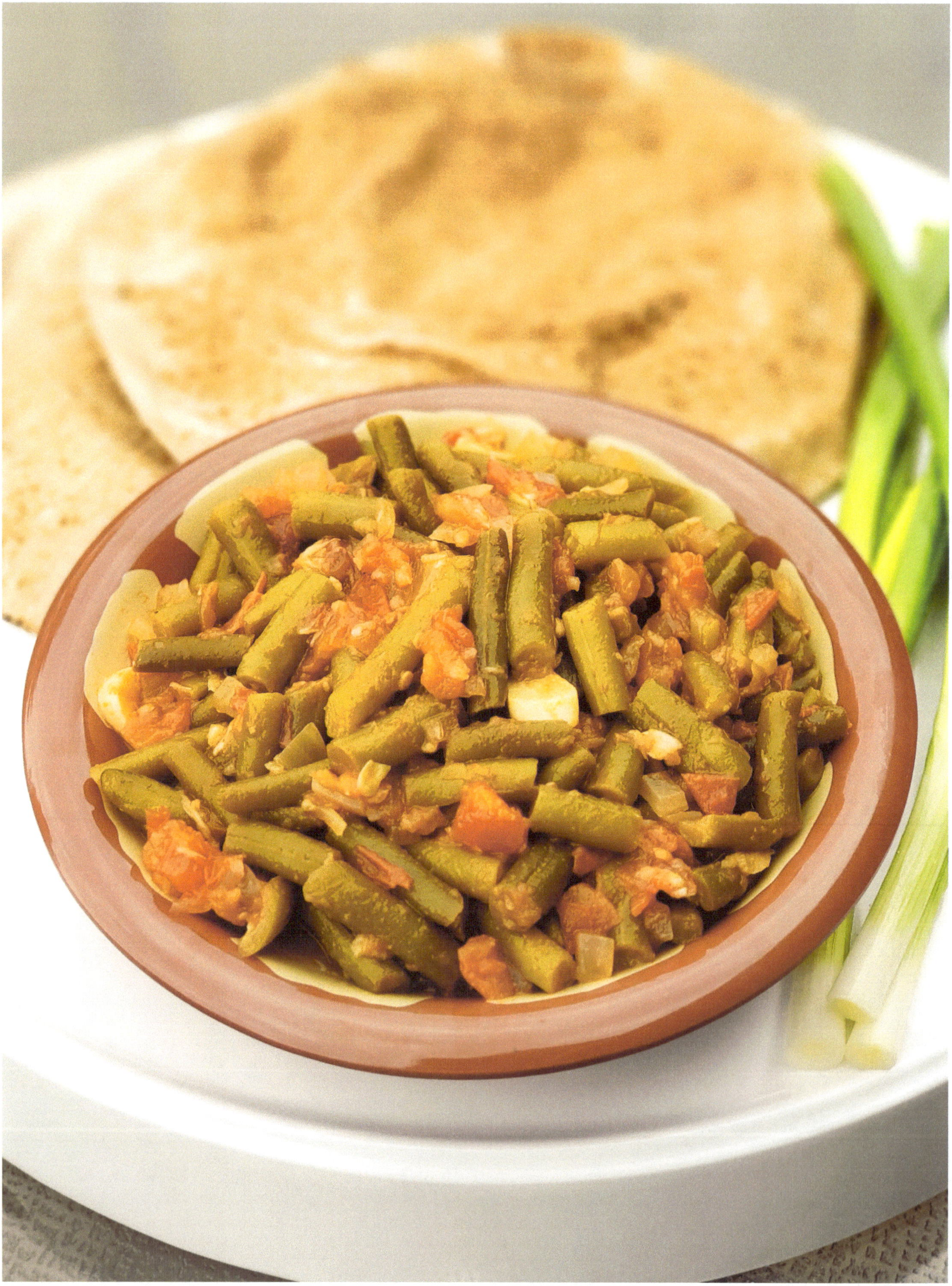

GREEN BEANS IN OIL

Lubyieh bi Zait لوبية بزيت

This juicy and flavorful vegetarian dish is famous and widely loved among the Lebanese cuisine. Though traditionally made with fresh Romano beans (which are broad and flat green beans), French green beans (also known as string or snap beans) can also be used, as these have a very similar flavor and texture as Romano beans (which are usually not available in the US, except in summertime at some farmers' markets and a few Middle Eastern grocery stores). This delicious dish comes together with only a handful of other basic fresh ingredients - tomatoes, onions, and garlic - and is eaten with Arabic pita bread. I go easy on the olive oil and use a lot of ripe and juicy tomatoes to add flavor and moistness to the dish.

RECIPE YIELD 15 cups

DF GF EF V FF

INGREDIENTS

Frozen cut green beans (1.8 kg)
10 medium red tomatoes, diced (1.3 kg)
2 medium yellow onions, diced (320 g)
¼ cup garlic, crushed (56 g)
10 medium whole garlic cloves, sliced into circles (50 g)
3 tbsp unsalted tomato paste
4 tbsp olive oil
2 tsp salt
black pepper, to taste
chili pepper powder, optional

NOTE

Fresh beans may take longer to cook, thus, the cooking time in step 4 may need to be bumped up to 40 to 45 minutes.

INSTRUCTIONS

1. Thaw the frozen beans on the counter for about 1 hour. Rinse well with warm water until all ice is melted. Let sit to drain well.
2. In a large pot, covered, cook the onions with the olive oil on low heat for 20 minutes, stirring occasionally.
3. Gently press down on the beans, draining away any excess water before adding to the onions, then cook, covered, on low for another 20 minutes, stirring occasionally.
4. Stir in the tomatoes, sliced garlic, and tomato paste, then let cook, covered, on low for 30 minutes, stirring occasionally.
5. Add the crushed garlic and salt, then let cook, covered, on low for another 20 minutes, stirring occasionally.
6. Let cool before serving. Best served lukewarm or cold out of the refrigerator.
7. Serve with whole wheat pita bread and green onions if desired.

NUTRITION FACTS PER CUP

108 Kcal	3.6 g Protein	4 g Fat	17 g Carbs	5 g Fiber	6 g Sugar

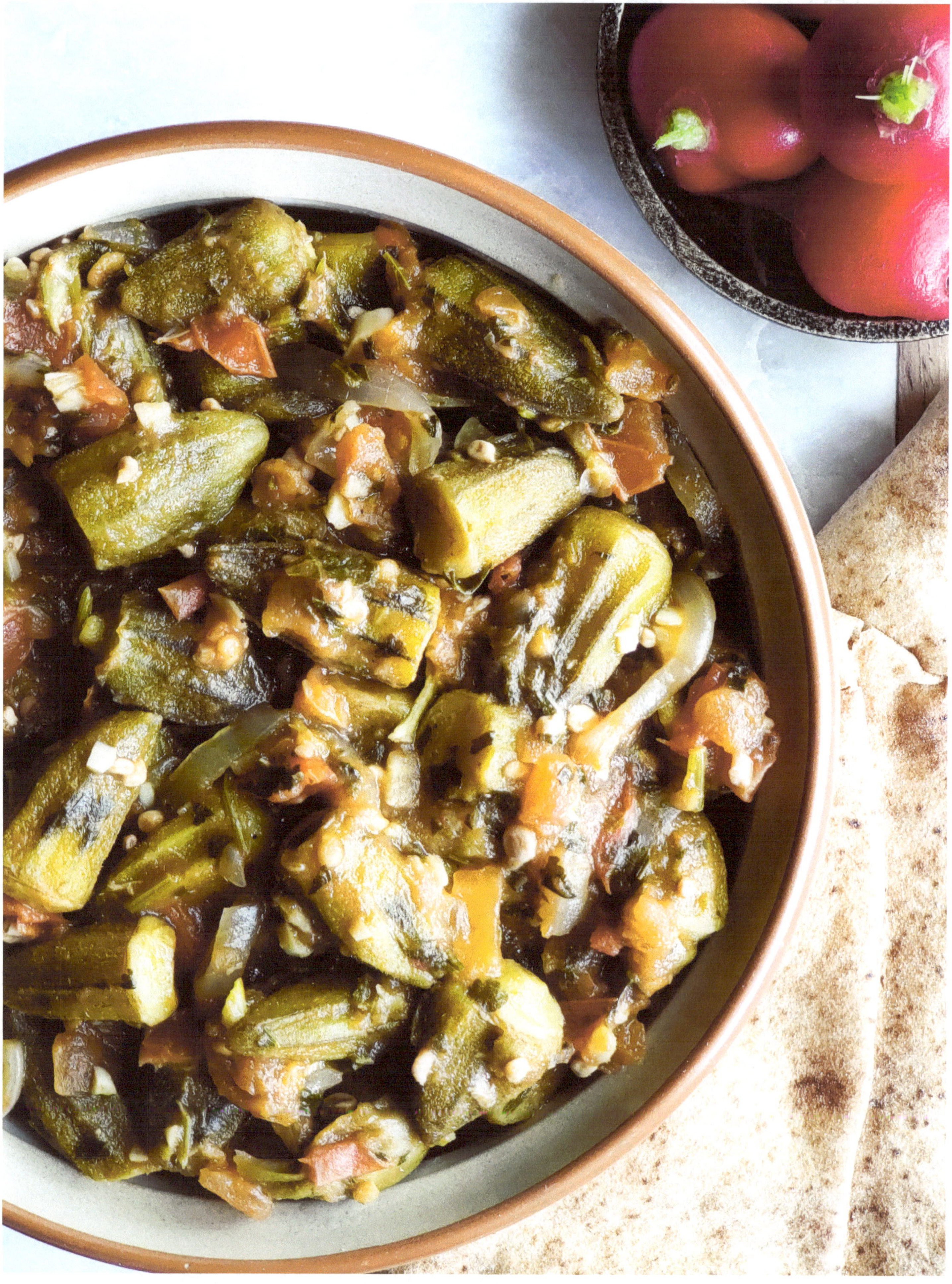

OKRA IN OIL

Baimyieh bi Zait باميه بزيت

Somewhat similar to the green beans in oil dish (on the previous page), this dish is simple to make but very flavorful and nutritious. It is traditionally prepared with small fresh okra, but I prefer making it with frozen okra to speed up the preparation time. Not to mention that I also prefer small okra over the larger okra variety common here in the West, since one can't really slice them up for the dish without turning the sauce into a gooey texture. While traditionally this recipe is prepared with caramelized onions and quite a bit of olive oil, I skip the caramelization and keep the amount of oil added to a minimum.

RECIPE YIELD 15 cups

DF GF EF V FF

INGREDIENTS

Frozen small okra (2 kg)
10 medium red tomatoes, diced (1.3 kg)
2 medium yellow onions, sliced into short strips (320 g)
1 bunch coriander, finely chopped (85 g)
½ cup garlic, minced (75 g)
3 tbsp unsalted tomato paste
1 tsp pomegranate molasses
4 tbsp olive oil
2 tsp salt
black pepper, to taste
chili pepper powder, optional

NOTE

Fresh okra may take longer to cook, thus, the cooking time in step 4 may need to be bumped up to 40 to 45 minutes.

INSTRUCTIONS

1. Thaw the frozen okra on the counter for about 30 minutes. Rinse well with warm water until all ice is melted. Let sit to drain well.
2. In a large pot, covered, cook the onions with the olive oil on low heat for 20 minutes, stirring occasionally.
3. Gently press down on the okra, draining away any excess water before adding to the onions, then cook, covered, on low for another 20 minutes, stirring occasionally.
4. Stir in the tomatoes, tomato paste, garlic, and salt, then let cook for 30 minutes, stirring occasionally.
5. Add the coriander, then let cook for another 20 minutes, stirring occasionally.
6. Add the pomegranate molasses, then stir to mix.
7. Let cool before serving. Best served lukewarm or cold out of the refrigerator.
8. Serve with whole wheat pita bread and radishes if desired.

NUTRITION FACTS PER CUP

108 Kcal	4 g Protein	4 g Fat	17 g Carbs	5 g Fiber	8 g Sugar

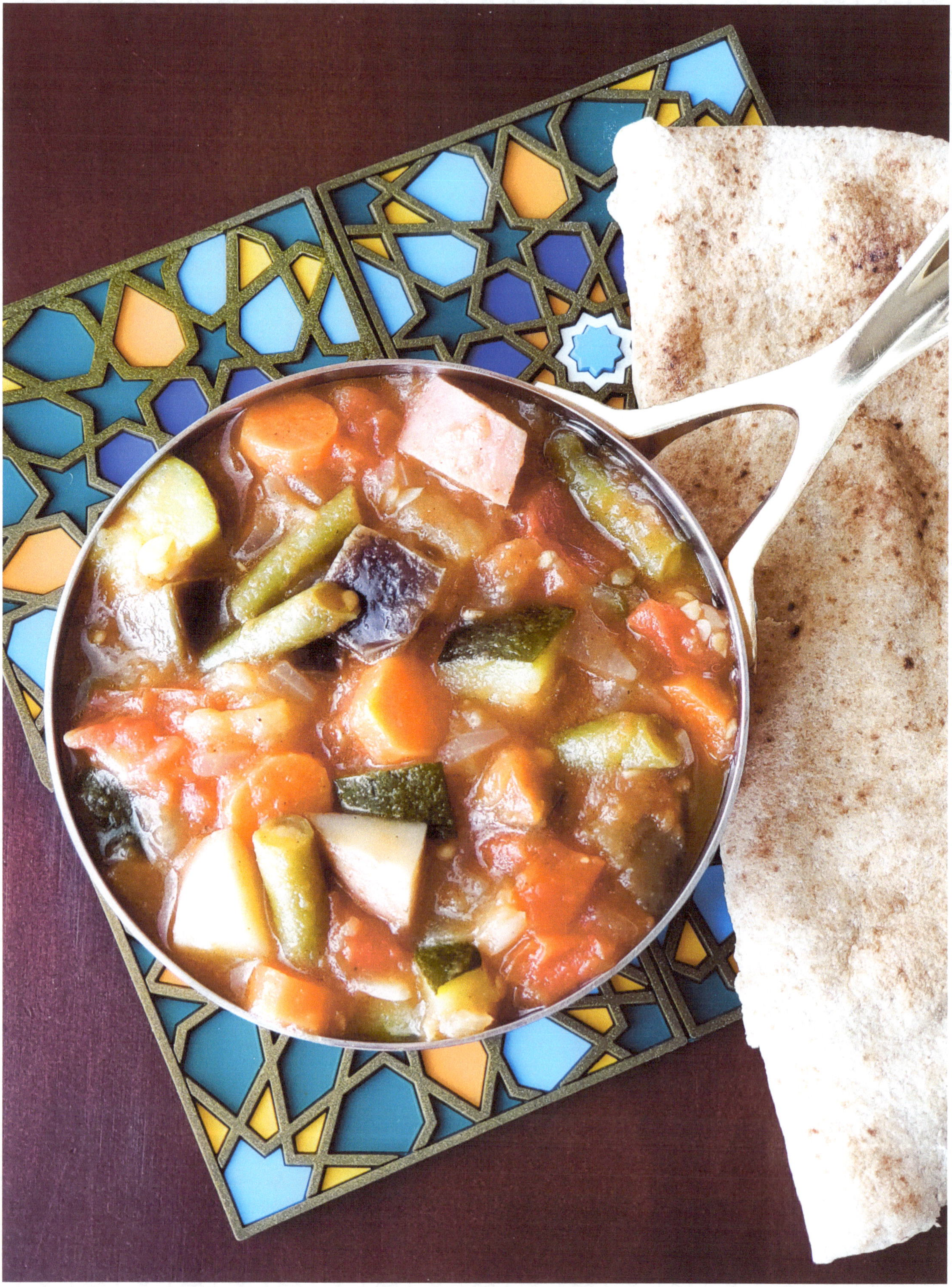

MIXED VEGGIES IN OIL

Makhlootit Khudra bi Zait مخلوطة خُضرة بزيت

This is a very simple Lebanese vegan dish commonly prepared with different combinations of vegetables, with some adding bell peppers and garlic to the mix as well. Though simple, this dish is both hearty and very nutritious, offering a load of fiber and nutrients. As with other dishes cooked with olive oil, I like to control the amount of oil added to keep the calories and fat content at a moderate level.

RECIPE YIELD 12 cups

DF GF EF V FF

INGREDIENTS

10 medium red tomatoes, cubed (1.3 kg)
7 small red potatoes (with skin), cubed (473 g)
4 medium zucchinis, cubed (450 g)
1 medium Italian eggplant (with skin, no end), cubed (363 g)
2 medium yellow onions, diced (320 g)
4 medium carrots (no skin), sliced into circles (240 g)
1 cup frozen cut green beans (115 g), thawed, rinsed, drained well
1 tbsp unsalted tomato paste
2 tbsp olive oil
¼ tsp allspice
1 ½ tsp salt
black pepper, to taste
chili pepper powder, optional

INSTRUCTIONS

1. In a large pot, covered, cook the onions with the olive oil on low heat for 20 minutes, stirring occasionally.
2. Add the tomatoes, eggplant, tomato paste, and spices, then stir to mix. Cook, covered, on low heat for another 15 minutes, stirring occasionally.
3. Stir in the carrots, then cover and let cook for 5 minutes before adding the potatoes, zucchini, and green beans. Cook, covered, on low heat for another 25 minutes.
4. Let cool before serving. Best served lukewarm or cold out of the refrigerator.
5. Serve with whole wheat pita bread and green onions if desired.

NUTRITION FACTS PER CUP

104 Kcal	3 g Protein	3 g Fat	18.6 g Carbs	4.6 g Fiber	8 g Sugar

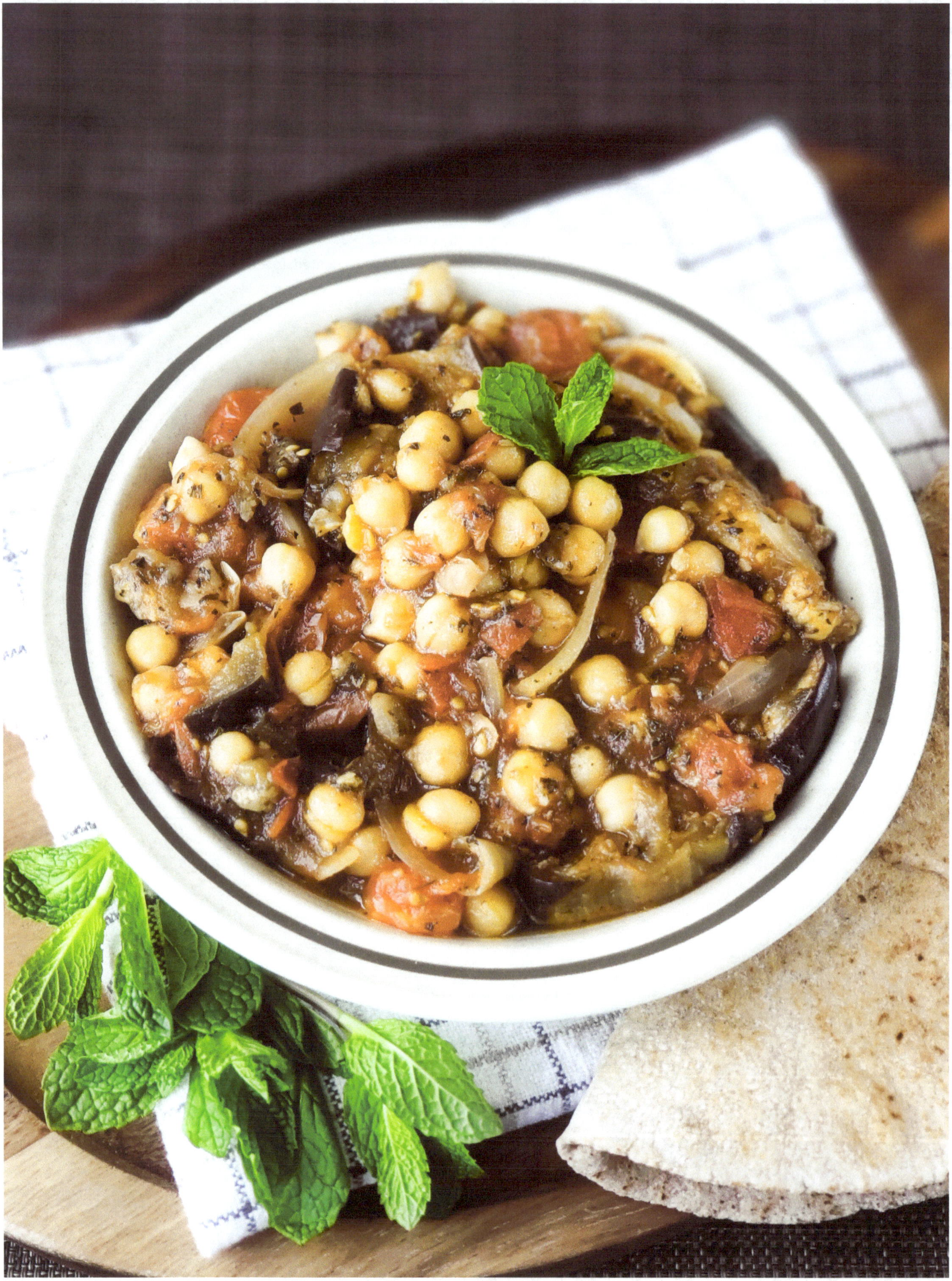

CHICKPEAS AND EGGPLANT

Maghmoor مغمور

This popular Lebanese vegan dish is unique, hearty, and super flavorful. Traditionally made with fried eggplant and peeled chickpeas, I prefer baking my eggplants and keeping the chickpeas whole, for a healthier and more nutritious profile, while making sure not to go overboard with the amount of oil added to the dish.

RECIPE YIELD 12 cups

DF GF EF V FF

INGREDIENTS

1 ½ cups dry chickpeas (278 g)
4 medium Italian eggplants (with skin, no ends), sliced (1,450 g)
10 medium red tomatoes, diced (1.3 kg)
2 medium yellow onions, sliced into short strips (320 g)
1 tbsp garlic, crushed
3 tbsp unsalted tomato paste
2 tbsp olive oil
4 tbsp dry mint leaves
1 ½ tsp salt
1 tsp baking soda

INSTRUCTIONS

1. Soak the chickpeas and baking soda in water for 12 hours. Drain and rinse, discarding any bad pieces.

2. Transfer the chickpeas to a pot, cover with water, then bring to a boil. Skim off the white foam that floats to the surface, then cook, covered, on low heat for 45 minutes. Uncover and place the lid ajar.

3. Place the finger-sized eggplant slices on 2 large sheet pans (recommended dimensions: 30 cm x 40 cm or similar) lined with parchment paper (make sure the slices are spread out and not laying on top of one another), then bake in a preheated oven at 400 °F for 45 minutes (or until tender). Cover with foil to keep warm until serving.

4. In a large pot, covered, cook the onions with the olive oil on low heat for 20 minutes, stirring occasionally.

5. Add the tomatoes, garlic, tomato paste, herbs, and spices, then stir to mix. Cook, covered, on low heat for another 15 minutes.

6. Drain the chickpeas well, then add to the pot and stir to mix.

7. Add the baked eggplant, then fold in.

8. Let cool before serving. Best served lukewarm or cold out of the refrigerator.

9. Serve with whole wheat pita bread and fresh mint leaves if desired.

NUTRITION FACTS PER CUP

180 Kcal	8 g Protein	4 g Fat	31 g Carbs	10 g Fiber	11.4 g Sugar

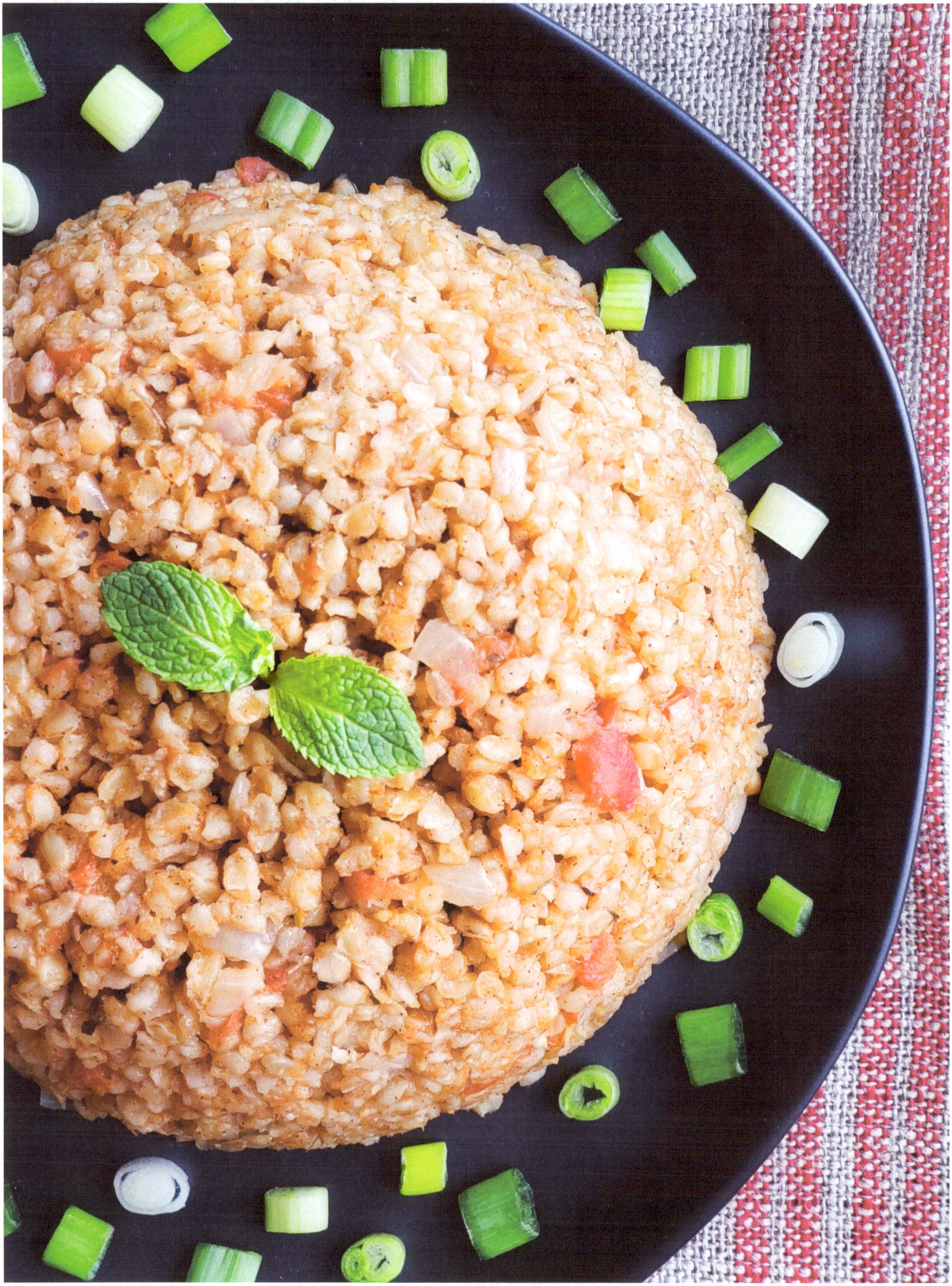

TOMATO BULGUR PILAF

Burghul a Banadoora   برغل عبندورة

This simple but flavorful Lebanese dish requires only a handful of main ingredients: bulgur, onions, and tomatoes. While traditionally made with caramelized onions, this dish tastes just as delicious with onions lightly cooked in some olive oil just until tender. And while many make this dish with only tomatoes (no tomato paste) and some warm spices like allspice, cinnamon, and/or 7-spices, I like adding some tomato paste, as well as some garlic, dry mint, and pomegranate molasses for a nice twist.

RECIPE YIELD 14 cups

DF EF V FF

INGREDIENTS

3 cups dry coarse bulgur (grade 4) (480 g)
6 medium red tomatoes, diced (800 g)
3 medium yellow onions, minced (480 g)
1 tbsp garlic, crushed
4 tbsp unsalted tomato paste
1 tsp pomegranate molasses
3 tbsp olive oil
3 cups water
1 ½ tsp dry mint leaves
1 ½ tsp allspice
2 ½ tsp salt
black pepper, to taste

NOTE

I am not a big fan of freezing bulgur, as I believe the texture of freshly cooked bulgur is much better than thawed frozen bulgur. But if one wants to freeze this dish, be sure to let it thaw completely in the refrigerator, before reheating it. I would suggest heating it in a baking dish covered with foil in the oven versus in a pot on the stove top.

INSTRUCTIONS

1. Rinse the bulgur well, then drain. Set aside.
2. In a large pot, covered, cook the onions with the olive oil on low heat for 20 minutes, stirring occasionally.
3. Add the water, bulgur, tomatoes, garlic, tomato paste, herbs, and spices, then stir to mix. Bring to a boil, then cook, covered, on low heat, for 15 minutes (do not stir during this time).
4. Stir in the pomegranate molasses, then cover and let sit for 5 minutes.
5. Uncover, stir again, then let rest, uncovered, for an additional 10 to 15 minutes (the bulgur will further fluff up as it cools). Stir again before serving.
6. Garnish with fresh mint and serve with green onions.

NUTRITION FACTS PER CUP

177 Kcal	4 g Protein	3.4 g Fat	33 g Carbs	5.4 g Fiber	4 g Sugar

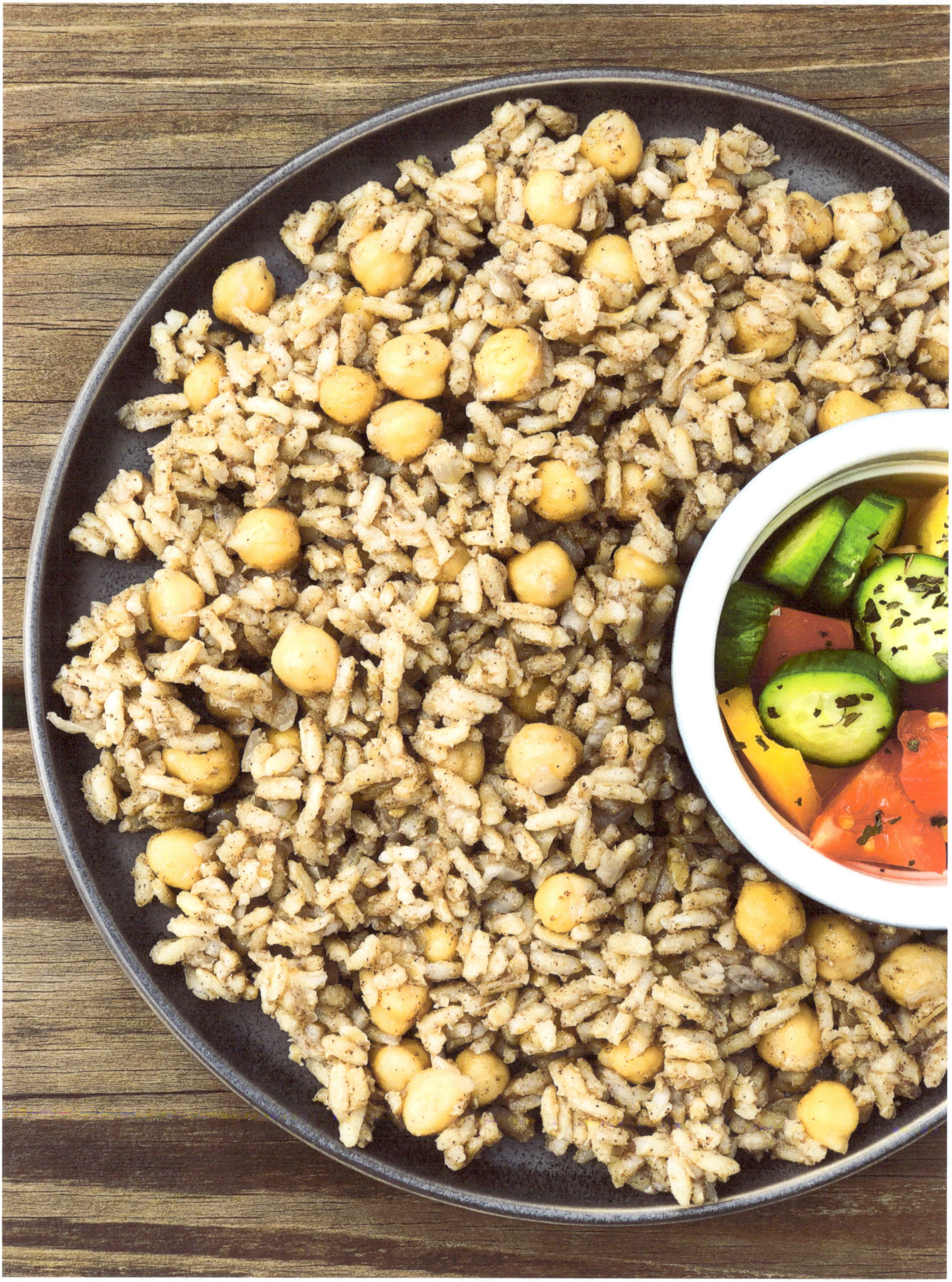

CHICKPEA RICE PILAF

Riz a Hummus رز عحمّص

This simple-to-make dish is full of flavor and rich in fiber and nutrients. For this dish, as with others, onions are traditionally fried in a lot of oil until caramelized. However, I simply cook them in a small amount of oil until they turn soft and translucent. While many like adding minced beef to this dish, I like keeping it vegetarian, enjoying the flavor of chickpeas and spices without the interference of meat. This dish is also traditionally made with fresh or dry broad fava beans instead of chickpeas.

RECIPE YIELD 18 cups

DF GF EF V FF

INGREDIENTS

2 cups dry chickpeas (370 g)
3 cups dry parboiled brown rice (546 g)
4 medium yellow onions, minced (640 g)
3 tbsp olive oil
2 cups water
2 ½ cups chickpea water
2 tbsp cumin
2 tsp cinnamon
1 ½ tsp allspice
1 tsp caraway
2 ¾ tsp salt
black pepper, to taste
1 tsp baking soda

NOTE

I am not a big fan of freezing rice, as I believe the texture of freshly cooked rice is much better than thawed frozen rice. But if one wants to freeze this dish, be sure to let it thaw completely in the refrigerator, before reheating it. I would suggest heating it in a baking dish covered with foil in the oven versus in a pot on the stove top.

INSTRUCTIONS

1. Soak the chickpeas and baking soda in water for 12 hours. Drain and rinse, discarding any bad pieces.
2. Transfer the chickpeas to a pot, cover with water, then bring to a boil. Skim off the white foam that floats to the surface, then cook, covered, on low heat for 30 minutes (or until tender). Drain away the chickpea water into a bowl.
3. Pick over the rice, removing any bad pieces. Rinse well, then drain. Set aside.
4. In a large pot, covered, cook the onions with the olive oil on low heat for 20 minutes, stirring occasionally.
5. Add the water, chickpea water, rice, and spices, then stir to mix. Bring to a boil, then cook, covered, on low heat, for 25 minutes (do not stir during this time).
6. Stir, then cover and let sit for 5 minutes.
7. Stir the rice again, then gently fold in the chickpeas. Keep uncovered, then let rest for an additional 10 to 15 minutes (the rice will further fluff up as it cools). Stir again before serving.
8. Serve with a garlicy and lemony salad, or a small serving of skim yogurt.

NUTRITION FACTS PER CUP

241 Kcal	8 g Protein	5 g Fat	41 g Carbs	6 g Fiber	5 g Sugar

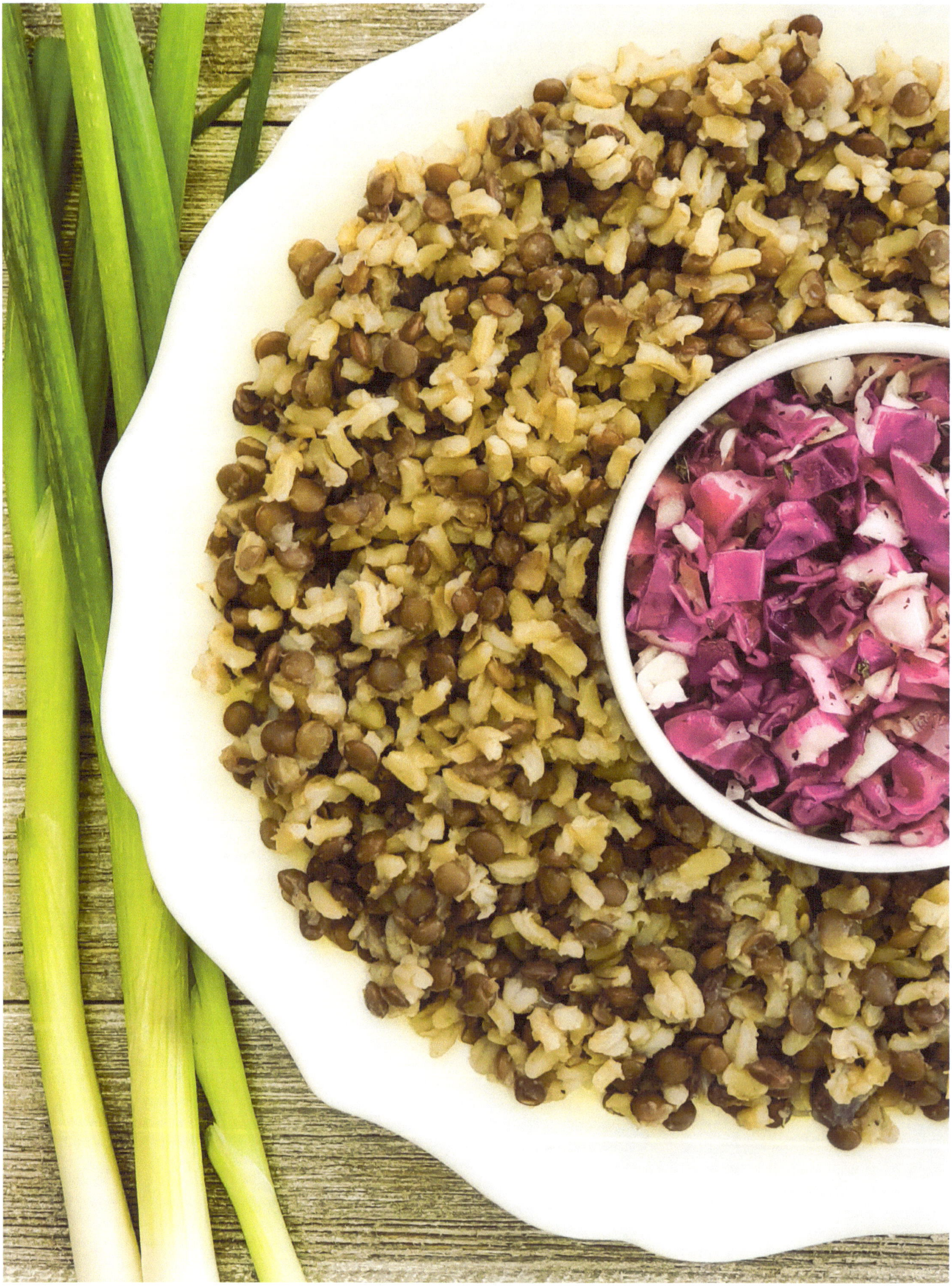

BROWN LENTIL RICE PILAF

Mdardara مدردرة

A flavorful and healthy vegan dish, this lentil and rice pilaf is traditionally made with white rice and some lentils (green or brown). The ratio of lentils to rice may vary between households, with some adding less lentils and others making it with more. I like using equal quantities of brown lentils and rice, and I prefer using brown rice for a more nutritious meal. For this dish, onions are traditionally deeply caramelized, and many will fry additional onion strips for garnish. I have found that adding cardamom and cumin to this dish completely compensates for the missing flavor of the browned onions.

RECIPE YIELD 18 cups

DF GF EF V FF

INGREDIENTS

2 ½ cups dry brown lentils (488 g)
2 ½ cups dry parboiled brown rice (455 g)
2 large red onions, minced (750 g)
3 tbsp olive oil
3 ¾ cups water
1 tbsp cumin
2 ¾ tsp salt
black pepper, to taste
10 cardamom pods

NOTE

❁ I am not a big fan of freezing rice, as I believe the texture of freshly cooked rice is much better than thawed frozen rice. But if one wants to freeze this dish, be sure to let it thaw completely in the refrigerator, before reheating it. I would suggest heating it in a baking dish covered with foil in the oven versus in a pot on the stove top.

INSTRUCTIONS

1. Pick over the lentils and rice, removing any bad pieces. Rinse well, then drain. Set aside (separately).
2. In a large pot, covered, cook the onions with the olive oil on low heat for 45 minutes.
3. Add the water, rice, spices, and cardamom pods, then stir to mix. Bring to a boil, then cook, covered on low heat, for 25 minutes (do not stir during this time).
4. While the rice is cooking, place the lentils in a separate pot and cover with water. Bring to a boil, then cook, covered, on low heat for 20 minutes, or until the lentils are cooked, but still look firm. Drain away any excess water.
5. Once the rice is done, stir, then keep covered and let sit for 5 minutes.
6. Pick out the cardamom pods, then gently fold in the lentils.
7. Keep uncovered, then let rest for an additional 10 to 15 minutes (the rice will further fluff up as it cools). Stir again before serving.
8. Enjoy with a garlicy and lemony salad or with a side of vegetables, olives, and pickles.

NUTRITION FACTS PER CUP

212 Kcal	9 g Protein	3.5 g Fat	41 g Carbs	7.4 g Fiber	2.5 g Sugar

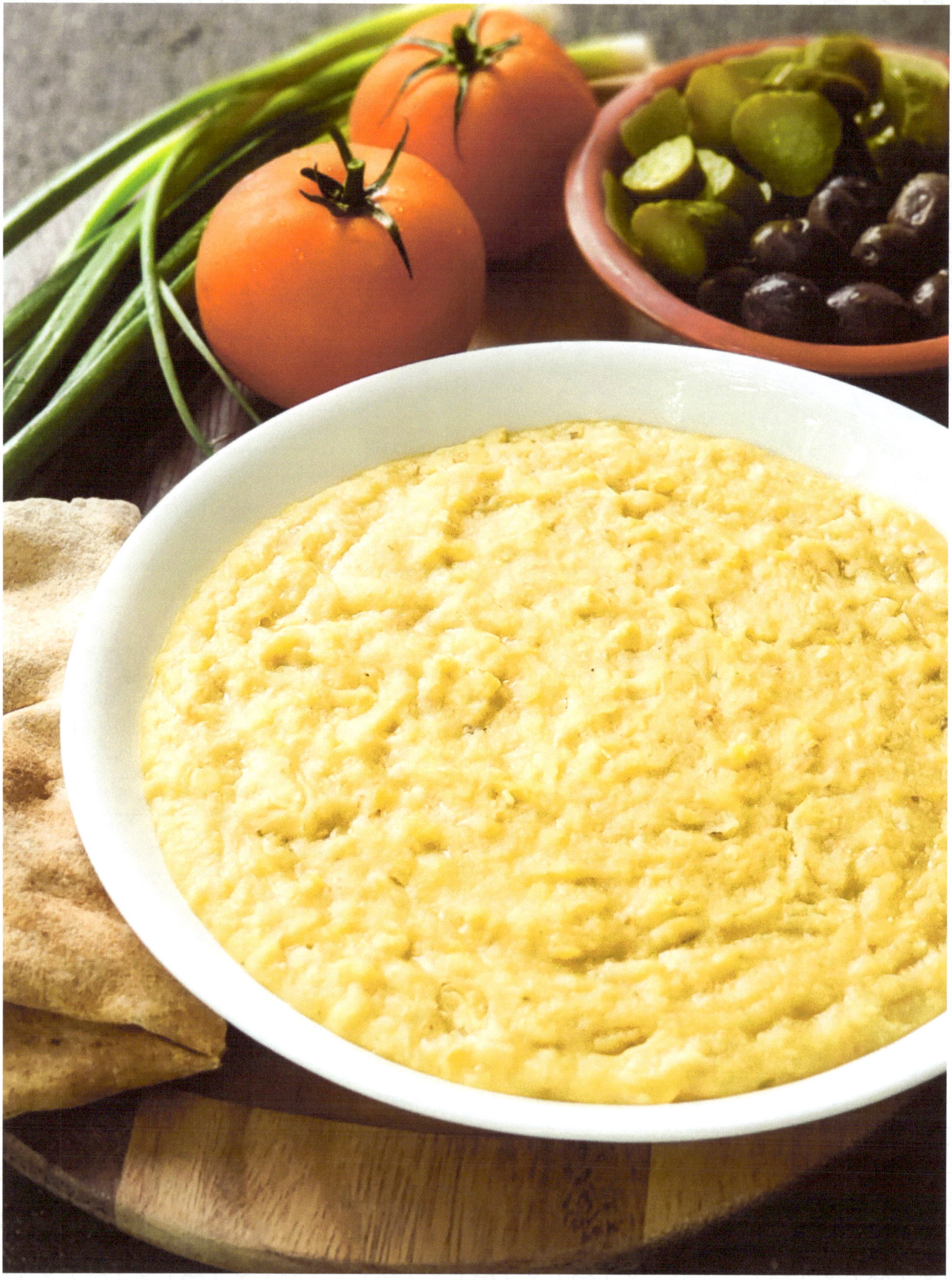

YELLOW LENTIL PORRIDGE

Mjaddara Safra مجدّرة صفراء

This savory dish is unique and a bit similar in ingredients to the lentil rice pilaf on the previous page. However, it contains much more lentils than rice, and is cooked until the ingredients have melted into a thick paste or porridge, to be scooped up and eaten with pita bread. Any lentil type can be used for this dish, though I love the flavor of red lentils. For *mjaddara* made with brown or green lentils, onions are traditionally fried in oil until deeply caramelized and browned, while for *mjaddara* made with red lentils, onions are cooked just until translucent. Some will often fry additional onion strips for placing on the surface before serving. I have come to love adding some cumin to this lentil dish which helps compensate for the missing caramelized onion flavor, as well as some turmeric for enhanced color and health benefits.

RECIPE YIELD 10 cups

DF GF EF V FF

INGREDIENTS

3 cups dry red (orange) lentils (530 g)
1/3 cup dry parboiled brown rice (61 g)
3 medium yellow onions, minced (480 g)
2 tbsp olive oil
6 cups water
1 tsp cumin
1/3 tsp turmeric
2 tsp salt

RECIPE ALTERNATIVE

- A 1/3 cup coarse bulgur (grade 4) can be used instead of the rice in the making of this dish.

INSTRUCTIONS

1. Pick over the lentils and rice, removing any bad pieces. Rinse well, then drain. Set aside.
2. In a large pot, covered, cook the onions with the olive oil on low heat for 20 minutes.
3. Add the water, lentils, rice, and spices, then stir to mix. Bring to a boil, then cook, covered on low heat, for 50 minutes, stirring occasionally (bump up the stirring in the last 20 minutes to prevent any scorching).
4. Pour into bowls or glass storage containers. Let cool before covering.
5. Can serve warm or cold out of the refrigerator. Enjoy with a side of green onions, tomatoes, black olives, or pickles if desired, or serve with a garlicy and lemony salad.

NUTRITION FACTS PER CUP

260 Kcal	14 g Protein	4 g Fat	41.5 g Carbs	15.5 g Fiber	4 g Sugar

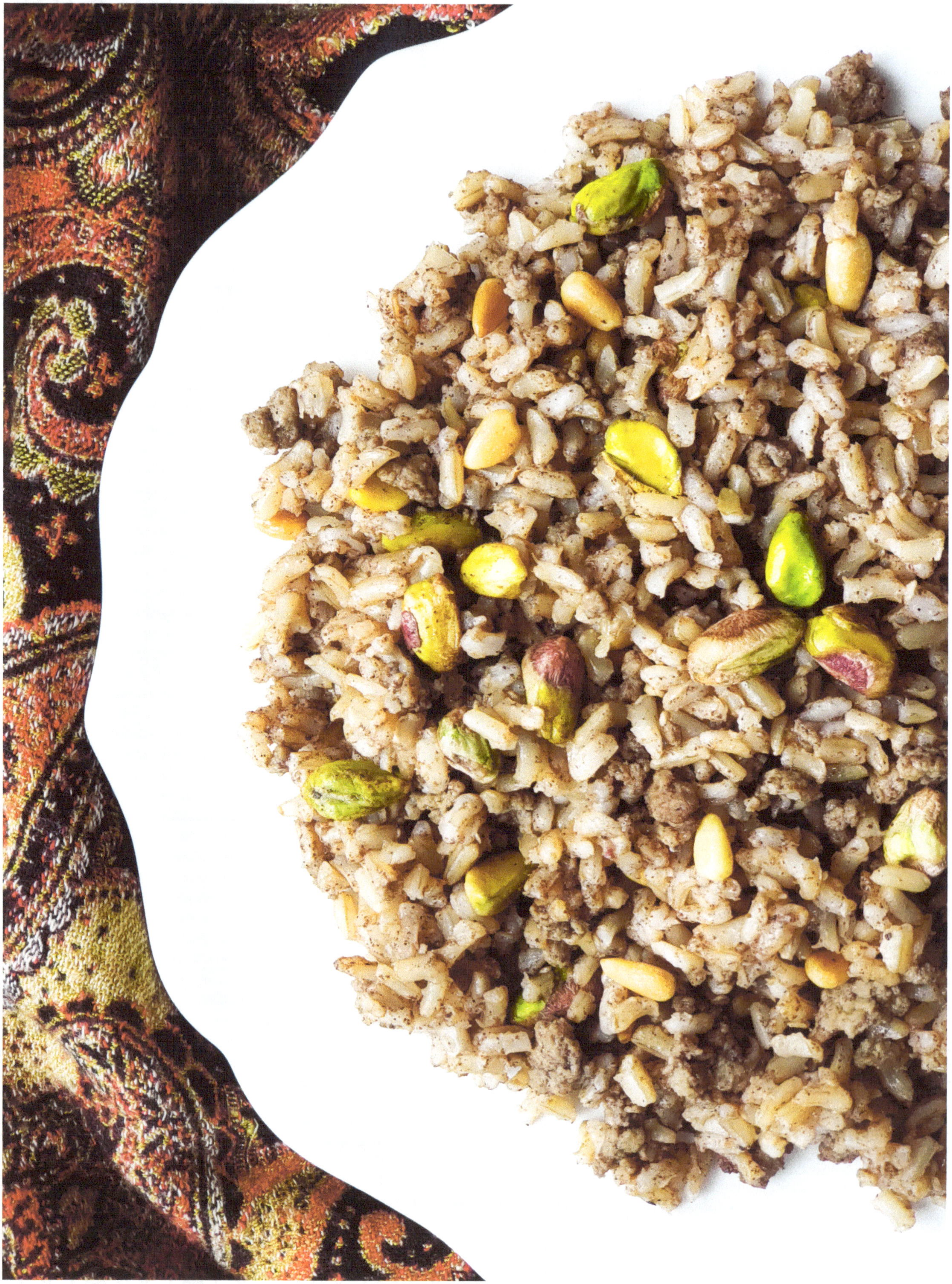

ARABIAN RICE WITH BEEF

Riz bi Lahmeh   رز بلحمة

This spiced rice and beef dish is a simple Middle Eastern classic with a few variations and presentations. It is very common for this dish to be used as a chicken stuffing, whereas it is also very common to be prepared as a main dish on its own with boiled/roasted chicken pieces mixed in with it. Some add onions and other vegetables, mainly peas and carrots, while others go without any vegetables. Fried nuts are almost always added as garnish to this dish, especially pine nuts and almonds. In the ingredients below, I have shared the simplest and most basic recipe of the dish (I like adding an onion, whereas traditionally, no onions are included), with some of the alternative variations presented below in the notes.

RECIPE YIELD 14 cups

DF GF EF FF

INGREDIENTS

Raw extra lean beef, ground (500 g)
3 cups dry parboiled brown rice (546 g)
1 medium yellow onion, minced (160 g)
2 tbsp olive oil
4 ½ cups water
1 tbsp cinnamon
1 ½ tsp allspice
1 ½ tsp 7-spices
2 ½ tsp salt
black pepper, to taste
1 cinnamon stick
2 bay leaves

INSTRUCTIONS

1. Pick over the rice, removing any bad pieces. Rinse well, then drain. Set aside.
2. In a medium pan or skillet, covered, cook the onions with 1 tbsp olive oil on low heat for 20 minutes.
3. Add the meat with the cinnamon stick and bay leaves, stirring frequently until browned. Cover and cook on low heat for 15 minutes, stirring occasionally. Remove the bay leaves and cinnamon stick.
4. To a large pot, pour in the water, 1 tbsp olive oil, and spices, then whisk well. Stir in the rice, then bring to a boil. Cook, covered on low heat, for 25 minutes (do not stir during this time).
5. Stir, then cover and let sit for 5 minutes.
6. Gently fold in the meat and onions.
7. Keep uncovered and let rest for an additional 10 to 15 minutes (the rice will further fluff up as it cools). Stir again before serving.
8. Garnish with dry roasted nuts if desired.

See next page for notes »

NUTRITION FACTS PER CUP

215 Kcal	11 g Protein	4.6 g Fat	31 g Carbs	2 g Fiber	0.7 g Sugar

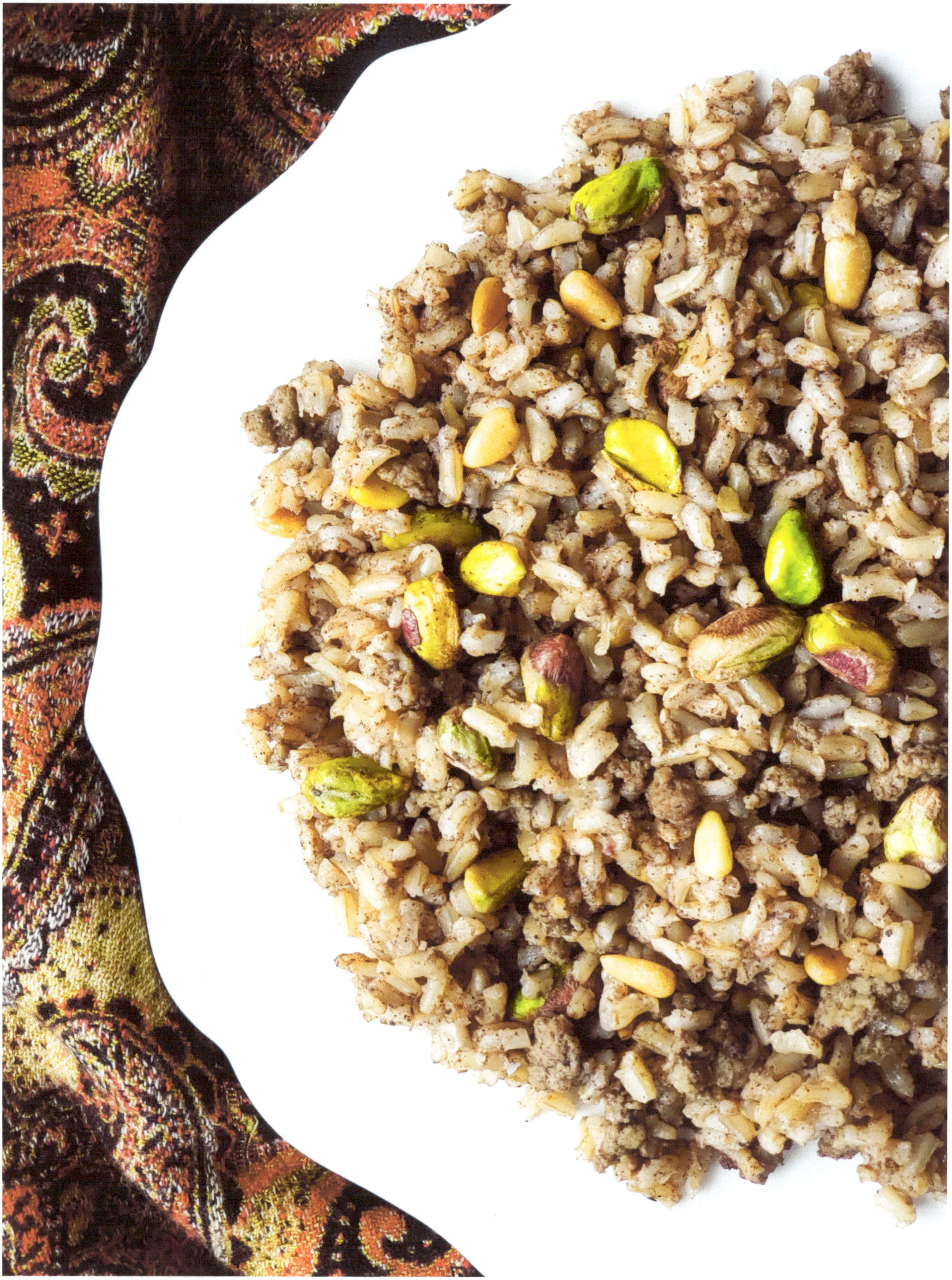

INGREDIENTS

Raw extra lean beef, ground (500 g)
3 cups dry parboiled brown rice (546 g)
1 medium yellow onion, minced (160 g)
2 tbsp olive oil
4 ½ cups water
1 tbsp cinnamon
1 ½ tsp allspice
1 ½ tsp 7-spices
2 ½ tsp salt
black pepper, to taste
1 cinnamon stick
2 bay leaves

NOTE

- I am not a big fan of freezing rice, as I believe the texture of freshly cooked rice is much better than thawed frozen rice. But if one wants to freeze this dish, be sure to let it thaw completely in the refrigerator, before reheating it. I would suggest heating it in a baking dish covered with foil in the oven versus in a pot on the stove top.

RECIPE ALTERNATIVES

- Adding 1 cup dry roasted nuts to the dish once it is done really accents this dish. I like adding a combination of ⅓ cup almond slivers, ⅓ cup pine nuts, and ⅓ cup pistachios.

- Instead of nuts (or in addition to nuts), one can add 500 g frozen peas and carrots (rinse and drain, then add to the rice when ready to cook). This version of the dish is often referred to as *ouzi*. The salt quantity will need to be bumped up to 3 tsp.

- If one would like to add boiled/roasted chicken to the dish, add 250 g cooked chicken meat. This version of the dish is often referred to as *riz bi djaij*, i.e. rice with chicken. Make sure to use unsalted chicken broth instead of water for the cooking of the rice to further accent the chicken flavor. The salt quantity will need to be bumped up to 3 tsp.

INSTRUCTIONS

1. Pick over the rice, removing any bad pieces. Rinse well, then drain. Set aside.

2. In a medium pan or skillet, covered, cook the onions with 1 tbsp olive oil on low heat for 20 minutes.

3. Add the meat with the cinnamon stick and bay leaves, stirring frequently until browned. Cover and cook on low heat for 15 minutes, stirring occasionally. Remove the bay leaves and cinnamon stick.

4. To a large pot, pour in the water, 1 tbsp olive oil, and spices, then whisk well. Stir in the rice, then bring to a boil. Cook, covered on low heat, for 25 minutes (do not stir during this time).

5. Stir, then cover and let sit for 5 minutes.

6. Gently fold in the meat and onions.

7. Keep uncovered and let rest for an additional 10 to 15 minutes (the rice will further fluff up as it cools). Stir again before serving.

8. Garnish with dry roasted nuts if desired.

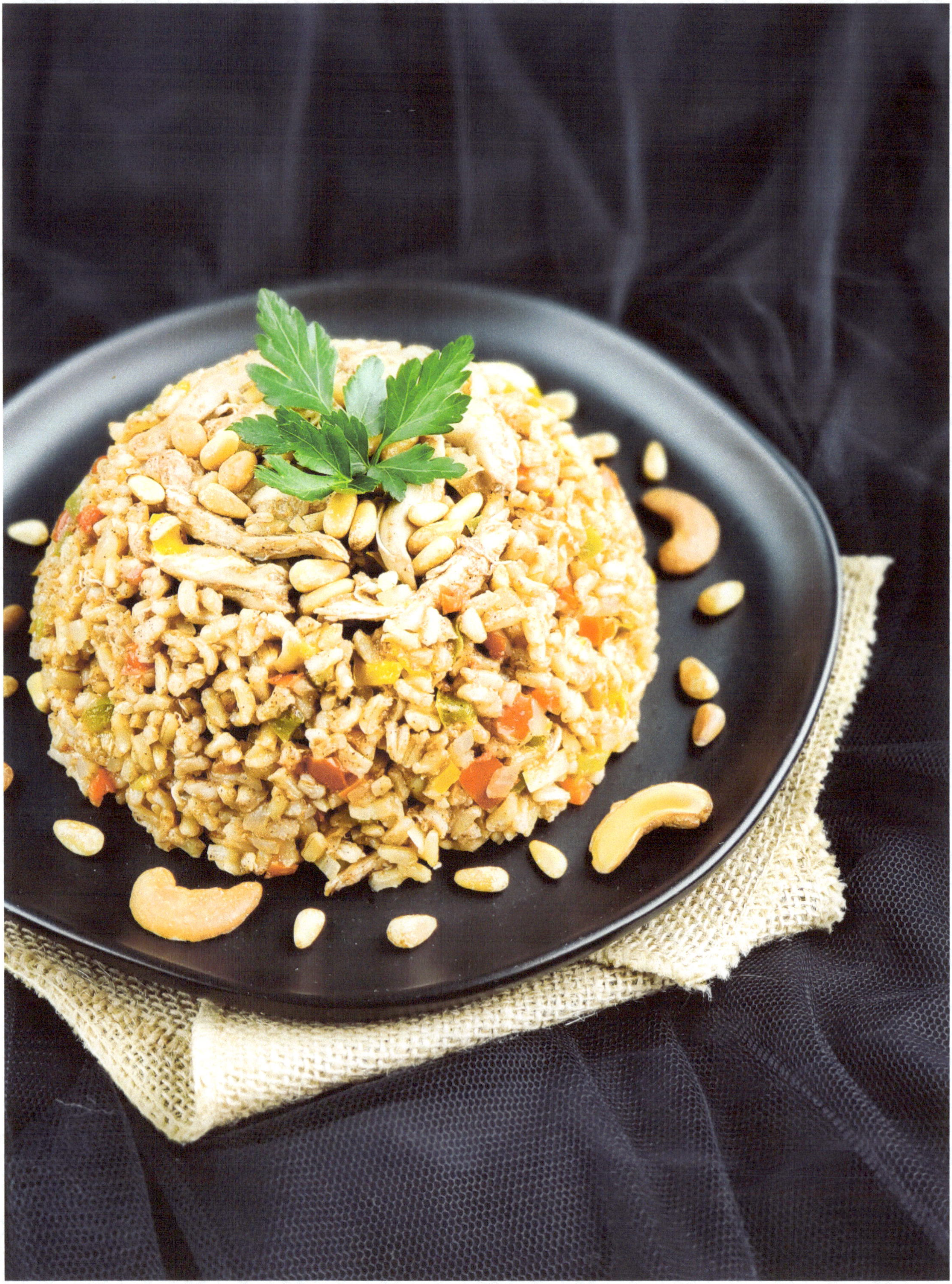

ARABIAN RICE WITH CHICKEN

Kabseh a Djaij كبسة عدجاج

Traditionally Saudi Arabian, this dish is prepared in many countries around the Middle Eastern region. Recipes differ slightly between countries, and even between households, mostly differing in the blend of spices used (with many using pre-mixed spice blends) and/or vegetables included (some only include onions and tomatoes). Here is my simple, flavorful, and healthy version of chicken *kabseh* that includes brown rice, added sweet peppers, and healthy olive oil.

RECIPE YIELD 18 cups

DF GF EF FF

INGREDIENTS

1 small boiled chicken (no skin, no bones), picked over by hand (500 g)
3 cups dry parboiled brown rice (546 g)
3 medium bell peppers (1 green, 1 red, 1 yellow), diced (495 g)
3 medium yellow onions, minced (480 g)
3 medium red tomatoes, diced (400 g)
3 tbsp unsalted tomato paste
2 tbsp olive oil
± 3 ½ cups water
2 tsp cinnamon
2 tsp allspice
2 tsp coriander
½ tsp cumin
2 ¾ tsp salt
⅛ tsp black pepper
30 cardamom pods
1 dried lime

INSTRUCTIONS

1. Pick over the rice, removing any bad pieces. Rinse well, then drain. Set aside.
2. In a large pot, covered, cook the onions with 1 tbsp olive oil on low heat for 20 minutes.
3. Add the sweet peppers and tomatoes, then cook, covered, on low for another 20 minutes.
4. Transfer the vegetables into a bowl, draining the vegetable broth (~ 1 cup) into a smaller bowl.
5. To the large pot, pour in the water (adjust the amount of water depending on how much vegetable broth is obtained, i.e. make sure total liquid equals 4.5 cups), then add the vegetable broth, 1 tbsp olive oil, tomato paste, and spices. Whisk well.
6. Stir in the rice and add the cardamom pods and dried lime, then bring to a boil. Cook, covered on low heat, for 25 minutes (do not stir during this time).
7. Stir, then cover and let sit for 5 minutes.
8. Pick out the cardamom pods and dried lime, then gently fold in the chicken and vegetables.
9. Keep uncovered and let rest for an additional 10 to 15 minutes (the rice will further fluff up as it cools). Stir again before serving.
10. Garnish with dry roasted pine nuts and/or almond slivers if desired.

See next page for notes »

NUTRITION FACTS PER CUP

217 Kcal	12 g Protein	6 g Fat	28.4 g Carbs	3 g Fiber	3 g Sugar

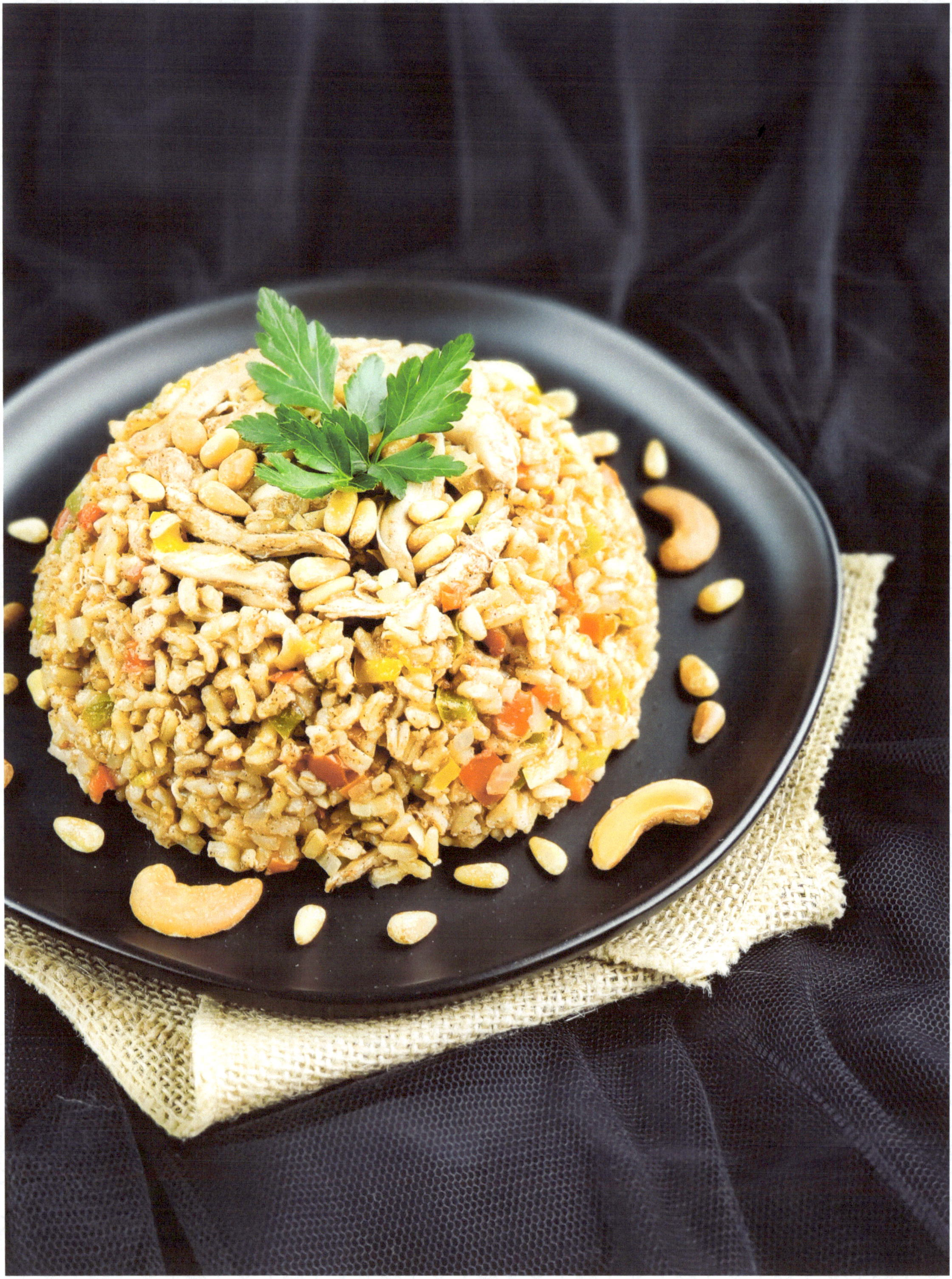

INGREDIENTS

1 small boiled chicken (no skin, no bones), picked over by hand (500 g)
3 cups dry parboiled brown rice (546 g)
3 medium bell peppers (1 green, 1 red, 1 yellow), diced (495 g)
3 medium yellow onions, minced (480 g)
3 medium red tomatoes, diced (400 g)
3 tbsp unsalted tomato paste
2 tbsp olive oil
± 3 ½ cups water
2 tsp cinnamon
2 tsp allspice
2 tsp coriander
½ tsp cumin
2 ¾ tsp salt
⅛ tsp black pepper
30 cardamom pods
1 dried lime

NOTES

- For a stronger chicken flavor, one can use unsalted chicken broth instead of water for the cooking of the rice.
- If a spicy hot flavor is desired, garnish with ground cayenne pepper or red pepper flakes.
- To make removing the many cardamom pods from the cooked rice less tedious, one can wrap them in a cooking sachet (using a piece of cheesecloth or coffee filter paper) from the start, then insert them as such into the pot of water and rice.
- I am not a big fan of freezing rice, as I believe the texture of freshly cooked rice is much better than thawed frozen rice. But if one wants to freeze this dish, be sure to let it thaw completely in the refrigerator, before reheating it. I would suggest heating it in a baking dish covered with foil in the oven versus in a pot on the stove top.

INSTRUCTIONS

1. Pick over the rice, removing any bad pieces. Rinse well, then drain. Set aside.
2. In a large pot, covered, cook the onions with 1 tbsp olive oil on low heat for 20 minutes.
3. Add the sweet peppers and tomatoes, then cook, covered, on low for another 20 minutes.
4. Transfer the vegetables into a bowl, draining the vegetable broth (~ 1 cup) into a smaller bowl.
5. To the large pot, pour in the water (adjust the amount of water depending on how much vegetable broth is obtained, i.e. make sure total liquid equals 4.5 cups), then add the vegetable broth, 1 tbsp olive oil, tomato paste, and spices. Whisk well.
6. Stir in the rice and add the cardamom pods and dried lime, then bring to a boil. Cook, covered on low heat, for 25 minutes (do not stir during this time).
7. Stir, then cover and let sit for 5 minutes.
8. Pick out the cardamom pods and dried lime, then gently fold in the chicken and vegetables.
9. Keep uncovered and let rest for an additional 10 to 15 minutes (the rice will further fluff up as it cools). Stir again before serving.
10. Garnish with dry roasted pine nuts and/or almond slivers if desired.

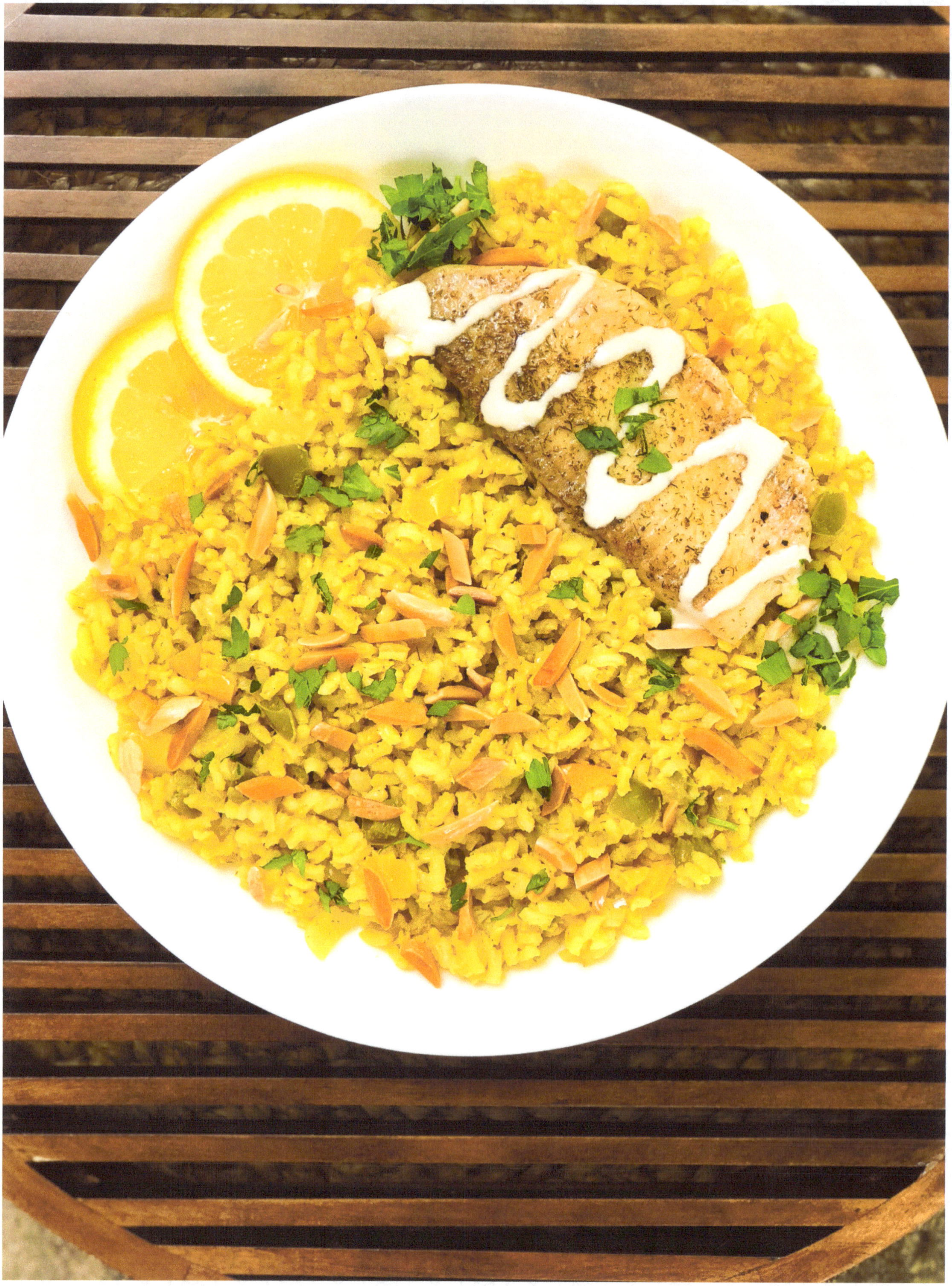

ARABIAN RICE WITH FISH

Sayyadiyeh صيّاديّة

This dish is commonly prepared in Lebanon and other countries of the Middle East. Recipes can differ slightly in and between countries, with the variables mostly being the blend of spices used (some add saffron, thus making it reminiscent of an Indian biryani dish) and vegetables included (many just include onions, lightly caramelizing them, and sometimes adding fried onions as garnish). My version is light, healthy, and very flavorful.

RECIPE YIELD 18 cups

DF GF EF FF

INGREDIENTS

Raw white fish fillets (no skin, no bones) (500 g)
3 cups dry parboiled brown rice (546 g)
4 medium bell peppers (2 green, 2 yellow), diced (660 g)
3 medium yellow onions, minced (480 g)
2 tbsp garlic, crushed
2 tbsp olive oil
± 4 cups water
2 ½ tsp ginger
2 tsp curry
½ tsp turmeric
2 ¼ tsp dill weed
3 tsp salt
⅛ tsp black pepper

INSTRUCTIONS

1. Pick over the rice, removing any bad pieces. Rinse well, then drain. Set aside.
2. In a large pot, covered, cook the onions with 1 tbsp olive oil on low heat for 20 minutes.
3. Add the sweet peppers and garlic, then cook, covered, on low for another 20 minutes.
4. Transfer the vegetables into a bowl, draining the vegetable broth (~ ½ cup) into a smaller bowl.
5. To the large pot, pour in the water (adjust the amount of water depending on how much vegetable broth is obtained, i.e. make sure total liquid equals 4.5 cups), then add the vegetable broth, 2 tsp olive oil, and spices (minus the ¼ tsp dill, ¼ tsp salt, and the black pepper). Whisk well.
6. Stir in the rice, bring to a boil, then cook, covered on low heat, for 25 minutes (do not stir during this time).
7. In the meantime, place the fish fillets on a lightly greased sheet pan (recommended dimensions: 25 cm x 35 cm or similar), brush with 1 tsp olive oil, then sprinkle with the remaining dill and salt, as well as the black pepper.

Instructions continued on the next page »

NUTRITION FACTS PER CUP

176 Kcal	8 g Protein	3 g Fat	28 g Carbs	3 g Fiber	3 g Sugar

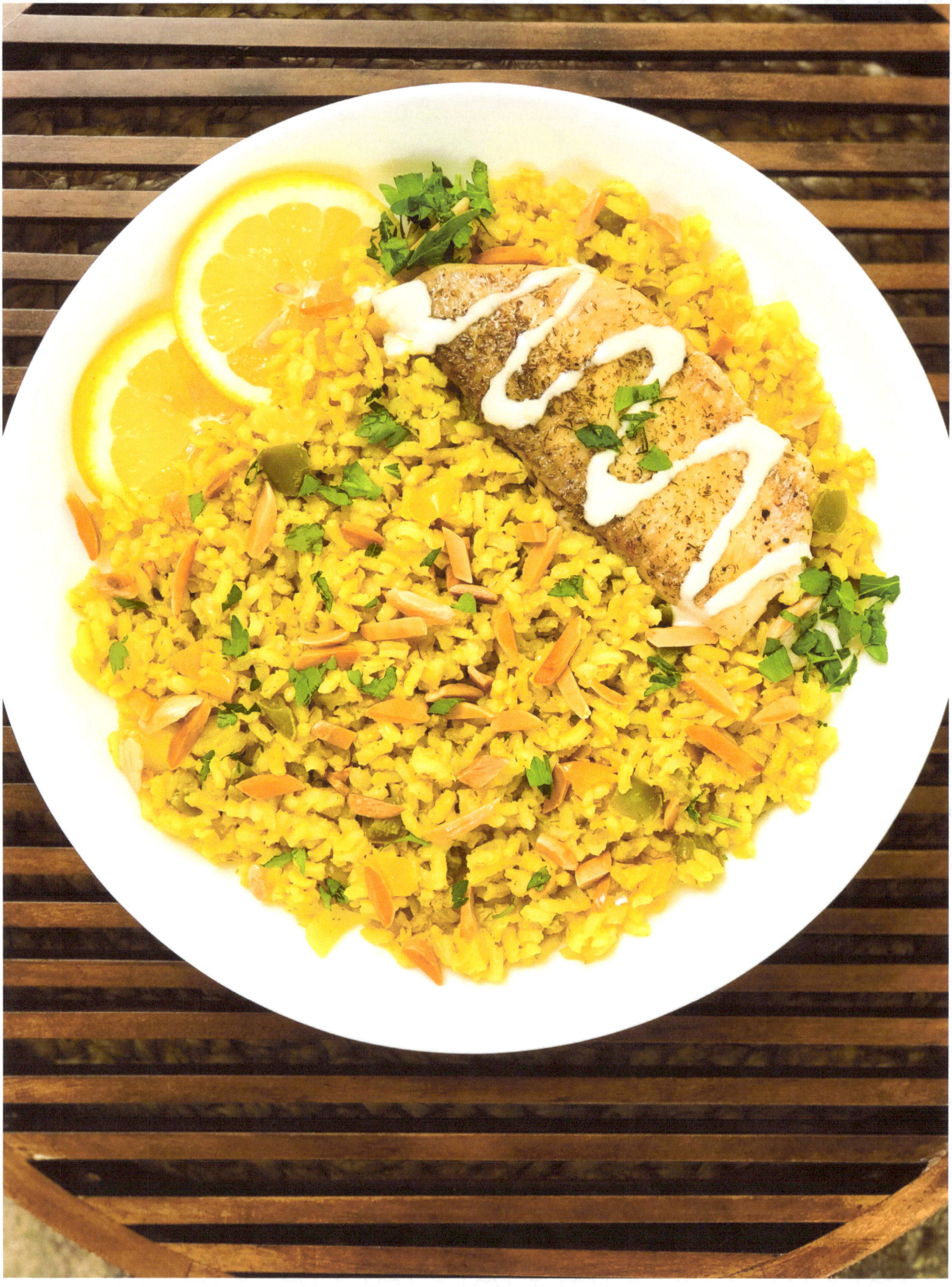

INGREDIENTS

Raw white fish fillets (no skin, no bones) (500 g)
3 cups dry parboiled brown rice (546 g)
4 medium bell peppers (2 green, 2 yellow), diced (660 g)
3 medium yellow onions, minced (480 g)
2 tbsp garlic, crushed
2 tbsp olive oil
± 4 cups water
2 ½ tsp ginger
2 tsp curry
½ tsp turmeric
2 ¼ tsp dill weed
3 tsp salt
⅛ tsp black pepper

NOTES

❋ For a stronger fish flavor, one can save the fish broth and use it instead of some water for the cooking of the rice.

❋ I am not a big fan of freezing rice, as I believe the texture of freshly cooked rice is much better than thawed frozen rice. But if one wants to freeze this dish, be sure to let it thaw completely in the refrigerator, before reheating it. I would suggest heating it in a baking dish covered with foil in the oven versus in a pot on the stove top.

INSTRUCTIONS

1. Pick over the rice, removing any bad pieces. Rinse well, then drain. Set aside.

2. In a large pot, covered, cook the onions with 1 tbsp olive oil on low heat for 20 minutes.

3. Add the sweet peppers and garlic, then cook, covered, on low for another 20 minutes.

4. Transfer the vegetables into a bowl, draining the vegetable broth (~ ½ cup) into a smaller bowl.

5. To the large pot, pour in the water (adjust the amount of water depending on how much vegetable broth is obtained, i.e. make sure total liquid equals 4.5 cups), then add the vegetable broth, 2 tsp olive oil, and spices (minus the ¼ tsp dill, ¼ tsp salt, and the black pepper). Whisk well.

6. Stir in the rice, bring to a boil, then cook, covered on low heat, for 25 minutes (do not stir during this time).

7. In the meantime, place the fish fillets on a lightly greased sheet pan (recommended dimensions: 25 cm x 35 cm or similar), brush with 1 tsp olive oil, then sprinkle with the remaining dill and salt, as well as the black pepper.

8. Bake the fish in a preheated oven at 375°F for about 15 minutes (if using refined olive oil, one can bake the fish in a hotter oven, at a broil setting of 450 °F for about 10 minutes, on one level higher than the middle oven rack). Different white fish varieties may vary slightly in the way they bake, so adjust accordingly. Pick over the fish and break/shred into the desired size (the whole fish fillet in the picture is for display purposes only).

9. Once the rice is done, stir, then cover and let sit for 5 minutes.

10. Gently fold in the fish and vegetables, then keep uncovered and let rest for an additional 10 to 15 minutes (the rice will further fluff up as it cools). Stir again before serving.

11. Garnish with fresh parsley and/or dry roasted almond slivers, and serve with *tahini* sauce (recipe on page 139) if desired.

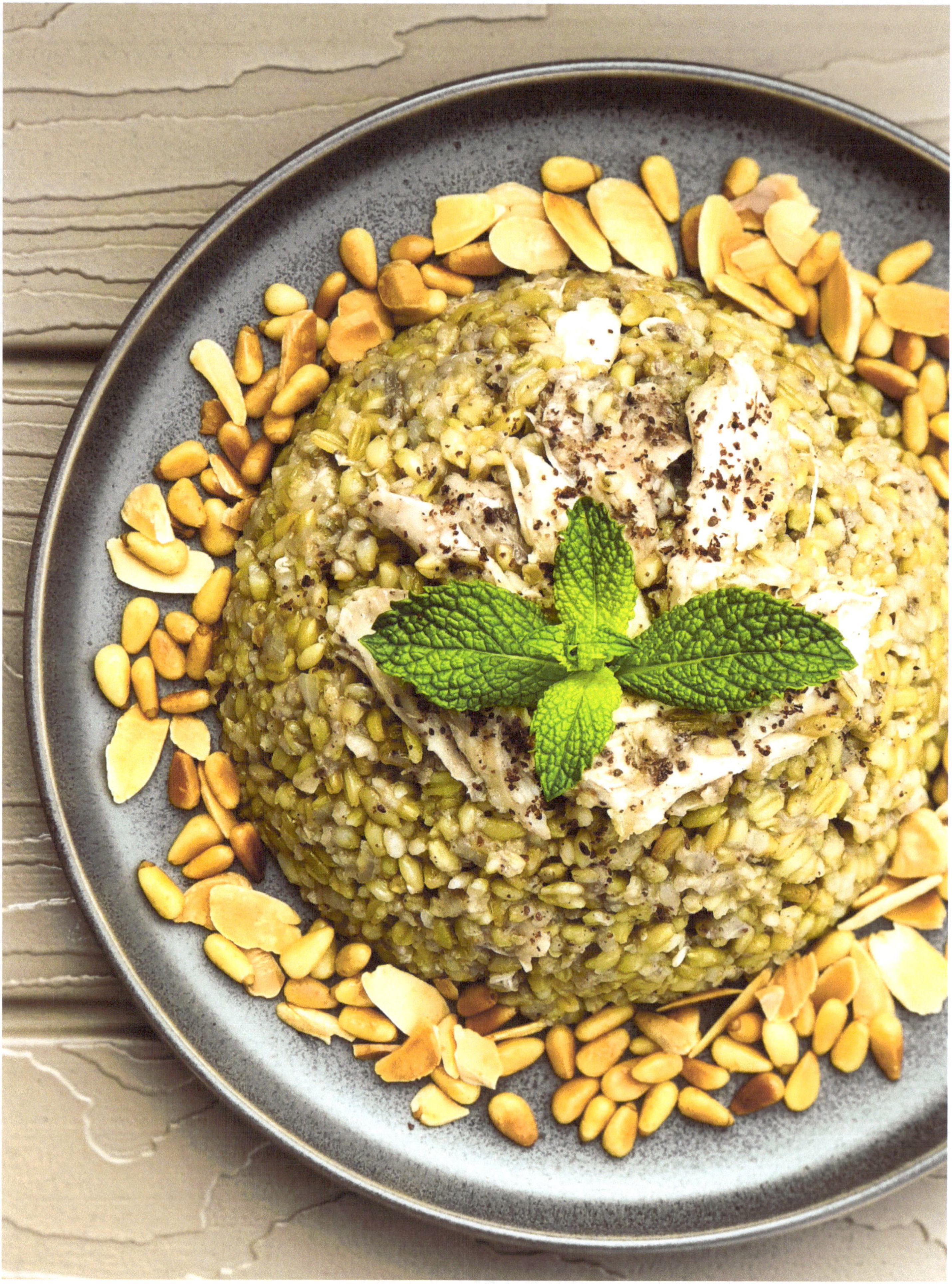

ARABIAN GREEN WHEAT WITH CHICKEN

Freekeh bi Djaij فريكة بدجاج

This simple yet hearty and healthy Middle Eastern dish is commonly made in many countries of the region. Freekeh, which is young green wheat that is roasted then dried, captures the center of this dish along with just a handful of other ingredients, mainly chicken and onions. As with many other traditional dishes containing onions, onions for this dish are commonly browned for the caramelized flavor, and nuts are roasted in oil to garnish the dish. My simple modifications to this dish entail skipping the browning of the onions, while making up for the caramelized flavor by adding a variety of spices from cumin to cinnamon, as well as adding a slight pungency by including some sumac.

RECIPE YIELD 18 cups

DF EF FF

INGREDIENTS

1 small boiled chicken (no skin, no bones), picked over by hand (500 g)
4 ½ cups dry coarse cracked green wheat (800 g)
4 medium yellow onions, minced (640 g)
2 tbsp olive oil
3 cups water
4 cups unsalted chicken broth
1 ½ tsp cinnamon
½ tsp allspice
1 tbsp cumin
1 tbsp sumac
2 ¾ tsp salt
⅓ tsp black pepper

INSTRUCTIONS

1. Pick over the wheat, removing any bad pieces. Rinse well, then drain.
2. In a large pot, covered, cook the onions with the olive oil on low heat for 20 minutes.
3. Add the wheat, chicken broth, water, and spices, then stir to mix. Bring to a boil, then cook, covered, on low for another 30 minutes (do not stir during this time).
4. Stir, then gently fold in the chicken. Cover and let sit for 5 minutes.
5. Uncover, then let rest for an additional 10 to 15 minutes (the wheat will further fluff up as it cools). Stir again before serving.
6. Sprinkle extra black pepper or sumac, garnish with pomegranate seeds or dry roasted pine nuts and/or almond slivers, or serve with a salad if desired.

See next page for notes »

NUTRITION FACTS PER CUP

262 Kcal	16 g Protein	6.4 g Fat	35.5 g Carbs	9 g Fiber	3 g Sugar

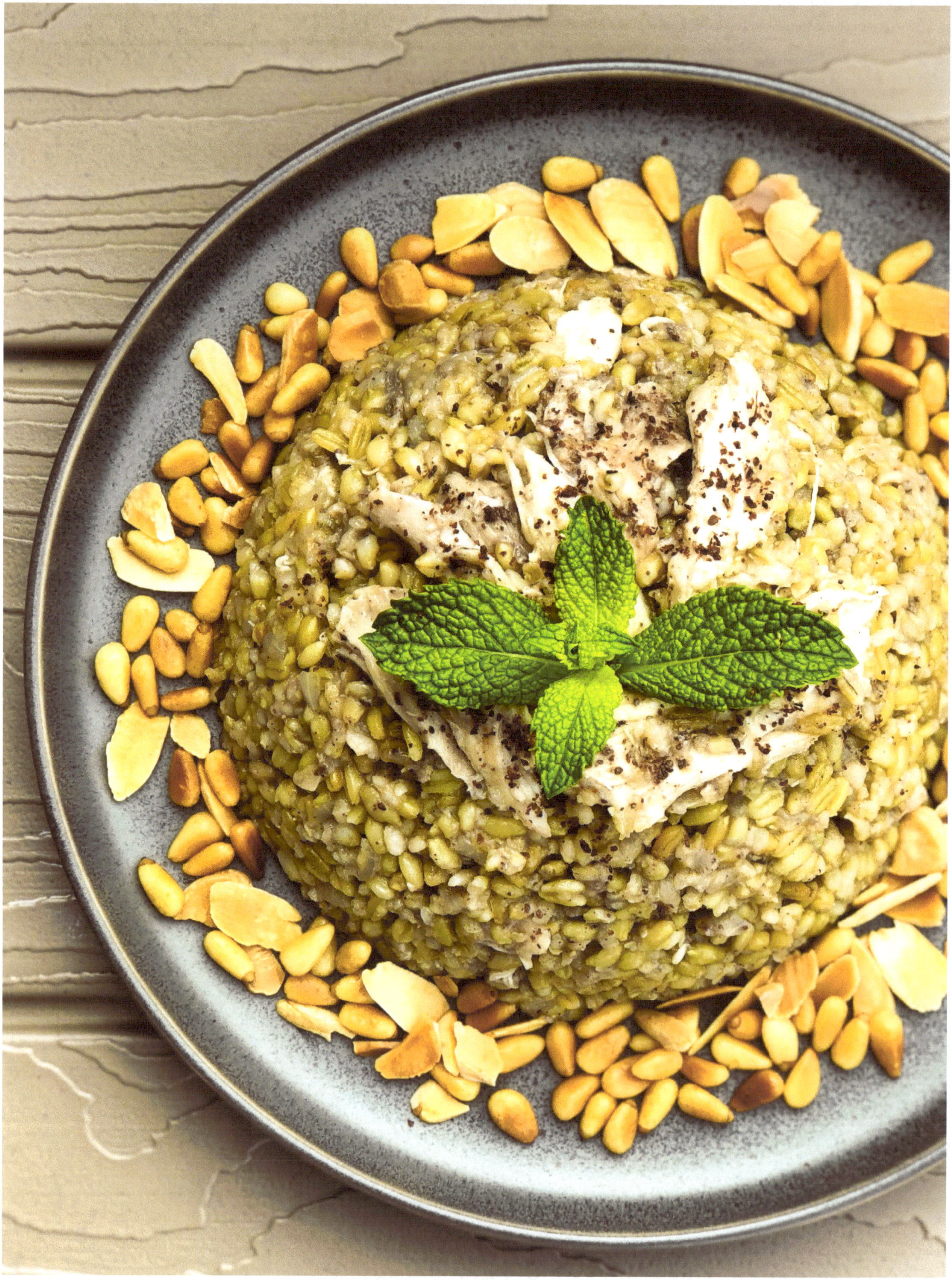

INGREDIENTS

1 small boiled chicken (no skin, no bones), picked over by hand (500 g)
4 ½ cups dry coarse cracked green wheat (800 g)
4 medium yellow onions, minced (640 g)
2 tbsp olive oil
3 ½ cups water
4 cups unsalted chicken broth
1 ½ tsp cinnamon
½ tsp allspice
1 tbsp cumin
1 tbsp sumac
2 ¾ tsp salt
⅓ tsp black pepper

NOTES

- Whole green wheat kernels can be used for this dish, but will require a longer cooking time as well as additional liquid.
- For a stronger chicken flavor, one can use more unsalted chicken broth instead of the water.
- I am not a big fan of freezing wheat, as I believe the texture of freshly cooked wheat is much better than thawed frozen wheat. But if one wants to freeze this dish, be sure to let it thaw completely in the refrigerator, before reheating it. I would suggest heating it in a baking dish covered with foil in the oven versus in a pot on the stove top.

ALTERNATIVE COOKING METHOD

- Instead of cooking the green wheat in the pot with the onions, broth, and water, one can boil the wheat in a similar way to pasta, adding it to a pot of boiling water and cooking, on high heat, for 20 minutes. Drain well, then add to the pot of onions (cooked for at least 40 minutes) and spices. Eliminate the chicken broth and water from the ingredients.

INSTRUCTIONS

1. Pick over the wheat, removing any bad pieces. Rinse well, then drain.

2. In a large pot, covered, cook the onions with the olive oil on low heat for 10 minutes.

3. Add the wheat, chicken broth, water, and spices, then stir to mix. Bring to a boil, then cook, covered, on low for another 30 minutes (do not stir during this time).

4. Stir, then gently fold in the chicken. Cover and let sit for 5 minutes.

5. Uncover, then let rest for an additional 10 to 15 minutes (the wheat will further fluff up as it cools). Stir again before serving.

6. Sprinkle extra black pepper or sumac, garnish with pomegranate seeds or dry roasted pine nuts and/or almond slivers, or serve with a salad if desired.

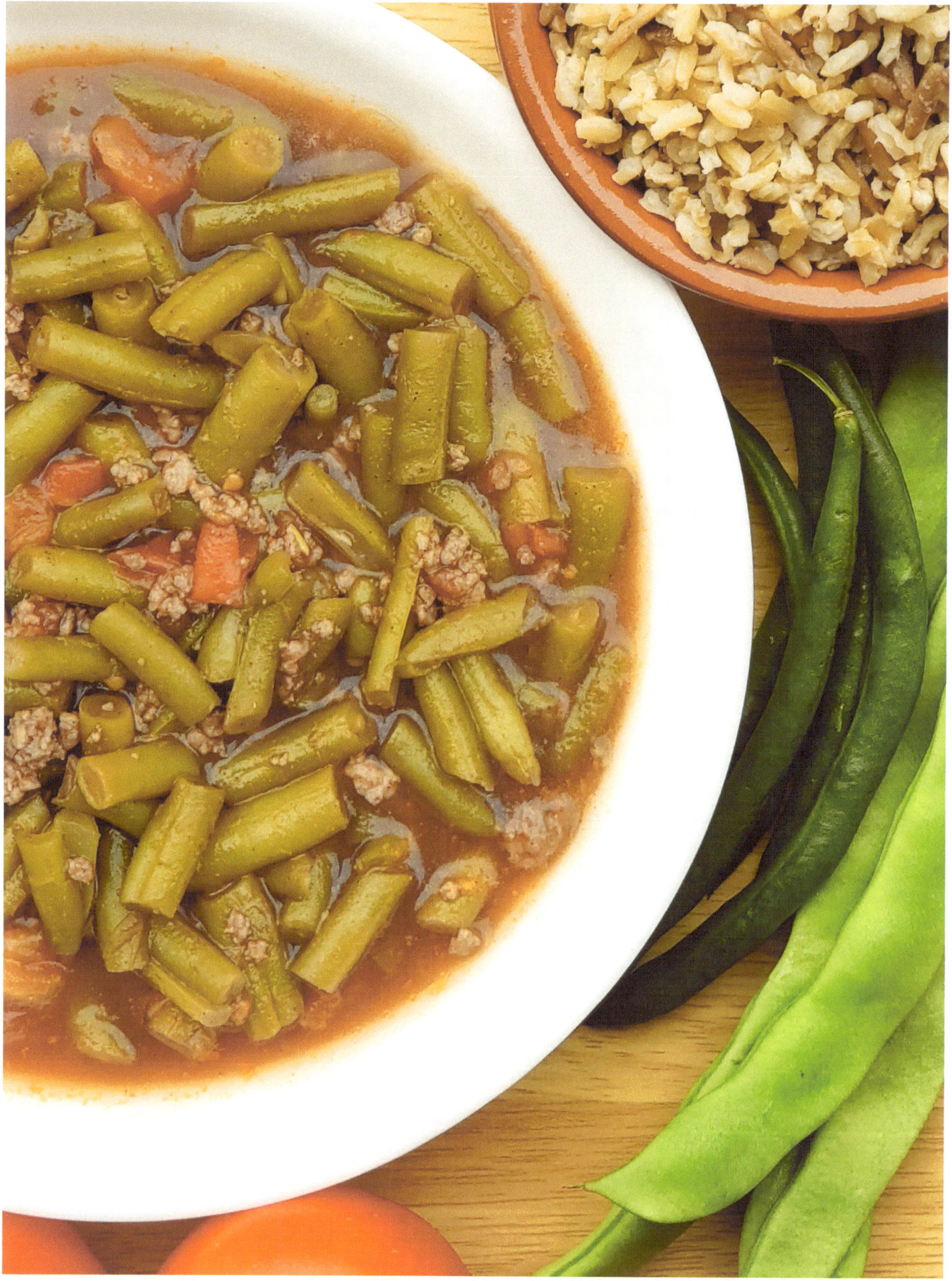

GREEN BEAN STEW

Yakhnit Lubyieh bi Lahmeh يخنة لوبية بلحمة

Stews are an integral part of the Lebanese cuisine as well as other Middle Eastern countries. They are comprised of a vegetable and a meat source (usually beef or lamb) cooked in a flavorful tomato-based sauce, and eaten with rice (commonly white rice) or bulgur to the side. This green bean stew is the most basic of all stews. Fresh Romano beans (broad and flat) are traditionally used, however, living in the US, I have often been unable to find this green bean as it is only available in the summertime at some farmers' markets and a few Middle Eastern grocery stores. For convenience purposes, I have thus resorted to using frozen French green beans (string beans or snap beans) that give the same great flavor and texture as Romano beans. While traditionally this recipe is made with fatty beef (or lamb) chunks, I use a small amount of extra lean ground beef instead.

RECIPE YIELD 18 cups

DF GF EF FF

INGREDIENTS

Raw extra lean beef, ground (500 g)
Frozen cut green beans (1.8 kg)
4 medium red tomatoes, diced (540 g)
⅔ cup unsalted tomato paste (160 g)
2 tsp olive oil
8 cups water
2 tsp cinnamon
2 tsp allspice
2 ¾ tsp salt
black pepper, to taste
1 cinnamon stick
2 dry bay leaves

NOTE

❁ If fresh green beans are to be used for this dish, one would need about 2 kg.

INSTRUCTIONS

1. Thaw the frozen beans on the counter for about 1 hour. Rinse well with warm water until all ice is melted. Let sit to drain well.
2. Whisk the water, oil, tomato paste, and spices in a large pot, then bring to a boil. Boil, covered, on low heat, for 10 minutes.
3. Gently press down on the beans, draining away any excess water before adding to the boiling sauce, then cook, covered, on low heat for 20 minutes.
4. Add the tomatoes, then let cook for another 15 minutes, or until the beans are tender.
5. In a medium pan or skillet, sauté the meat, stirring frequently until browned. Add the cinnamon stick and bay leaves, then cover and cook on low heat for 15 minutes, stirring occasionally. Remove the bay leaves and cinnamon stick.
6. Add the meat to the pot of stew and stir to mix.
7. Serve the stew with a side of brown rice (recipe on page 129) or bulgur (recipe on page 131).

NUTRITION FACTS PER CUP

86.5 Kcal	8 g Protein	2 g Fat	11 g Carbs	3.5 g Fiber	3 g Sugar

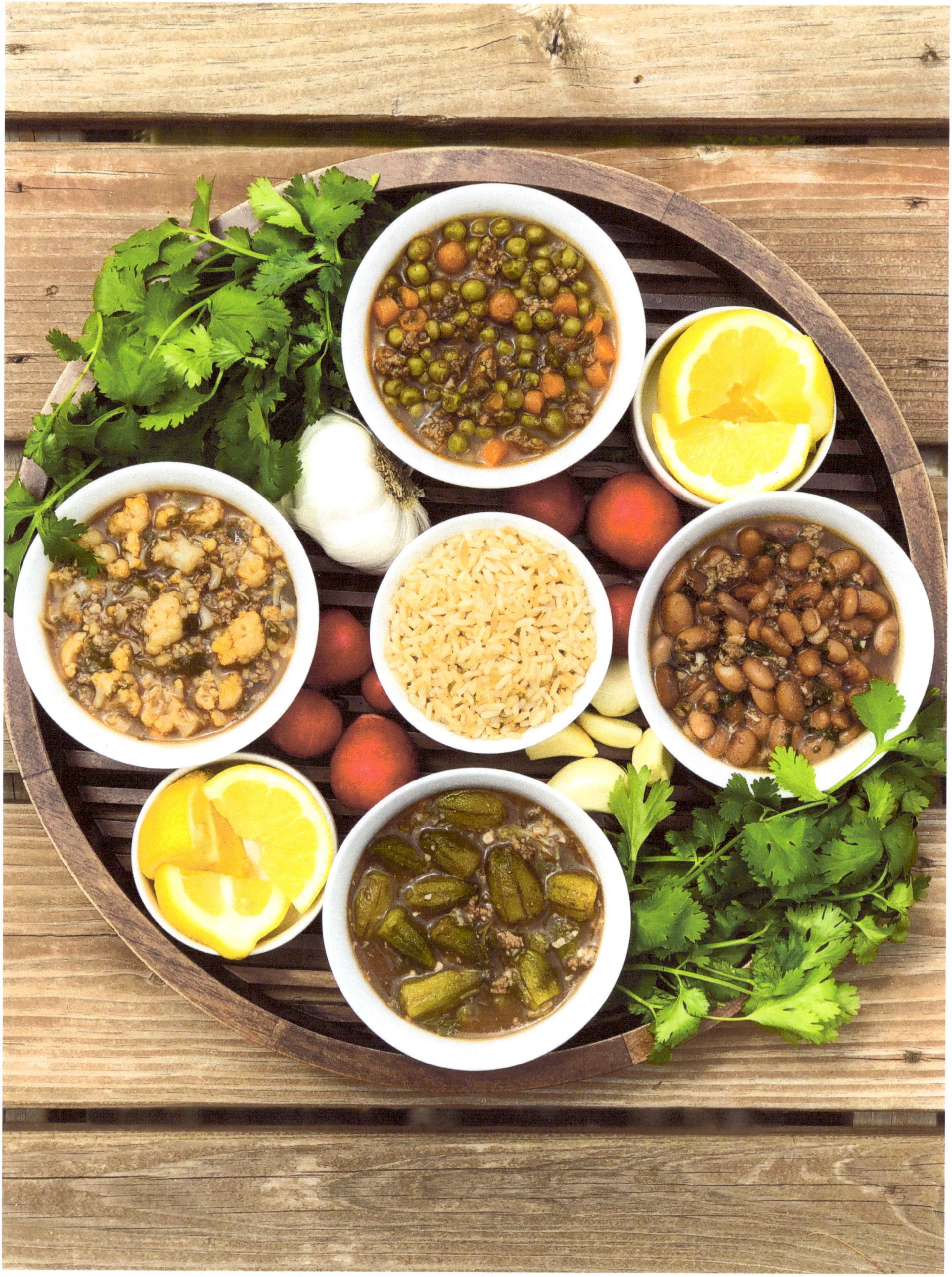

FOUR-IN-ONE VEGETABLE STEWS

Yakhnit Bazailla wa Jazar/ Baimyieh/ Arnabeet/ Fasoolia bi Lahmeh

يخنة بازيلا وجزر / بامية / أرنبيط/ فاصوليا بلحمة

Starting with the stew sauce used for the green bean stew (on the previous page), while simply adding fresh garlic and coriander, results in a new sauce traditionally used for four different stews varying simply in the kind of vegetable added (either peas with carrots, okra, cauliflower, or beans). Cauliflower in this stew is traditionally deep fried, but I simply boil it in the stew sauce, giving the same great flavor of the traditional stew. For the bean stew, dried beans are traditionally used, usually broad lima beans or small white beans. However, red kidney beans, pinto beans, and even black-eyed peas all work wonderfully well, maintaining the same great flavor of the traditional stew. As with the green bean stew, to cut down on the fat content, I use extra lean ground beef.

RECIPE YIELD 18 cups

DF GF EF FF

INGREDIENTS

Raw extra lean beef, ground (500 g)
Frozen peas and carrots (1.8 kg) ***or***
Frozen small okra (1.8 kg) ***or***
2 large cauliflower heads (no stalks), broken/ chopped into small florets (1.8 kg) ***or***
~ 5 cups dry pinto beans (850 g)
2 bunches coriander, finely chopped (170 g)
⅓ cup garlic, crushed (75 g)
1 cup unsalted tomato paste (240 g)
2 tsp olive oil
9 cups water
2 tsp cinnamon
2 tsp allspice
2 ¾ tsp salt
black pepper, to taste
1 ½ tsp baking soda
1 cinnamon stick
2 dry bay leaves

INSTRUCTIONS

1. Thaw the frozen vegetables on the counter for about 30 minutes to 1 hour. Rinse well with warm water until all ice is melted. Let sit to drain well.
2. Whisk the water, oil, tomato paste, and spices in a large pot and bring to a boil. Boil, covered, on low heat, for 10 minutes.
3. Add the desired vegetable to the boiling sauce. Bring to a boil, then cook, covered, on low heat for 15 minutes for the cauliflower stew, 20 minutes for the okra stew, and 20 minutes for the pea and carrot stew (add the coriander and garlic before the last 15 minutes of the total cooking time for each stew).
4. For the bean stew, soak the beans in water with baking soda for 12 hours. Rinse and let drain. Boil the beans separately (for 30 to 45 minutes or until tender), drain, then set aside. Let the stew sauce boil for 10 minutes before adding the garlic and coriander, then cook for 15 minutes. Stir in the cooked beans.

Instructions continued on the next page »

NUTRITION FACTS PER CUP

Pea and Carrot Stew		Okra and Cauliflower Stews		Bean Stew	
112 Kcal	16 g Carbs	86.5 Kcal	10.4 g Carbs	220.5 Kcal	37 g Carbs
10 g Protein	4 g Fiber	8.5 g Protein	3 g Fiber	17 g Protein	8 g Fiber
2 g Fat	3 g Sugar	2 g Fat	3 g Sugar	3 g Fat	1 g Sugar

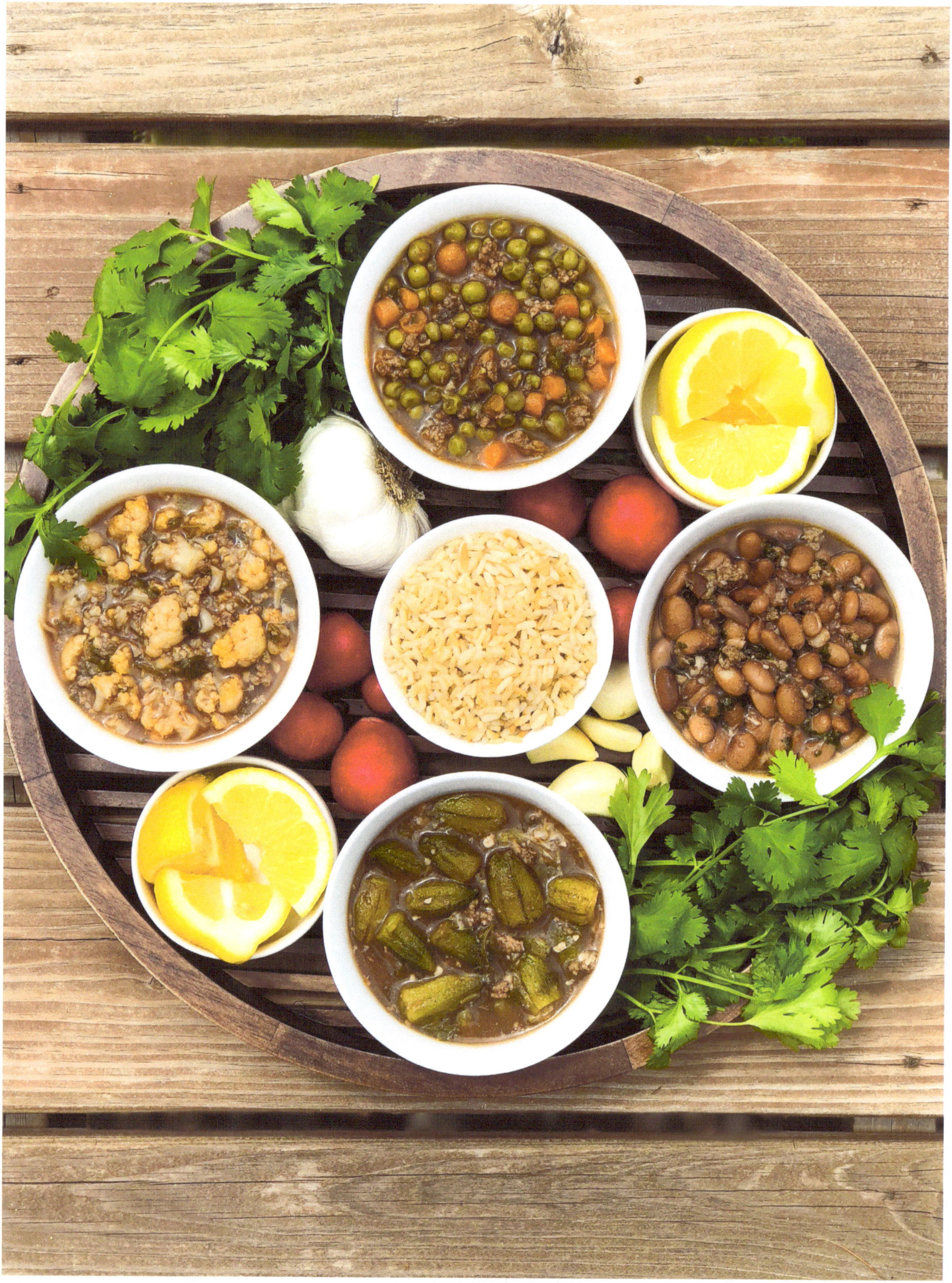

INGREDIENTS

Raw extra lean beef, ground (500 g)
Frozen peas and carrots (1.8 kg) ***or***
Frozen small okra (1.8 kg) ***or***
2 large cauliflower heads (no stalks), broken/ chopped into small florets (1.8 kg) ***or***
~ 5 cups dry pinto beans (850 g)
2 bunches coriander, finely chopped (170 g)
⅓ cup garlic, crushed (75 g)
1 cup unsalted tomato paste (240 g)
2 tsp olive oil
9 cups water
2 tsp cinnamon
2 tsp allspice
2 ¾ tsp salt
black pepper, to taste
1 ½ tsp baking soda
1 cinnamon stick
2 dry bay leaves

NOTES

- Fresh okra can be used for this stew instead of frozen okra. Care must be given though when slicing the top off of the okra and making sure that the inside of the vegetable is not exposed or else the stew will become gooey.
- For the bean stew, any of the following beans will yield pretty much the same flavor: broad lima beans, cannellini white beans, great northern beans, kidney beans, and black-eyed peas. Each type of bean will measure up differently in a cup given the difference in size and weight of each bean, so I would stick to the weight (850 g) called for rather than the number of cups (850 g of pinto beans measures up to be just under 5 cups).
- For garlic lovers, use ½ cup crushed garlic instead of ⅓ cup.
- A sister dish to the above stews is a potato stew prepared with coriander and garlic, with or without tomato paste.
- Since the okra and cauliflower stews have only slight differences in nutritional value, the numbers were averaged between them.

INSTRUCTIONS

1. Thaw the frozen vegetables on the counter for about 30 minutes to 1 hour. Rinse well with warm water until all ice is melted. Let sit to drain well.
2. Whisk the water, oil, tomato paste, and spices in a large pot and bring to a boil. Boil, covered, on low heat, for 10 minutes.
3. Add the desired vegetable to the boiling sauce. Bring to a boil, then cook, covered, on low heat for 15 minutes for the cauliflower stew, 20 minutes for the okra stew, and 20 minutes for the pea and carrot stew (add the coriander and garlic before the last 15 minutes of the total cooking time for each stew).
4. For the bean stew, soak the beans in water with baking soda for 12 hours. Rinse and let drain. Boil the beans separately (for 30 to 45 minutes or until tender), drain, then set aside. Let the stew sauce boil for 10 minutes before adding the garlic and coriander, then cook for 15 minutes. Stir in the cooked beans.
5. In a medium pan or skillet, sauté the meat, stirring frequently until browned. Add the cinnamon stick and bay leaves, then cover and cook on low heat for 15 minutes, stirring occasionally. Remove the bay leaves and cinnamon stick.
6. Add the meat to the pot of stew and stir to mix.
7. Serve the stews with a side of brown rice (recipe on page 129) or bulgur (recipe on page 131) as well as lots of lemon juice.

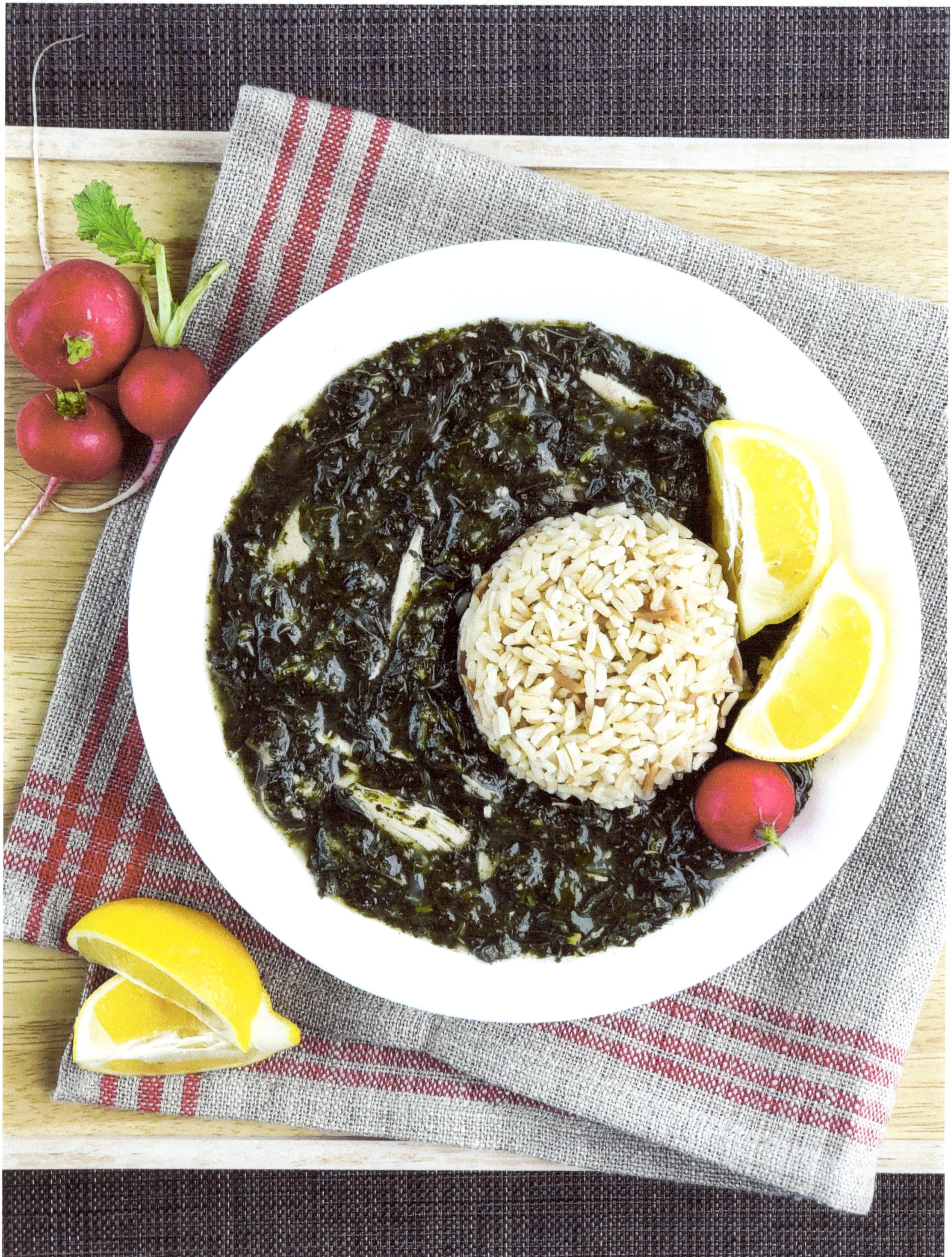

JEW'S MALLOW STEW

Yakhnit Mloukhiyeh يخنة ملوخية

This tasty stew made with Jew's mallow is unique to Lebanon and the surrounding Middle Eastern countries. While some countries, like Egypt, Palestine, and Jordan, traditionally make the stew with minced Jew's mallow leaves, the stew is made with whole leaves in Lebanon. I have actually come to like making it with a mix of both, liking the effect that minced leaves give to thickening up the stew broth a bit. This stew is also traditionally made with both red meat and chicken, but I prefer sticking to only chicken and using my flavorful low-fat homemade chicken broth.

RECIPE YIELD 18 cups

DF GF EF FF

INGREDIENTS

1 small boiled chicken (no skin, no bones), picked over by hand (500 g)
Frozen Jew's mallow (3 bags whole leaves, 2 bags minced leaves) (2 kg)
1 medium yellow onion, minced (160 g)
2 bunches coriander, finely chopped (170 g)
⅓ cup garlic, crushed (75 g)
1 tbsp olive oil
8 cups unsalted chicken broth
⅓ cup lemon juice
1 tsp coriander
1 tsp allspice
2 ½ tsp salt
¼ tsp black pepper
cayenne pepper, to taste

NOTES

- In Lebanon and other countries of the Middle East, it is common for fresh Jew's mallow leaves to be used for this dish, as well as dry Jew's mallow leaves. If fresh leaves are to be used, one would need about 2.2 kg for this recipe. If dry leaves are to be used, one would only need about 500 g (the leaves expand in volume quite a bit once rehydrated in water and cooked in the broth).
- Fresh and dry Jew's mallow leaves may take a bit longer to cook than frozen leaves.

INSTRUCTIONS

1. In a large pot, covered, cook the onions with the olive oil on low heat for 20 minutes, stirring occasionally.
2. Add the chicken broth and frozen Jew's mallow, then stir occasionally, over high heat, until all the Jew's mallow has thawed and the stew comes to a boil.
3. Cook, covered, on low heat for 15 minutes, stirring occasionally.
4. Add the garlic, coriander, and spices, then cook, covered, on low for another 15 minutes.
5. Fold in the chicken, then stir on high heat for a few minutes.
6. Stir in the lemon juice.
7. Serve with a side of brown rice (recipe on page 129) and add more lemon juice if desired.

NUTRITION FACTS PER CUP

137.6 Kcal	16.4 g Protein	4.5 g Fat	11 g Carbs	3 g Fiber	2 g Sugar

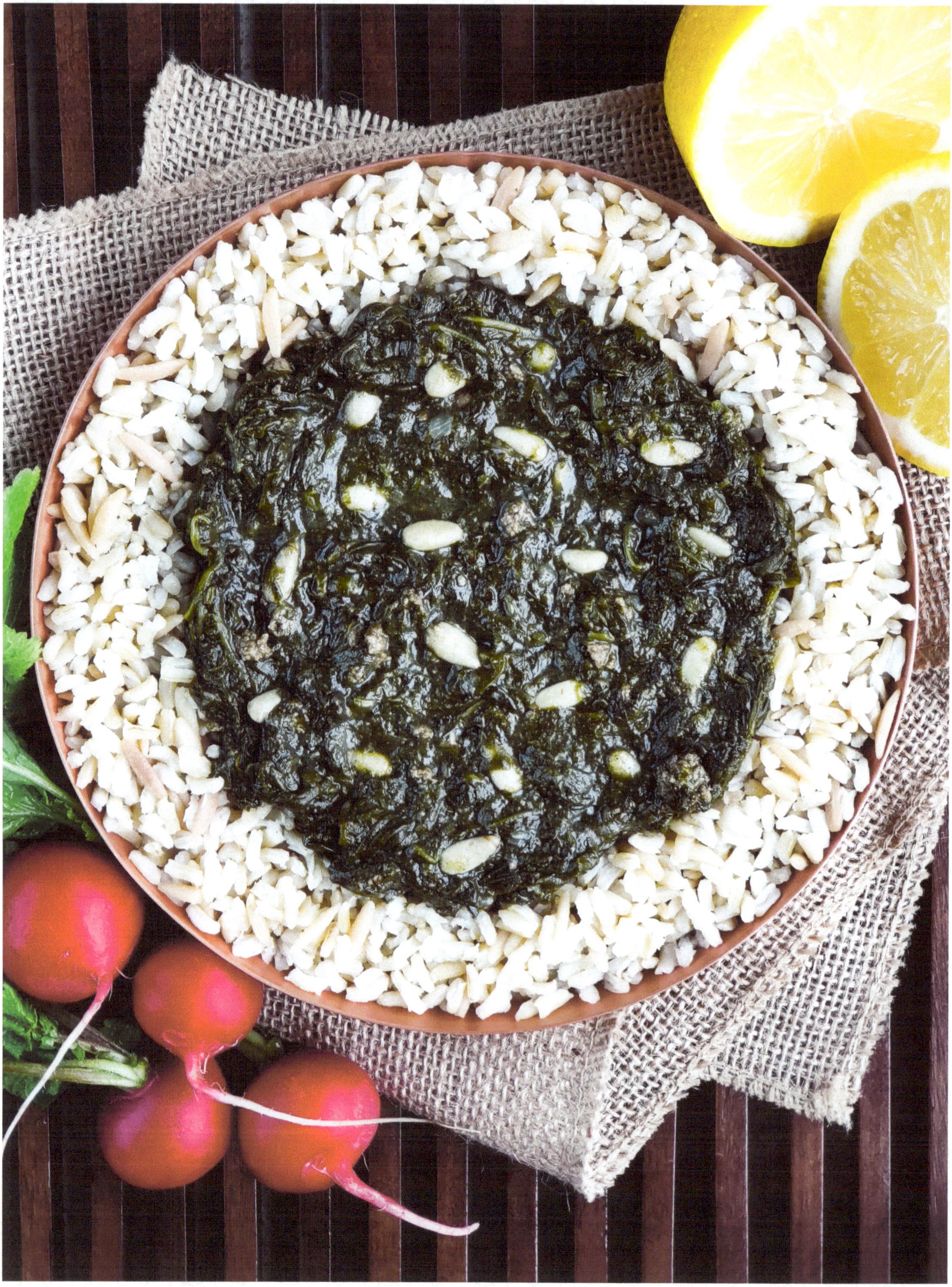

SPINACH STEW

Yakhnit Sbainikh يخنة سبانخ

This traditional stew is both nutritious and super flavorful! As with other stews, I use extra lean ground beef instead of the fattier beef/lamb cuts traditionally used. One will feel very awkward walking out of the grocery store with the amount of spinach needed for this recipe, but you will be surprised how much the volume of spinach shrinks once cooked!

RECIPE YIELD 18 cups

DF GF EF FF

INGREDIENTS

Raw extra lean beef, ground (500 g)
Fresh baby spinach, whole (2,200 g)
2 medium yellow onions, minced (320 g)
2 bunches coriander, finely chopped (170 g)
⅓ cup garlic, crushed (75 g)
½ cup pine nuts (68 g)
2 tsp olive oil
7 cups water
¼ cup lemon juice
2 tsp allspice
1 ½ tsp sumac
1 tsp dry mint leaves
2 ½ tsp salt
⅛ tsp black pepper
1 cinnamon stick
2 dry bay leaves

NOTE

This dish can be made from frozen spinach if desired. In this case, one would need about 1,750 g of frozen spinach.

INSTRUCTIONS

1. In a large pot, covered, cook the onions with the olive oil on low heat for 20 minutes, stirring occasionally.
2. Over high heat, add the spinach little by little, breaking them by hand as desired before throwing into the pot. Stir until the spinach has shrunk enough to add another bunch. Continue this process until all the spinach has been added to the pot.
3. Add the water, herbs, and spices, then stir to mix.
4. Bring to a boil, then cook, covered, on low heat for 20 minutes, stirring occasionally (the spinach will try to float, so one needs to push it down and stir, until it starts cooking, when it will sink).
5. Add the garlic, coriander, and pine nuts, then boil, covered, on low for another 15 minutes.
6. In a medium pan or skillet, sauté the meat, stirring frequently until browned. Add the cinnamon stick and bay leaves, then cover and cook on low heat for 15 minutes, stirring occasionally. Remove the bay leaves and cinnamon stick.
7. Add the meat and lemon juice to the pot of stew and stir to mix.
8. Serve with a side of brown rice (recipe on page 129) and add more lemon juice if desired.

NUTRITION FACTS PER CUP

110 Kcal	10.6 g Protein	4.4 g Fat	9 g Carbs	4 g Fiber	2 g Sugar

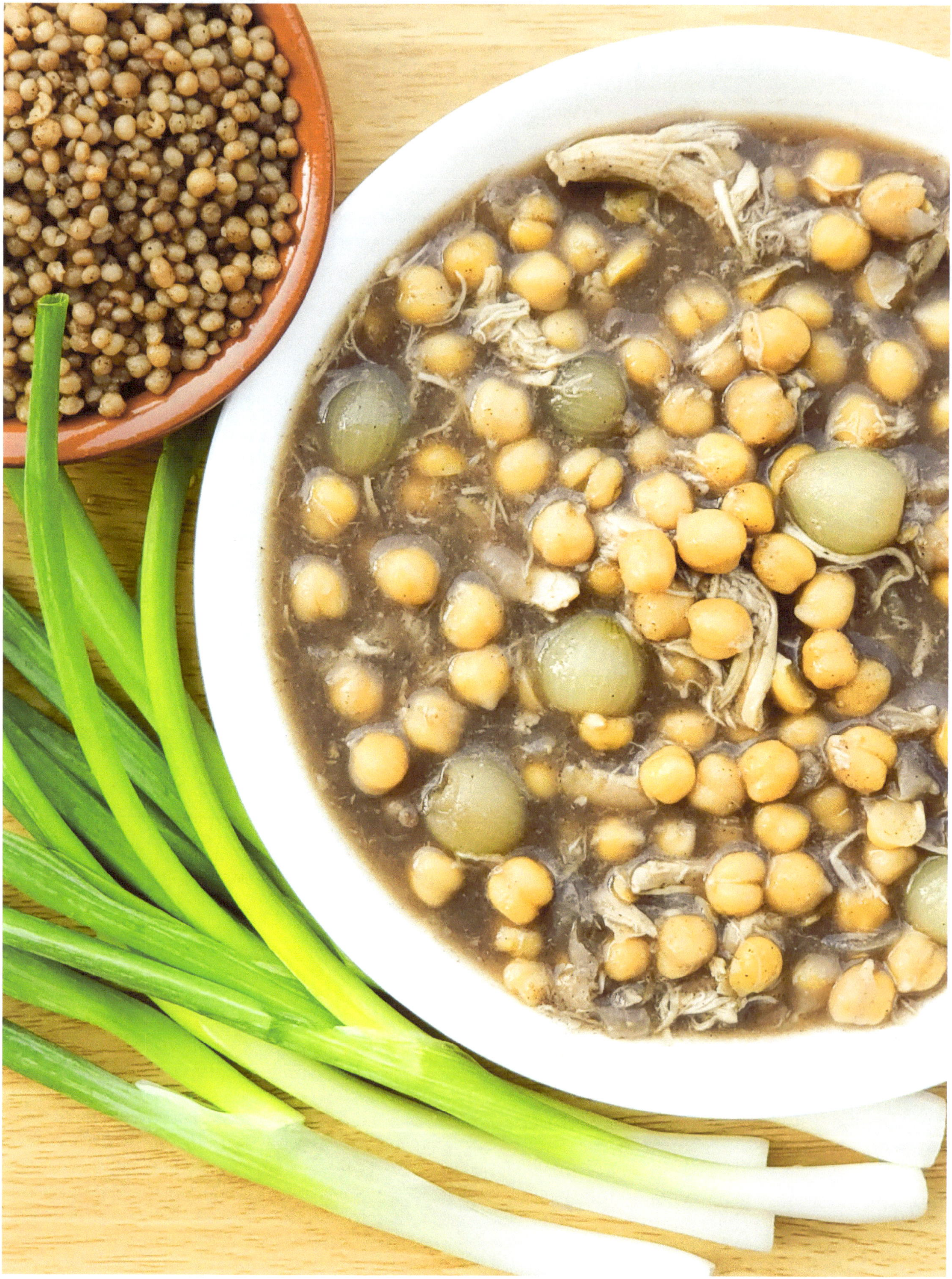

CHICKPEA STEW

Moghrabiyeh/Maftool مغربيّة / مفتول

Moghrabiyeh is both the name of a dish commonly made in Lebanon, as well as the name of the rolled wheat side dish it is eaten with. The word *moghrabiyeh* translates into 'from Morocco', possibly indicating the origin of the dish or the concept of rolled wheat. While the dish is referred to as *moghrabiyeh* in Lebanon and Syria, it is called *maftool* in Jordan and Palestine. This dish is considered a stew of chickpeas, pearl onions, and chicken (although some make it with chicken and beef or lamb). The base of the stew is chicken broth that is beautifully flavored with the sweetness of pearl onions and a lot of fragrant and warm spices. I rely on my low-fat chicken broth for a lighter stew and add some heart-healthy olive oil. I grew up eating *moghrabiyeh* with the traditional side the dish is supposed to be served with (Lebanese couscous, see page 13), but I have turned to serving it with Palestinian couscous, for a more whole side dish.

RECIPE YIELD 18 cups

DF GF EF FF

INGREDIENTS

1 small boiled chicken (no skin, no bones), picked over by hand (500 g)
3 ½ cups dry chickpeas (650 g)
50 medium white pearl onions (no skin) (500 g)
1 tbsp olive oil
5 cups chickpea water
5 cups unsalted chicken broth
3 tbsp caraway
2 tbsp cumin
2 tbsp cinnamon
1 tsp allspice
2 ½ tsp salt
¼ tsp black pepper
2 tsp baking soda

NOTES

- If both dark and light caraway spice is available, then use 2 tbsp light caraway and 1 tbsp dark caraway.
- The water obtained from the boiling of chickpeas is known as aquafaba, which becomes viscous upon cooling. This liquid is often saved and used as a replacement for egg whites.

INSTRUCTIONS

1. Soak the chickpeas and baking soda in water for 12 hours. Drain and rinse, discarding any bad pieces.
2. Transfer the chickpeas to a pot, cover with water, then bring to a boil. Skim off the white foam that floats to the surface, then cook, covered, on low heat for 30 minutes (or until tender). Drain away the chickpea water into a bowl.
3. In a large pot, pour in the chicken broth and required amount of chickpea water, then whisk in the olive oil and spices. Cover and bring to a boil.
4. Cook, covered, on low heat for 10 minutes, then add the pearl onions, and continue cooking for another 10 minutes.
5. Fold in the chicken and chickpeas, then let sit, covered, for 10 minutes before serving.
6. Stir well before serving, since some of the spices in the stew will sediment to the bottom of the pot. Serve with a side of Palestinian couscous (recipe on page 133).

NUTRITION FACTS PER CUP

253 Kcal	18.5 g Protein	7 g Fat	29 g Carbs	8.5 g Fiber	7 g Sugar

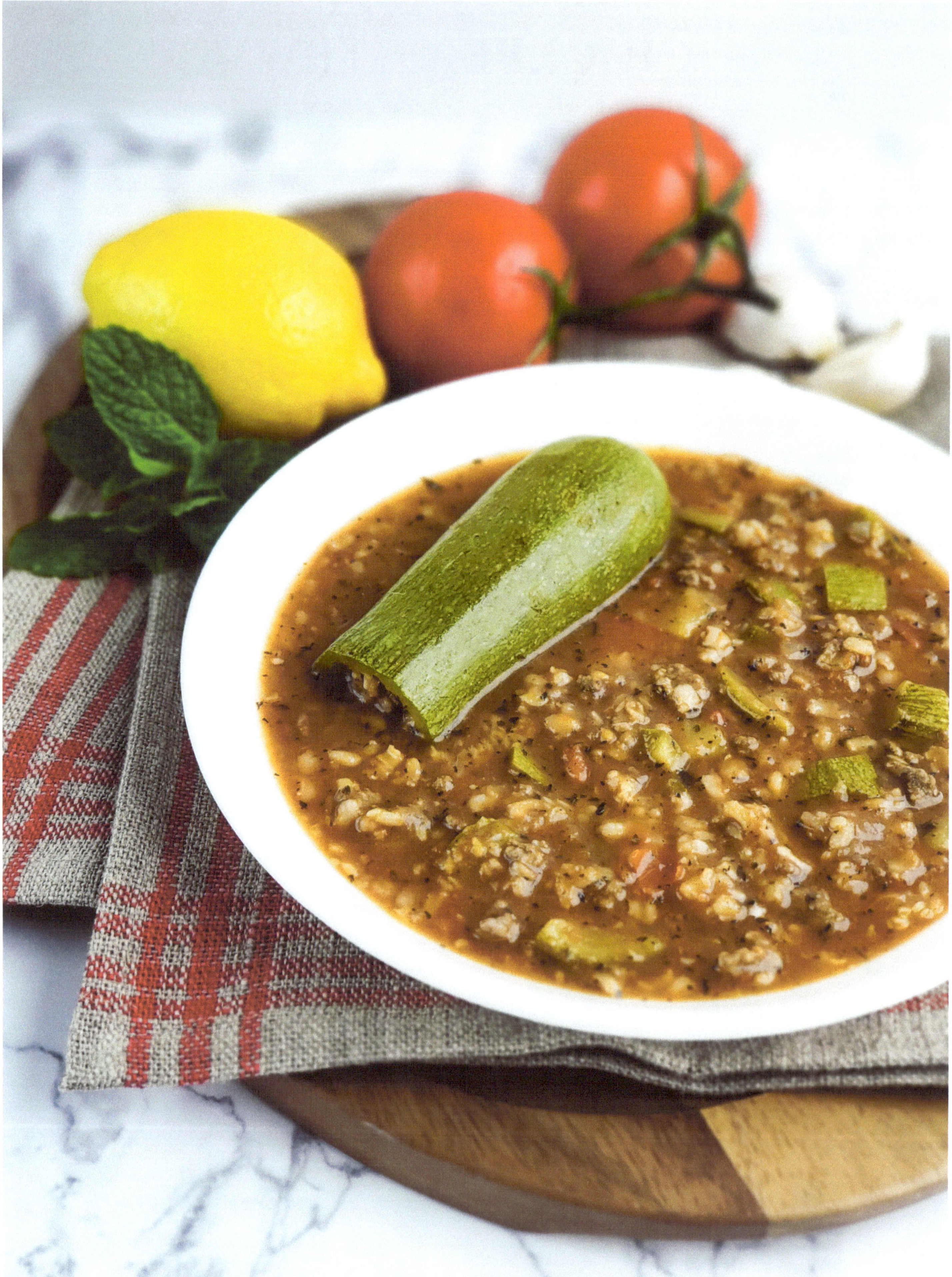

STUFFED ZUCCHINI À LA STEW STYLE

Kusa Mihsheh كوسة محشي

This recipe is a big twist to the famous Middle Eastern dish: stuffed zucchini. Carving out the insides of zucchini (also known as 'coring') has never been my favorite activity because it requires a lot of practice, patience, and time - not to mention the additional time required to stuff each cored zucchini with a white rice, meat, and vegetable stuffing. To add simplicity and convenience to the preparation of this delicious dish, I have turned to chopping up the zucchinis and cooking them in the tomato-based sauce with all the other required ingredients, thereby making it into a stew. Unlike traditional Middle Eastern stews, however, I cook the rice inside the stew, so as to mimic the flavors and texture of the traditional dish, i.e. somewhat overcooked rice that has soaked up the flavors of the other ingredients. To make this dish healthier and more whole, I use brown rice and extra lean ground beef, with some heart-healthy olive oil.

RECIPE YIELD 20 cups

DF GF EF FF

INGREDIENTS

Raw extra lean beef, ground (500 g)
1 cup dry parboiled brown rice (182 g)
9 medium Mexican zucchinis, diced (1 kg)
6 medium red tomatoes, diced (800 g)
2 medium yellow onions, minced (320 g)
¼ cup garlic, crushed (56 g)
⅔ cup unsalted tomato paste (160 g)
1 tbsp olive oil
10 cups water
¼ cup lemon juice
4 tsp dry mint leaves
2 ½ tsp 7-spices
1 tsp cinnamon
2 tsp salt
black pepper, to taste
1 cinnamon stick
2 dry bay leaves

NOTES

- Since the rice will drink up some of the stew juice as the dish sits, one can make some extra sauce (water, tomato paste, salt and spices, heated over the stove), to pour onto individual bowls if desired.
- The actual stuffed zucchini in the picture is for display purposes to show the traditional dish.

INSTRUCTIONS

1. Pick over the rice, removing any bad pieces. Rinse well, then drain. Set aside.
2. In a large pot, covered, cook the onions with the olive oil on low heat for 20 minutes, stirring occasionally.
3. Add the water, tomato paste, and spices (except for the dry mint), then whisk well.
4. Mix in the zucchinis and rice, then bring to a boil. Cook, covered, on low heat, for 10 minutes.
5. Add the tomatoes, garlic, and mint, then stir to mix. Cook, covered, on low for another 15 minutes.
6. In a medium pan or skillet, sauté the meat, stirring frequently until browned. Add the cinnamon stick and bay leaves, then cover and cook on low heat for 15 minutes, stirring occasionally. Remove the bay leaves and cinnamon stick.
7. Add the meat and lemon juice to the pot of stew and stir to mix.
8. Once served, add more freshly squeezed lemon juice if desired.

NUTRITION FACTS PER CUP

106 Kcal	7.6 g Protein	2 g Fat	14.4 g Carbs	2 g Fiber	3 g Sugar

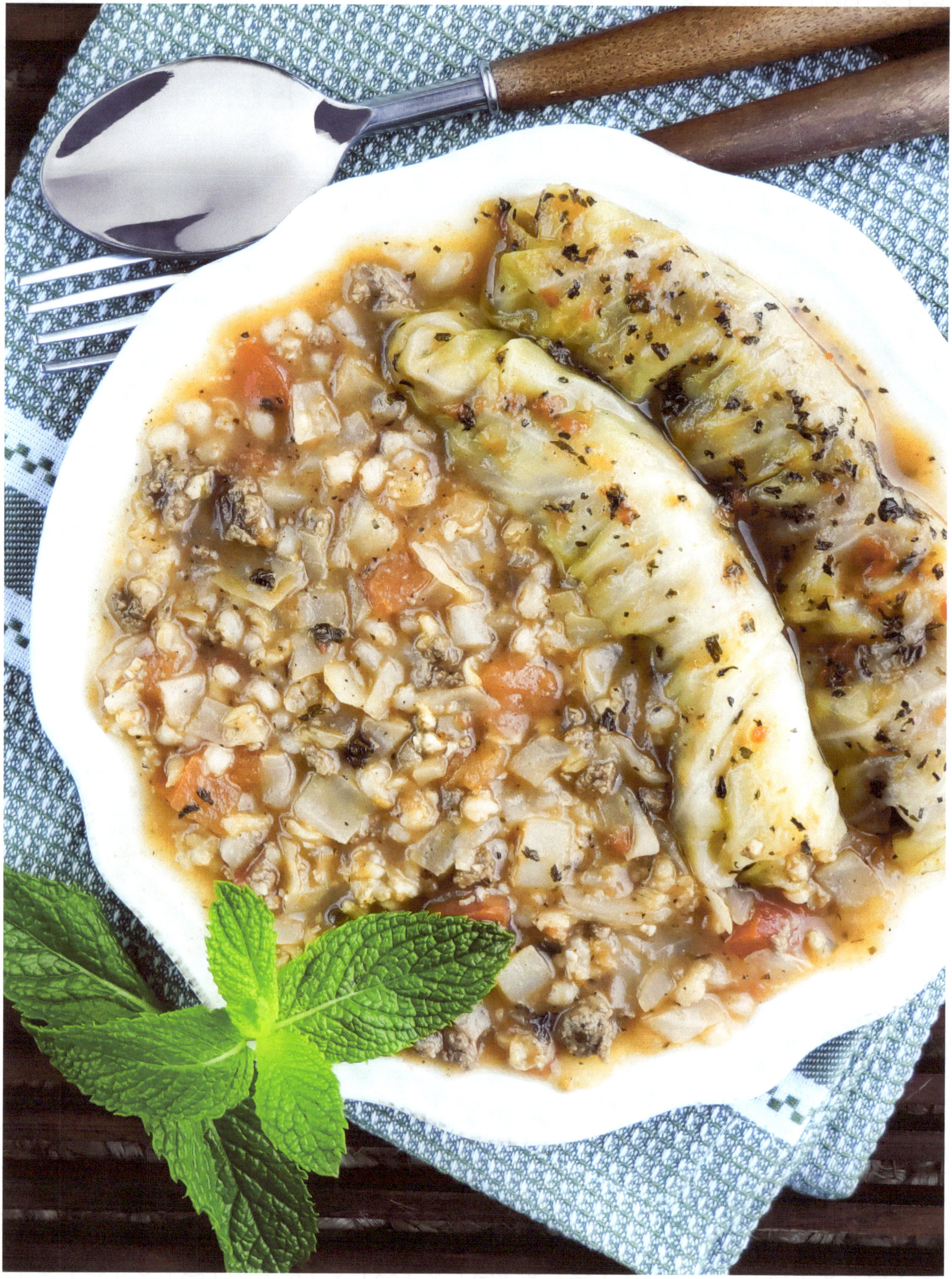

STUFFED CABBAGE ROLLS À LA STEW STYLE

Malfoof Mihsheh ملفوف محشي

My take on traditional stuffed cabbage rolls includes mixing all ingredients together in one large pot (the two cabbage rolls in the picture show what the traditional dish looks like), making it a lot more convenient to make, given the long preparation time it takes to separate cabbage leaves from one another followed by stuffing and rolling them. Traditionally made with not so lean meat and white rice, my healthier version is light and tastes just as good. Unlike traditional Middle Eastern stews, but similar to my stuffed zucchini recipe (on previous page), I cook the rice in the stew pot in order to mimic the flavors and texture of the traditional dish, i.e. somewhat overcooked rice that has soaked up the flavors of the other ingredients.

RECIPE YIELD 20 cups

DF GF EF FF

INGREDIENTS

Raw extra lean beef, ground (500 g)
1 ½ cups dry parboiled brown rice (273 g)
⅔ whole medium white cabbage, finely chopped (1 kg)
5 medium red tomatoes, diced (665 g)
1 medium yellow onion, minced (160 g)
⅓ cup garlic, crushed (75 g)
4 tbsp unsalted tomato paste
1 tbsp olive oil
11 cups water
½ cup lemon juice
1 tbsp dry mint leaves
1 ½ tsp 7-spices
½ tsp cinnamon
2 tsp salt
black pepper, to taste
1 cinnamon stick
2 dry bay leaves

INSTRUCTIONS

1. Pick over the rice, removing any bad pieces. Rinse well, then drain. Set aside.
2. In a large pot, covered, cook the onions with the olive oil on low heat for 20 minutes, stirring occasionally.
3. Add the water, tomato paste, and spices (except for the dry mint), then whisk well.
4. Mix in the cabbage, then bring to a boil. Cook, covered, on low heat, for 10 minutes.
5. Stir in the tomatoes and rice, then cook, covered, on low for another 20 minutes.
6. Add the garlic and mint, then continue cooking, covered, on low heat for another 10 minutes.
7. In a medium pan or skillet, sauté the meat, stirring frequently until browned. Add the cinnamon stick and bay leaves, then cover and cook on low heat for 15 minutes, stirring occasionally. Remove the bay leaves and cinnamon stick.
8. Add the meat and lemon juice to the pot of stew and stir
9. Once served, add more freshly squeezed lemon juice if desired.

See next page for notes »

NUTRITION FACTS PER CUP

120 Kcal	8 g Protein	2 g Fat	17.6 g Carbs	3 g Fiber	3 g Sugar

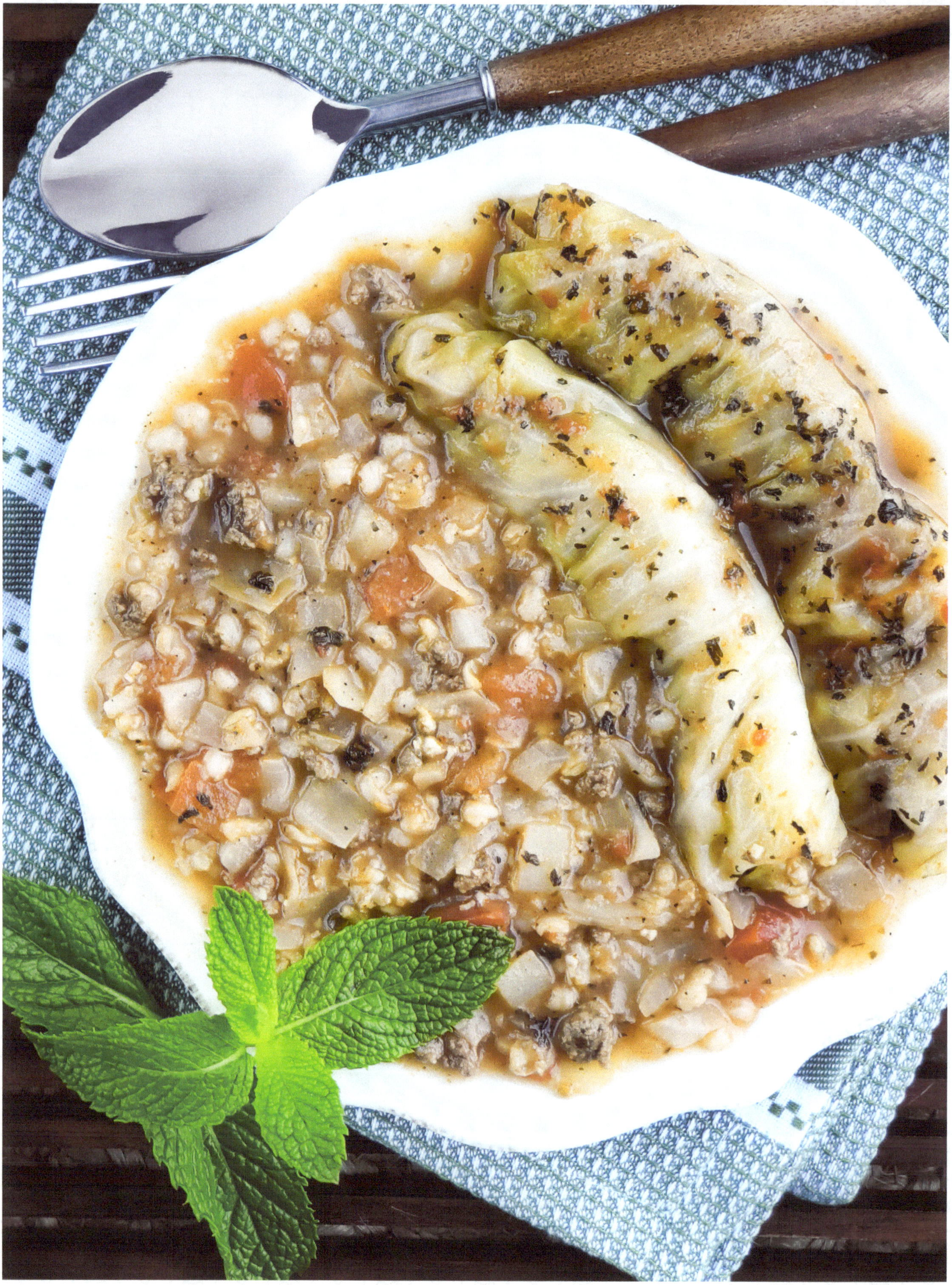

INGREDIENTS

Raw extra lean beef, ground (500 g)
1 ½ cups dry parboiled brown rice (273 g)
⅔ whole medium white cabbage, finely chopped (1 kg)
5 medium red tomatoes, diced (665 g)
1 medium yellow onion, minced (160 g)
⅓ cup garlic, crushed (75 g)
4 tbsp unsalted tomato paste
1 tbsp olive oil
11 cups water
½ cup lemon juice
1 tbsp dry mint leaves
1 ½ tsp 7-spices
½ tsp cinnamon
2 tsp salt
black pepper, to taste
1 cinnamon stick
2 dry bay leaves

NOTES

- Some make this dish without any tomato paste at all. More tomato paste can also be added if desired.
- Since the rice will drink up some of the stew juice as the dish sits, one can make some extra sauce (water, tomato paste, salt, and spices, heated over the stove), to pour onto individual bowls if desired.
- The actual stuffed cabbage rolls in the picture are for display purposes to show the traditional dish.

INSTRUCTIONS

1. Pick over the rice, removing any bad pieces. Rinse well, then drain. Set aside.
2. In a large pot, covered, cook the onions with the olive oil on low heat for 20 minutes, stirring occasionally.
3. Add the water, tomato paste, and spices (except for the dry mint), then whisk well.
4. Mix in the cabbage, then bring to a boil. Cook, covered, on low heat, for 10 minutes.
5. Stir in the tomatoes and rice, then cook, covered, on low for another 20 minutes.
6. Add the garlic and mint, then continue cooking, covered, on low heat for another 10 minutes.
7. In a medium pan or skillet, sauté the meat, stirring frequently until browned. Add the cinnamon stick and bay leaves, then cover and cook on low heat for 15 minutes, stirring occasionally. Remove the bay leaves and cinnamon stick.
8. Add the meat and lemon juice to the pot of stew and stir
9. Once served, add more freshly squeezed lemon juice if desired.

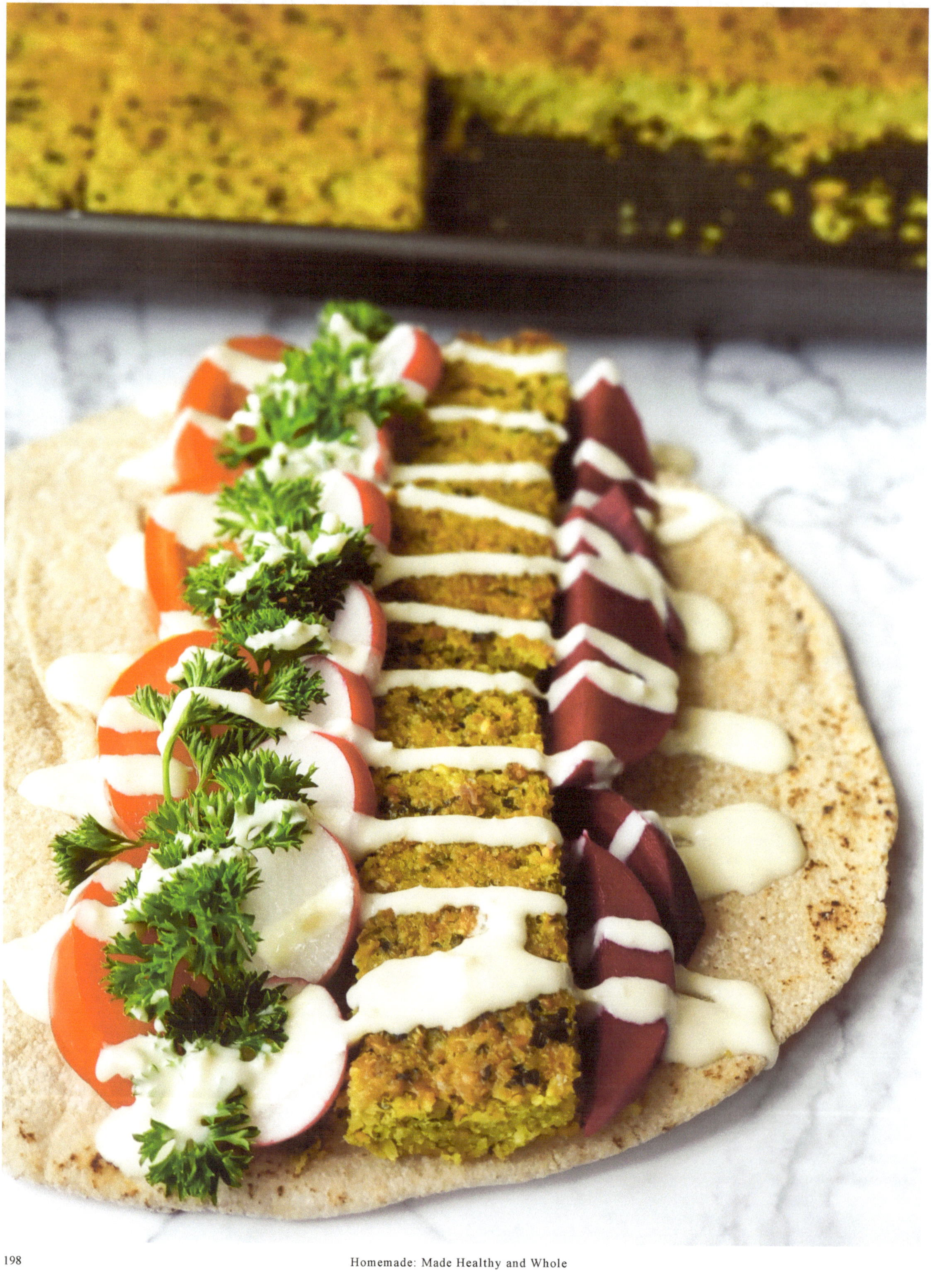

BAKED FALAFEL

Falafel bil Furn فلافل بالفرن

This vegan Middle Eastern street food, traditionally deep-fried, gets a healthy and convenient makeover by being flat-pressed into a pan and baked in the oven. While recipes differ between countries, with most calling for a combination of fava beans and chickpeas, I prefer using only chickpeas in my *falafel* - and I am sure those who are at risk of favism will be pleased!

RECIPE YIELD 15 slices

DF EF V FF

INGREDIENTS

3 cups dry chickpeas (555 g)
⅓ cup dry dark fine bulgur (grade 1) (47 g)
2 medium yellow onions, quartered (320 g)
2 bunches Italian parsley, coarsely chopped (210 g)
1 bunch coriander, coarsely chopped (85 g)
2 tbsp garlic, crushed
2 tbsp olive oil
3 tbsp water
3 ½ tsp cumin
1 ½ tsp turmeric
2 tsp salt
⅓ tsp black pepper
1 tbsp baking powder
1 ½ tsp baking soda
cayenne pepper, optional

RECIPE ALTERNATIVE

For a gluten-free *falafel* recipe, one can omit the bulgur and substitute it with a small boiled potato for better binding of the *falafel* dough.

INSTRUCTIONS

1. Soak the chickpeas and baking soda in water for 16 hours. Drain and rinse, discarding any bad pieces. Set aside.

2. Rinse the bulgur a couple times, then drain, pressing dry. Mix the bulgur and water in a small bowl, then stir in the olive oil, garlic, spices, and baking powder. Set aside.

3. In two batches, process the onions with the parsley and coriander in a large food processor until finely chopped, scraping down the sides as needed. Set aside in a large bowl.

4. Similarly, in two batches, process the hydrated chickpeas and bulgur mix in a food processor until a coarse paste is formed. Add to the bowl containing the onions and leafy greens, then mix well by hand.

5. Grease a large sheet pan (recommended dimensions: 30 cm x 40 cm or similar) with some olive oil. Spread the *falafel* dough onto the pan, gently patting down until the surface is even. Cover with aluminum foil. Bake in a preheated oven at 375 °F for one hour.

6. Switch to a broil setting at 500 °F, uncover the *falafel*, then bake for 10 to 15 minutes, or until the top turns a light golden color (it is optional to spread an extra 1 tbsp of olive oil on the surface for a crunchier top).

7. Enjoy a slice of *falafel* drizzled with *tahini* sauce (recipe on page 139) and eaten plain with tomatoes, parsley, radishes, and pickled turnips, or made into a sandwich on whole wheat pita bread.

NUTRITION FACTS PER SLICE

191 Kcal	9.4 g Protein	4.5 g Fat	31 g Carbs	9 g Fiber	6 g Sugar

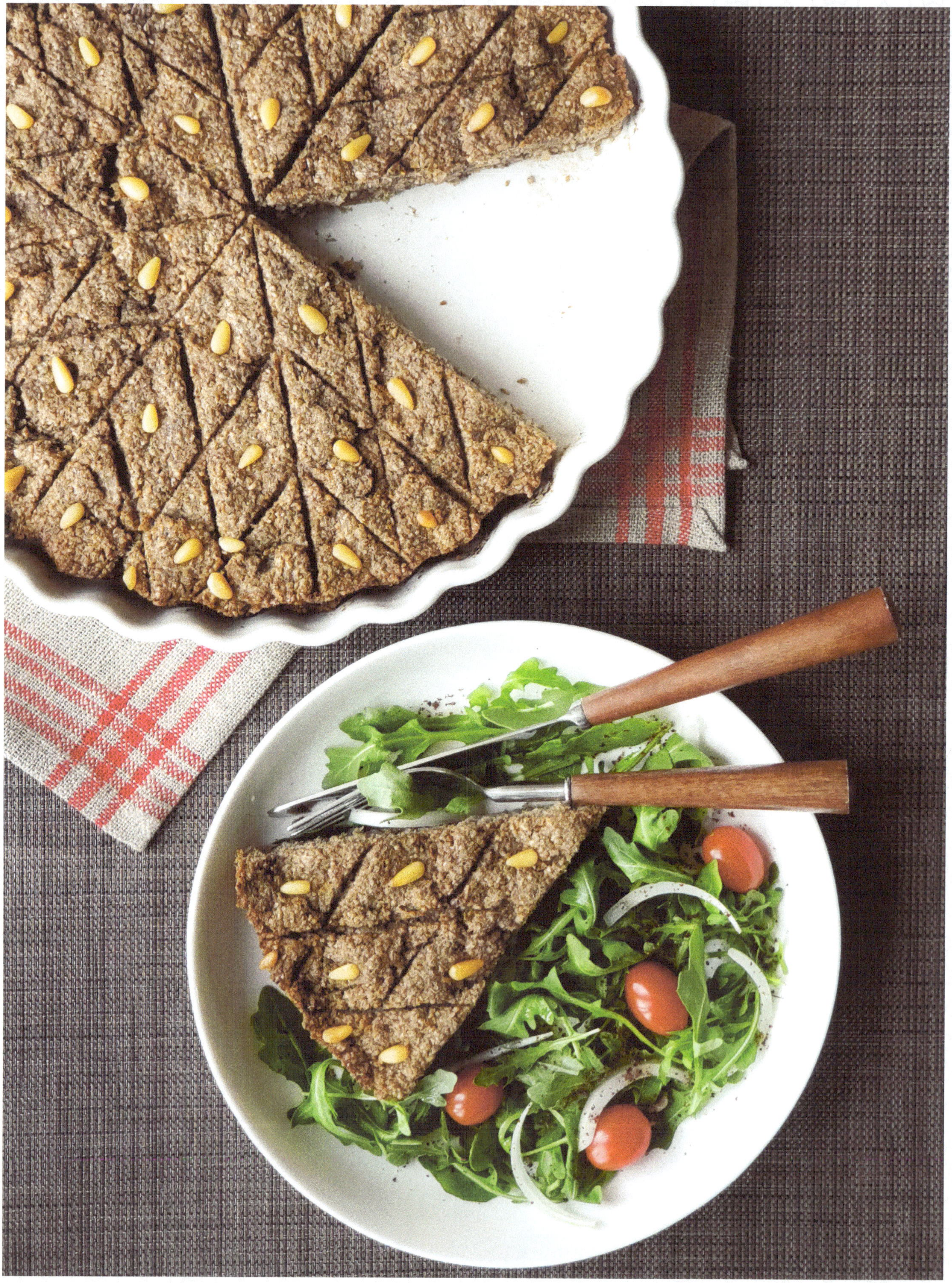

BAKED BEEF KIBBEH

Kibbit Lahmeh bis Sayniyyeh كبّة لحمة بالصّينيّة

Kibbeh is a traditional Middle Eastern dish prepared with four main ingredients: extra lean beef, bulgur, onions, and nuts. It is then flavored with many Middle Eastern spices, namely sumac, cumin, cinnamon, and allspice, as well as fresh herbs including mint, basil, and marjoram. While *kibbeh* is time consuming to prepare and requires some patience, it is definitely worth the effort. Baked *kibbeh* is healthier and much more convenient to prepare compared to *kibbeh* balls that are traditionally fried. My recipe is large, allowing one pan of *kibbeh* to be sent off to the freezer to save time later when a *kibbeh* craving hits!

RECIPE YIELD 20 slices

DF EF FF

INGREDIENTS

Filling

Raw extra lean beef, ground (500 g)
4 large red onions, minced (1,300 g)
⅓ cup pine nuts (45 g)
⅓ cup coarsely chopped walnuts (40 g)
2 ½ tsp pomegranate molasses
2 tbsp olive oil
7 tbsp sumac
3 ½ tsp cinnamon
3 ½ tsp allspice
⅔ tsp cloves
1 ¾ tsp salt
⅓ tsp black pepper
1 cinnamon stick
2 dry bay leaves

Dough

Raw extra lean beef, ground (1 kg)
6 cups dry dark fine bulgur (grade 1) (850 g)
3 medium yellow onions, quartered (480 g)
8 big fresh mint leaves
6 big fresh basil leaves
1 tbsp olive oil
1 cup water
1 tbsp dry marjoram leaves
1 tbsp 7-spices
5 tsp cumin
2 ½ tsp cinnamon
2 ½ tsp allspice
2 ½ tsp salt

INSTRUCTIONS

1. For the filling, cook the onions with the olive oil in a large deep pan or skillet, covered, on low heat for 45 minutes, stirring occasionally. Transfer to a bowl.
2. In the same pan, sauté the meat, stirring frequently until browned. Add the cinnamon stick and bay leaves, then cover and cook on low heat for 15 minutes, stirring occasionally. Remove the bay leaves and cinnamon stick, then transfer to the bowl with cooked onions.
3. Mix in the nuts, pomegranate molasses, and spices. Set aside.
4. For the dough, rinse and drain the bulgur, squeezing it dry. Place in a large bowl.
5. Add the water, olive oil, and spices, then stir to mix. Set aside.
6. In a large food processor, blend the onions and herbs until finely minced, scraping down the sides as needed. Transfer to the bowl of bulgur.
7. Add the meat to the bowl, then knead by hand, until all ingredients have been mixed.
8. In 6 batches, process the *kibbeh* dough in a food processor, scraping down the sides as needed, and blending well until smooth (this step will take some time and patience. The longer one processes the dough, the smoother it will get).

Instructions continued on the next page »

NUTRITION FACTS PER SLICE

339 Kcal	23 g Protein	9 g Fat	45 g Carbs	9 g Fiber	6 g Sugar

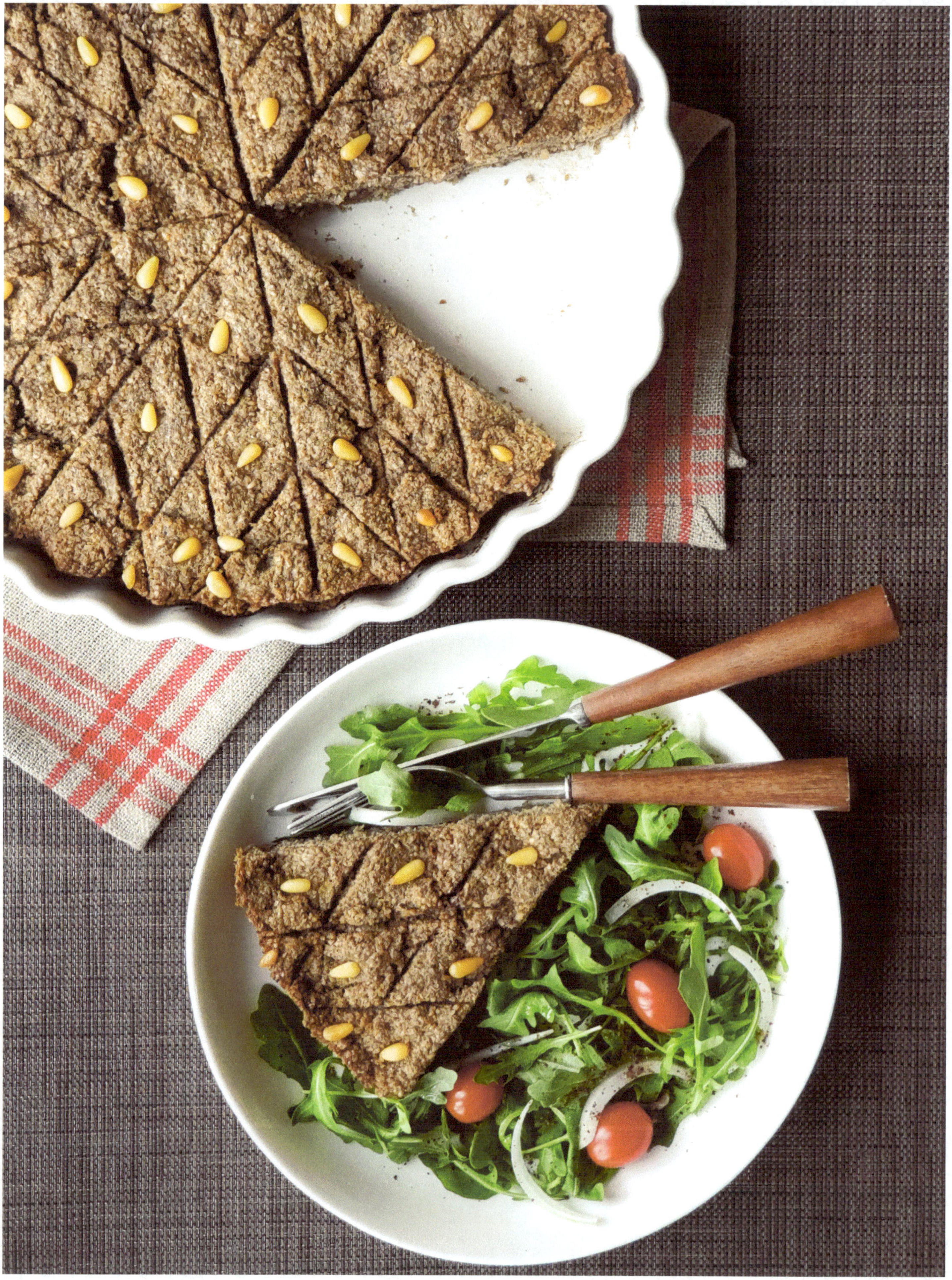

INGREDIENTS

Filling
Raw extra lean beef, ground (500 g)
4 large red onions, minced (1,300 g)
⅓ cup pine nuts (45 g)
⅓ cup coarsely chopped walnuts (40 g)
2 ½ tsp pomegranate molasses
2 tbsp olive oil
7 tbsp sumac
3 ½ tsp cinnamon
3 ½ tsp allspice
⅔ tsp cloves
1 ¾ tsp salt
⅓ tsp black pepper
1 cinnamon stick
2 dry bay leaves

Dough
Raw extra lean beef, ground (1 kg)
6 cups dry dark fine bulgur (grade 1) (850 g)
3 medium yellow onions, quartered (480 g)
8 big fresh mint leaves
6 big fresh basil leaves
1 tbsp olive oil
1 cup water
1 tbsp dry marjoram leaves
1 tbsp 7-spices
5 tsp cumin
2 ½ tsp cinnamon
2 ½ tsp allspice
2 ½ tsp salt

NOTE

❀ Cover the uncooked pan with foil, then place in the freezer. For future cooking of the frozen *kibbeh*: remove from the freezer 30 minutes before baking. Remove any ice on the under part of the foil as well as any formed ice crystals on the surface of the kibbeh. Brush with a bit of olive oil, then cover and bake at 375 °F for 50 minutes. Uncover, then bake for another 30 minutes. Broil at 500 °F for 5 minutes.

INSTRUCTIONS

1. For the filling, cook the onions with the olive oil in a large deep pan or skillet, covered, on low heat for 45 minutes, stirring occasionally. Transfer to a bowl.

2. In the same pan, sauté the meat, stirring frequently until browned. Add the cinnamon stick and bay leaves, then cover and cook on low heat for 15 minutes, stirring every 5 minutes. Remove the bay leaves and cinnamon stick, then transfer to the bowl with cooked onions.

3. Mix in the nuts, pomegranate molasses, and spices. Set aside.

4. For the dough, rinse and drain the bulgur, squeezing it dry. Place in a large bowl.

5. Add the water, olive oil, and spices, then stir to mix. Set aside.

6. In a large food processor, blend the onions and herbs until finely minced, scraping down the sides as needed. Transfer to the bowl of bulgur.

7. Add the meat to the bowl, then knead by hand, until all ingredients have been mixed.

8. In 6 batches, process the *kibbeh* dough in a food processor, scraping down the sides as needed, and blending well until smooth (this step will take some time and patience. The longer one processes the dough, the smoother it will get).

9. Grease the pans to be used for baking the *kibbeh*. My recommendation is 2 deep baking pans (25 cm x 35 cm dimension or similar), or 2 circular pans (100 cm diameter or similar).

10. Knead the processed dough by hand, blending the batches together, then divide the dough into equal batches depending on the number of pans to be used. Further divide each pan batch in half.

11. Spread half of the dough for each pan onto the greased surface, patting down with one's hands until the dough is evenly spread (dipping one's hands in water helps prevent the dough from sticking to the hands, and allows for smoother spreading).

12. Divide the *kibbeh* filling between the pans, spreading evenly onto the whole surface.

13. For the remaining *kibbeh* dough, flatten small patches between the hands and lay on top of the filling. With wetted hands, join the patches and mold them together, patting down gently, until a uniform surface is formed (the more one works with it the smoother it will turn out).

14. Score the top layer with the desired design using a sharp knife, lightly wetted with water. If desired, add pine nuts for garnish and brush some olive oil on the surface (to add more crunchiness during baking).

15. Cover with aluminum foil, then bake in a preheated oven at 375 °F for 30 minutes. Uncover, then bake for another 20 minutes. Broil at 500 °F for 5 minutes.

16. *Kibbeh* is traditionally served with either plain yogurt, a yogurt cucumber salad (recipe on page 87), or any vegetable salad.

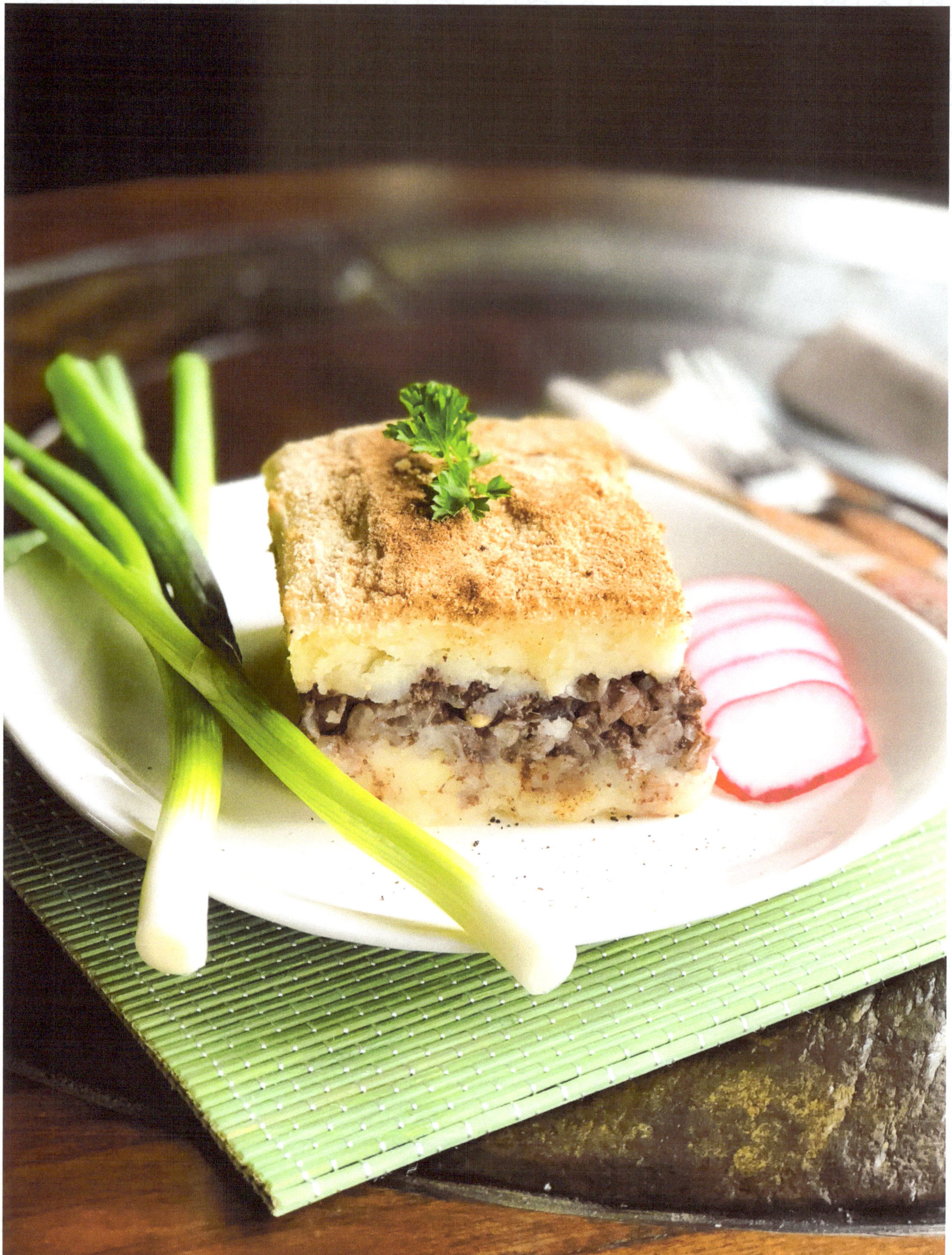

BAKED POTATO KIBBEH

Kibbit Batata wa Lahmeh bis Sayniyyeh كبّة بطاطا و لحمة بالصّينيّة

This dish is similar to an egg-free potato soufflé. It is a less-meaty traditional variation to the famous baked beef *kibbeh* (on the previous page); the filling contains similar ingredients, while the upper and lower layers of meat and bulgur are substituted with mashed potatoes (and sometimes bulgur). While mashed potatoes are often notorious for being rich in butter or cream, I keep my mashed potatoes light and simple with heart-healthy olive oil and no dairy. To add fiber to this dish, I like preparing the mashed potatoes with their skins, as well as using ground toasted whole wheat Arabic bread instead of ground *kaak* for sprinkling on top (as mentioned on page 13, *kaak* are simple breadsticks that are made from refined flour).

RECIPE YIELD 16 slices

DF EF

INGREDIENTS

Filling

Raw extra lean beef, ground (500 g)
4 large white onions, minced (1,280 g)
⅔ cup pine nuts (90 g)
1 tbsp olive oil
6 tbsp sumac
1 tbsp cinnamon
1 tbsp allspice
½ tsp cloves
1 ½ tsp salt
¼ tsp black pepper
1 cinnamon stick
2 dry bay leaves

Mashed Potato Layer

6 medium russet potatoes (with skin) (2.5 kg)
1 tbsp olive oil
1 ½ cups water
1 tsp garlic salt
2 tsp salt
¼ tsp black pepper
1 loaf whole wheat Arabic bread (medium size) (73 g)

INSTRUCTIONS

1. Separate the pita bread loaves into 2 individual halves. Place in a preheated oven at 350 °F, then toast for 7 to 10 minutes (until lightly browned and completely toasted). Let cool, then break up (by hand) into small pieces. Place in a food blender and process until ground up into fine breadcrumbs. Set aside.

2. For the filling, cook the onions with 1 tbsp olive oil in a large deep pan or skillet, covered, on low heat for 35 minutes, stirring occasionally. Transfer to a bowl.

3. In the same pan, sauté the meat, stirring frequently until browned. Add the cinnamon stick and bay leaves, then cover and cook on low heat for 15 minutes, stirring occasionally. Remove the bay leaves and cinnamon stick, then transfer to the bowl with the cooked onions.

4. Add the pine nuts and spices to the meat and onions, then stir to mix. Cover, and set aside.

5. For the potato layer, place the potatoes in a large pot of cold water with 1 tsp salt (make sure the water covers all the potatoes for even cooking), then bring to a boil. Cook, covered, on low heat for 40 to 45 minutes (until soft but not mushy). Drain away the water.

Instructions continued on the next page »

NUTRITION FACTS PER SLICE

270 Kcal	13 g Protein	7 g Fat	41.6 g Carbs	5.6 g Fiber	5 g Sugar

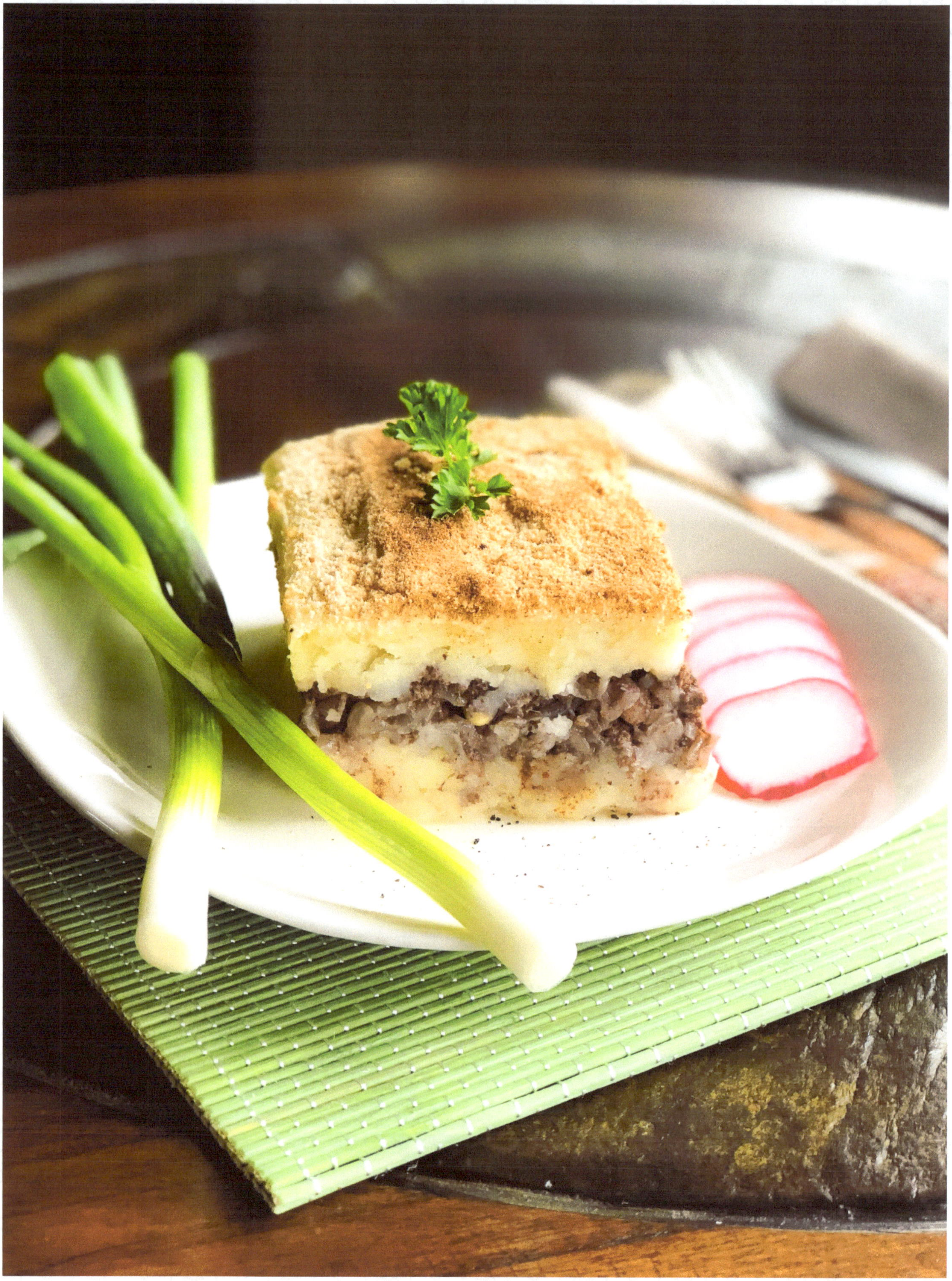

INGREDIENTS

Filling
Raw extra lean beef, ground (500 g)
4 large white onions, minced (1,280 g)
⅔ cup pine nuts (90 g)
1 tbsp olive oil
6 tbsp sumac
1 tbsp cinnamon
1 tbsp allspice
½ tsp cloves
1 ½ tsp salt
¼ tsp black pepper
1 cinnamon stick
2 dry bay leaves

Mashed Potato Layer
6 medium russet potatoes (with skin) (2.5 kg)
1 tbsp olive oil
1 ½ cups water
1 tsp garlic salt
2 tsp salt
¼ tsp black pepper
1 loaf whole wheat Arabic bread (medium size) (73 g)

NOTES

- Do not use a food processor, blender, or electric mixer while mashing up potatoes as this will mash them too aggressively, and they will end up being sticky and stretchy.
- For a thicker result, one can use a large deep baking pan (recommended dimensions: 28 cm x 37 cm or similar) instead of the 2 smaller pans.

INSTRUCTIONS

1. Separate the pita bread loaves into 2 individual halves. Place in a preheated oven at 350 °F, then toast for 7 to 10 minutes (until lightly browned and completely toasted). Let cool, then break up (by hand) into small pieces. Place in a food blender and process until ground up into fine breadcrumbs. Set aside.

2. For the filling, cook the onions with 1 tbsp olive oil in a large deep pan or skillet, covered, on low heat for 35 minutes, stirring occasionally. Transfer to a bowl.

3. In the same pan, sauté the meat, stirring frequently until browned. Add the cinnamon stick and bay leaves, then cover and cook on low heat for 15 minutes, stirring occasionally. Remove the bay leaves and cinnamon stick, then transfer to the bowl with the cooked onions.

4. Add the pine nuts and spices to the meat and onions, then stir to mix. Cover, and set aside.

5. For the potato layer, place the potatoes in a large pot of cold water with 1 tsp salt (make sure the water covers all the potatoes for even cooking), then bring to a boil. Cook, covered, on low heat for 40 to 45 minutes (until soft but not mushy). Drain away the water.

6. Using a knife, slice up the boiled potatoes, then add the water, olive oil, spices, and the remaining 1 tsp salt.

7. Using a whisk or potato masher, gently mash the potatoes until the ingredients are blended and the potatoes are well mashed; some potato lumps are okay and will not matter for this dish.

8. Divide the mashed potato into two equal portions.

9. Grease 2 deep baking pans (recommended dimensions: 23.5 cm x 33.5 cm or similar). Divide the potato mixture in half, then spread each one quarter of the potato mixture onto the pan, lightly patting it down until it is evenly spread.

10. Divide the meat mixture between the 2 pans, spreading evenly over the mashed potatoes. Add the remaining potato mixture over the meat, then spread carefully and evenly, patting down with one's hands.

11. Sprinkle the breadcrumbs evenly over the entire top of the potato layers.

12. In a preheated oven at 350 °F, bake uncovered for 20 minutes. Switch the oven to a broil setting at 500 °F and broil for 10 minutes or until the top has turned light golden brown.

13. Let cool for 10 minutes before serving. Enjoy with fresh vegetables or a side of salad.

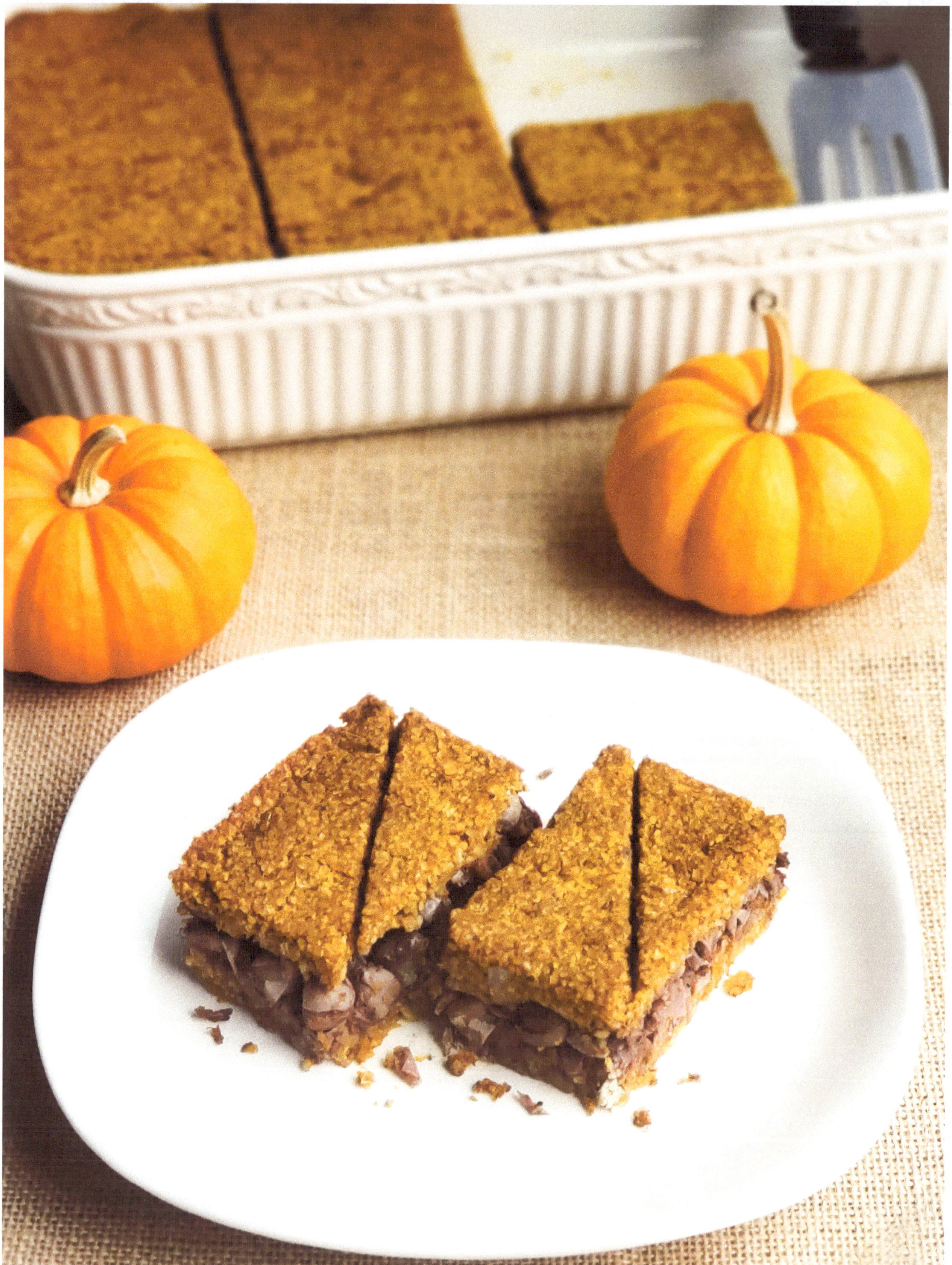

BAKED PUMPKIN KIBBEH

Kibbit Laqteen bis Sayniyyeh كبّة لقطين بالصّينيّة

This dish is a vegan version of the famous baked beef *kibbeh* (recipe on page 201), commonly made in Lebanon during the month of lent. Chickpeas substitute for meat in the filling, and pumpkin substitutes for the meat in the outer layers. This recipe is large, allowing for one pan to be sent off to the freezer to save time later when a pumpkin *kibbeh* craving hits!

RECIPE YIELD 20 slices

DF EF V FF

INGREDIENTS

Filling

2 cups dry chickpeas (370 g)
3 large red onions, minced (1,125 g)
⅔ cup pine nuts (90 g)
⅔ cup coarsely chopped walnuts (80 g)
2 tsp pomegranate molasses
3 tbsp olive oil
3 tbsp sumac
2 tsp cinnamon
2 tsp allspice
½ tsp cloves
1 ½ tsp salt
¼ tsp black pepper
1 tsp baking soda

Dough

4 cups dry dark fine bulgur (grade 1) (568 g)
6 cups pumpkin purée (canned) (1,350 g)
2 medium yellow onions, quartered (320 g)
1 tbsp olive oil
2 tbsp whole wheat flour
4 tsp cumin
2 tsp dry marjoram leaves
2 tsp 7-spices
2 tsp cinnamon
2 tsp allspice
2 tsp salt

INSTRUCTIONS

1. For the filling, soak the chickpeas and the baking soda in water for 12 hours. Drain and rinse, discarding any bad pieces.
2. Transfer the chickpeas to a pot, cover with water, then bring to a boil. Skim off the white foam that floats to the surface, then cook, covered, on low heat for 30 minutes (or until tender). Uncover and place the lid ajar.
3. Cook the onions in a large deep pan or skillet, covered, on low heat, for 45 minutes.
4. Drain the chickpeas, then add to the onions. Add the nuts, pomegranate molasses, and spices, then stir to mix. Set aside.
5. For the dough, rinse and drain the bulgur, squeezing it dry. Place in a large bowl.
6. Add the pumpkin purée, olive oil, flour, and spices. Mix and set aside.
7. In a large food processor, blend the onions until finely minced. Transfer to the bowl of bulgur and pumpkin.
8. Stir well to mix, until all ingredients have been blended.
9. Grease 2 deep baking pans (recommended dimensions: 23.5 cm x 33.5 cm or similar).

Instructions continued on the next page »

NUTRITION FACTS PER SLICE

322 Kcal	11 g Protein	10 g Fat	51 g Carbs	12.5 g Fiber	9 g Sugar

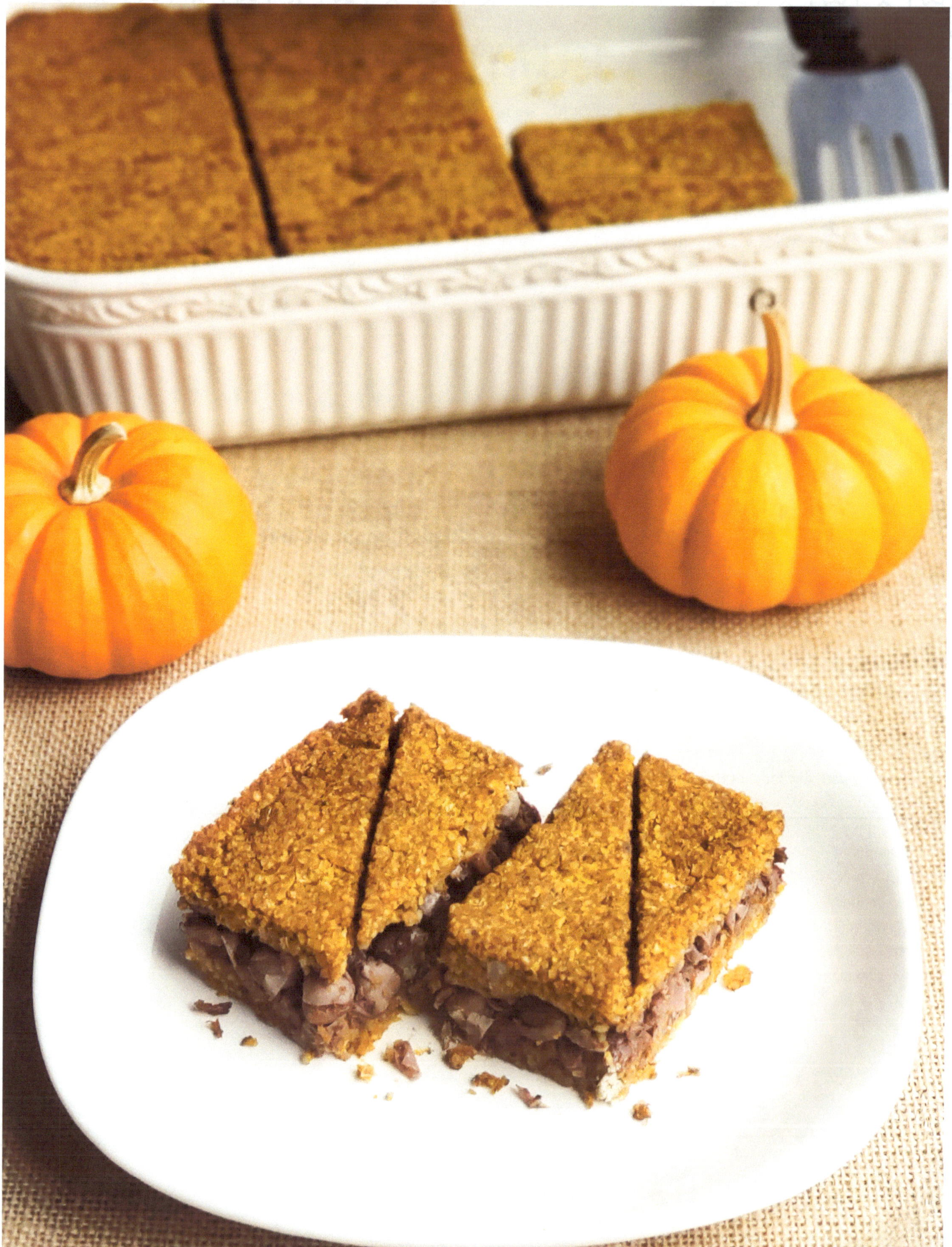

INGREDIENTS

Filling
2 cups dry chickpeas (370 g)
3 large red onions, minced (1,125 g)
⅔ cup pine nuts (90 g)
⅔ cup coarsely chopped walnuts (80 g)
2 tsp pomegranate molasses
3 tbsp olive oil
3 tbsp sumac
2 tsp cinnamon
2 tsp allspice
½ tsp cloves
1 ½ tsp salt
¼ tsp black pepper
1 tsp baking soda

Dough
4 cups dry dark fine bulgur (grade 1) (568 g)
6 cups pumpkin purée (canned) (1,350 g)
2 medium yellow onions, quartered (320 g)
1 tbsp olive oil
2 tbsp whole wheat flour
4 tsp cumin
2 tsp dry marjoram leaves
2 tsp 7-spices
2 tsp cinnamon
2 tsp allspice
2 tsp salt

NOTES

❁ In pumpkin season, it is great to make this dish from fresh pumpkins, but make sure to strain the cooked pumpkin of extra water to make a thick purée.

❁ Cover the uncooked pan with foil, then place in the freezer. For future cooking of the frozen *kibbeh*: remove from the freezer 30 minutes before baking. Remove any formed ice crystals on the surface of the *kibbeh*. Bake at 350 °F, uncovered, for 55 minutes, then broil at 500 °F for 5 minutes.

INSTRUCTIONS

1. For the filling, soak the chickpeas and the baking soda in water for 12 hours. Drain and rinse, discarding any bad pieces.

2. Transfer the chickpeas to a pot, cover with water, then bring to a boil. Skim off the white foam that floats to the surface, then cook, covered, on low heat for 30 minutes (or until tender). Uncover and place the lid ajar.

3. Cook the onions in a large deep pan or skillet, covered, on low heat, for 45 minutes.

4. Drain the chickpeas, then add to the onions. Add the nuts, pomegranate molasses, and spices, then stir to mix. Set aside.

5. For the dough, rinse and drain the bulgur, squeezing it dry. Place in a large bowl.

6. Add the pumpkin purée, olive oil, flour, and spices. Mix and set aside.

7. In a large food processor, blend the onions until finely minced. Transfer to the bowl of bulgur and pumpkin.

8. Stir well to mix, until all ingredients have been blended.

9. Grease 2 deep baking pans (recommended dimensions: 23.5 cm x 33.5 cm or similar).

10. Divide the dough into equal batches depending on the number of pans to be used. Further divide each pan batch in half.

11. Spread half of the dough for each pan onto the greased surface, smoothening out with one's hands until the dough is evenly spread.

12. Divide the *kibbeh* filling between the pans, spreading evenly onto the whole surface.

13. For the remaining *kibbeh* dough, drop small batches on top of the filling. Smoothen out until the dough is evenly spread.

14. Score the top layer with the desired design using a sharp knife, lightly wetted with water.

15. Bake in a preheated oven at 350 °F, uncovered, for 35 minutes, then broil at 500 °F for 5 minutes.

16. Serve with green onions or a side of salad.

RECIPE ALTERNATIVES

❁ For a less tangy *kibbeh* flavor and a warmer spice flavor, one can omit the sumac from the filling, bump up the cloves to 1 tsp, and add ⅓ tsp nutmeg.

❁ Many add a green leafy vegetable to the filling. I often add Swiss chard or spinach. Use about 175 g of the chopped vegetable and do the following modifications to the filling ingredients: bump up the cinnamon to 2 ¼ tsp, the allspice to 2 ¼ tsp, the salt to 1 ⅔ tsp, the black pepper to ⅓ tsp, and the pomegranate molasses to 1 tbsp. Add the vegetable to the onions at 35 minutes into cooking, then cook for 10 minutes.

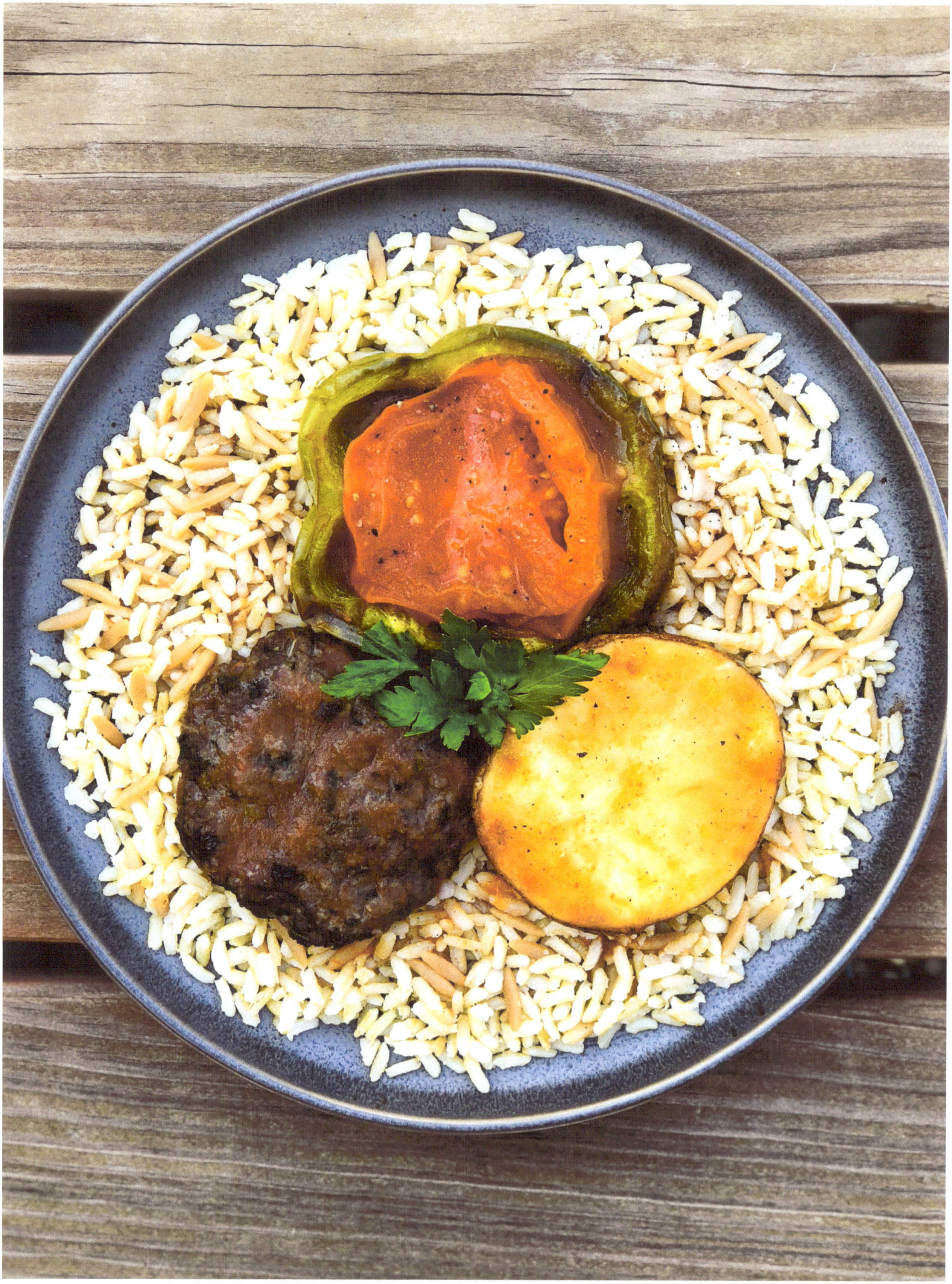

BAKED KAFTA IN TOMATO SAUCE

Kafta bis Sayniyyeh كفتة بالصّينيّة

Kafta is Middle Eastern spiced lean ground beef (some mix beef and lamb together, or just use lamb) combined with chopped parsley and onions. In warmer weather, *kafta* is commonly put on skewers and grilled outdoors. For a tomato sauce casserole, patties of *kafta* are layered with slices of potatoes, tomatoes, and bell peppers (some also add sliced onions), covered with a seasoned tomato sauce and baked in the oven, to be eaten with white rice. Traditionally, the meat patties as well as the potato slices are fried prior to layering with the vegetables. I pre-bake my patties and potatoes separately, before layering with green peppers and tomatoes, then top with a warm tomato sauce rich in cinnamon and allspice.

RECIPE YIELD 20 slices

DF GF EF FF

INGREDIENTS

Kafta

Raw extra lean beef, ground (1 kg)
1 large white onion, quartered (320 g)
6 medium green onion stalks, chopped (95 g)
2 bunches Italian Parsley, coarsely chopped (210 g)
1 tbsp olive oil
1 ½ tbsp cinnamon
1 ½ tbsp allspice
1 ½ tbsp 7-spices
2 ½ tsp salt

Vegetables

5 medium red tomatoes, sliced into circles (665 g)
4 medium green bell peppers, sliced into circles (660 g)
2 large russet potatoes (with skin), sliced into circles (1,180 g)

Sauce

± 5 cups water
1 cup + 2 tbsp unsalted tomato paste (270 g)
1 tbsp olive oil
3 ½ tsp cinnamon
1 ½ tsp allspice
½ tsp salt
⅛ tsp black pepper

INSTRUCTIONS

1. In 2 batches, process the *kafta* vegetables in a large food processor, scraping down the sides as needed, until minced.

2. Place the ground beef in a bowl, then add the *kafta* spices. Pour in the olive oil, add the minced vegetables, then knead until well mixed. Cover, then refrigerate for at least 30 minutes (to decrease stickiness while forming the patties).

3. Prepare the vegetables for the layering, slicing each tomato into 4 slices, each green pepper into 5 slices, and each potato into 10 slices (in order to yield 20 slices of each of the vegetables). Set the tomatoes aside.

4. Place the potato slices right on the middle oven rack and bake at 450 °F for 20 minutes. Set aside on a plate and cover.

5. Afterwards, place the bell pepper slices right on the middle oven rack and bake at the same temperature for 15 minutes. Set aside on a plate and cover.

6. Form 20 round *kafta* patties (using a slightly heaping ⅓ cup of *kafta* for each), then lay out onto 2 large sheet pans (recommended dimensions: 30 cm x 40 cm or similar). Bake in a preheated oven at 375 °F for 20 minutes.

Instructions continued on the next page »

NUTRITION FACTS PER SERVING

162 Kcal	13.4 g Protein	4 g Fat	20 g Carbs	4 g Fiber	3 g Sugar

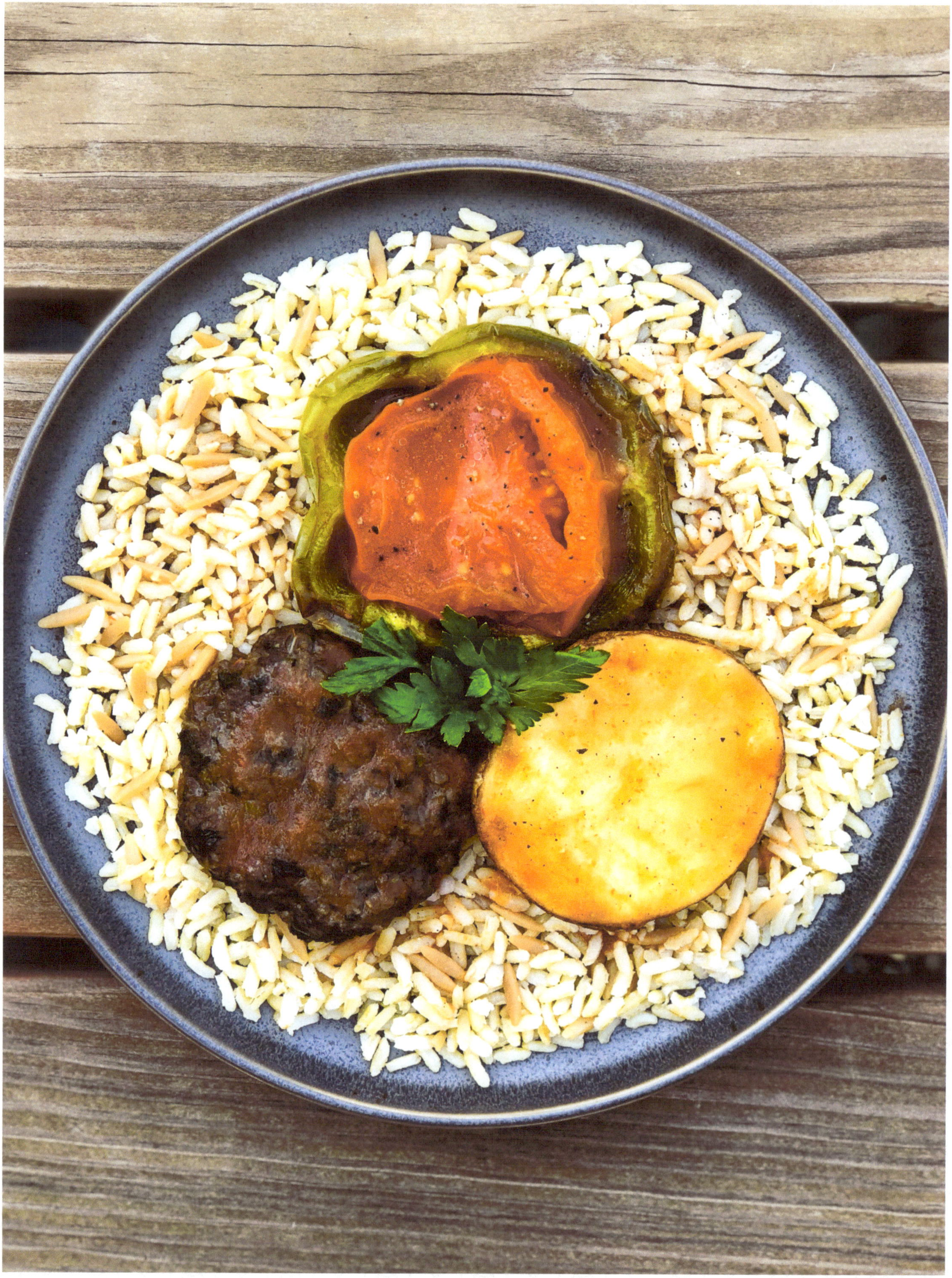

INGREDIENTS

Kafta
Raw extra lean beef, ground (1 kg)
1 large white onion, quartered (320 g)
6 medium green onion stalks, chopped (95 g)
2 bunches Italian Parsley, coarsely chopped (210 g)
1 tbsp olive oil
1 ½ tbsp cinnamon
1 ½ tbsp allspice
1 ½ tbsp 7-spices
2 ½ tsp salt

Vegetables
5 medium red tomatoes, sliced into circles (665 g)
4 medium green bell peppers, sliced into circles (660 g)
2 large russet potatoes (with skin), sliced into circles (1,180 g)

Sauce
± 5 cups water
1 cup + 2 tbsp unsalted tomato paste (270 g)
1 tbsp olive oil
3 ½ tsp cinnamon
1 ½ tsp allspice
½ tsp salt
⅛ tsp black pepper

NOTES

❁ Prepared *kafta* meat is freezer friendly raw or cooked.

❁ This dish can be sent off to the freezer soon after the prepared ingredients have been layered in the pan and topped with the prepared tomato sauce (allow the sauce to cool, though). Thus, instead of placing the ready ingredients in one pan, one can divide them up into 2 smaller pans, and send one off to the freezer (to be baked at a later time).

❁ Each serving consists of 1 *kafta* patty, 1 tomato slice, 1 green pepper slice, and 1 potato slice, topped with ~ 4 tbsp sauce.

INSTRUCTIONS

1. In 2 batches, process the *kafta* vegetables in a large food processor, scraping down the sides as needed, until minced.

2. Place the ground beef in a bowl, then add the *kafta* spices. Pour in the olive oil, add the minced vegetables, then knead until well mixed. Cover, then refrigerate for at least 30 minutes (to decrease stickiness while forming the patties).

3. Prepare the vegetables for the layering, slicing each tomato into 4 slices, each green pepper into 5 slices, and each potato into 10 slices (in order to yield 20 slices of each of the vegetables). Set the tomatoes aside.

4. Place the potato slices right on the middle oven rack and bake at 450 °F for 20 minutes. Set aside on a plate and cover.

5. Afterwards, place the bell pepper slices right on the middle oven rack and bake at the same temperature for 15 minutes. Set aside on a plate and cover.

6. Form 20 round *kafta* patties (using a slightly heaping ⅓ cup of *kafta* for each), then lay out onto 2 large sheet pans (recommended dimensions: 30 cm x 40 cm or similar). Bake in a preheated oven at 375 °F for 20 minutes.

7. Drain the meat broth (~ ⅔ cup) into a medium saucepan. Add the water (adjust the amount of water depending on how much meat broth is obtained, i.e. make sure total liquid equals 5 ⅔ cups), and the rest of the sauce ingredients, then whisk well. Cover, then bring to a boil. Cook, covered, on low heat for 20 minutes, stirring occasionally.

8. Using a deep baking pan (recommended dimensions: 28 cm x 37 cm or similar), pour some of the sauce on the bottom of the pan, lay out the *kafta* patties in one layer, then top with a layer of potatoes, then a layer of bell peppers, then add the tomatoes. Pour the rest of the sauce evenly over the top, then cover with foil. Bake in a preheated oven at 375 °F for 25 minutes.

9. Serve with a side of brown rice (recipe on page 129) (some enjoy eating it with pita bread instead of rice).

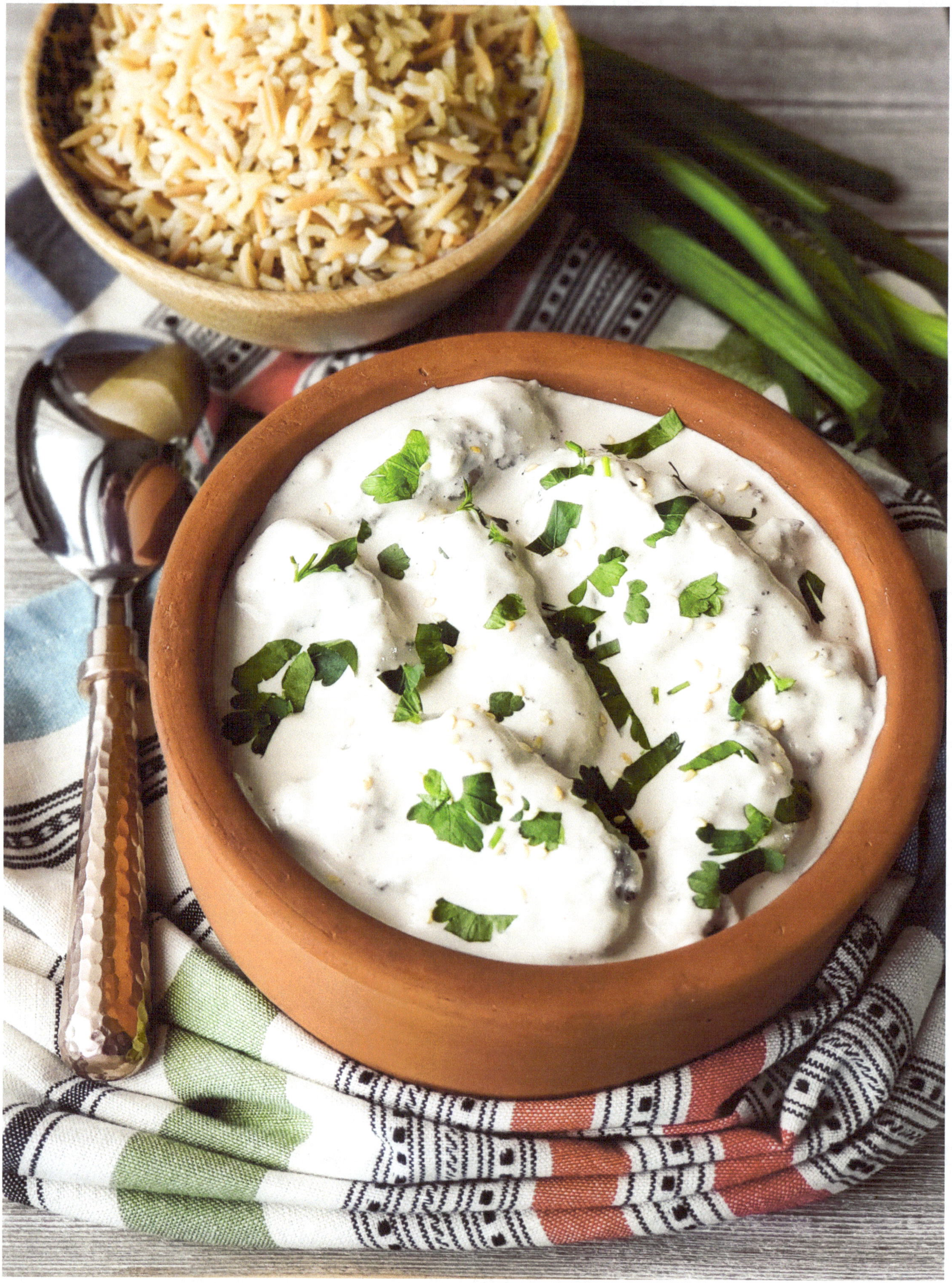

BAKED KAFTA IN TAHINI SAUCE

Kafta bit Tahini كفتة بالطّحينة

Kafta (as described in the previous recipe) is spiced lean ground beef combined with chopped parsley and onions. For this *kafta* casserole dish, *kafta* patties are covered with a flavorful garlic and lemon *tahini* sauce lightly flavored with warm spices. Traditionally, the meat patties are fried, and some add fried potato slices to the dish as well. As with all my other recipes, I avoid frying any ingredient, and rely solely on the baking process to bring out the flavors in the food.

RECIPE YIELD 15 servings

DF GF EF FF

INGREDIENTS

Kafta

Raw extra lean beef, ground (1 kg)
1 large white onion, quartered (320 g)
6 medium green onion stalks, chopped (95 g)
2 bunches Italian Parsley, coarsely chopped (210 g)
1 tbsp olive oil
1 ½ tbsp cinnamon
1 ½ tbsp allspice
1 ½ tbsp 7-spices
2 ½ tsp salt

Sauce

± 3 cups hot water
1 ½ cups tahini (360 g)
¾ cup lemon juice
1 tbsp garlic, crushed
⅓ tsp cinnamon
⅓ tsp allspice
⅓ tsp 7-spices
⅓ tsp salt

INSTRUCTIONS

1. In 2 batches, process the *kafta* vegetables in a large food processor, scraping down the sides as needed, until minced.

2. Place the ground beef in a bowl, then add the *kafta* spices. Pour in the olive oil, add the minced vegetables, then knead until well mixed. Cover, then refrigerate for at least 30 minutes (to decrease stickiness while forming the patties).

3. Form 30 oval *kafta* patties (using a ¼ cup of *kafta* for each), then lay out onto 2 large sheet pans (recommended dimensions: 30 cm x 40 cm or similar). Bake in a preheated oven at 375 °F for 20 minutes.

4. Drain the meat broth (~ ⅔ cup) into a bowl. Add the hot water (adjust the amount of water depending on how much meat broth is obtained, i.e. make sure total liquid equals 3 ⅔ cups), and the rest of the sauce ingredients, then whisk well. Process in 2 batches in a food blender until smooth and homogenous.

5. Using a deep baking pan (recommended dimensions: 25 cm x 35 cm or similar), pour some of the sauce on the bottom of the pan, lay out some of the *kafta* patties, then cover with another layer of sauce. Lay out some more patties, then cover with sauce. Repeat these steps until all the *kafta* patties and sauce have been used up (make sure the last layer of patties is well covered in sauce). Cover with foil, then bake in a preheated oven at 375 °F for 20 minutes.

6. Garnish with fresh parsley and serve with a side of brown rice (recipe on page 129) (some enjoy eating it with pita bread instead of rice), as well as fresh green onions or a salad if desired.

See next page for notes »

NUTRITION FACTS PER SERVING

259 Kcal	19 g Protein	17 g Fat	11 g Carbs	4 g Fiber	1.5 g Sugar

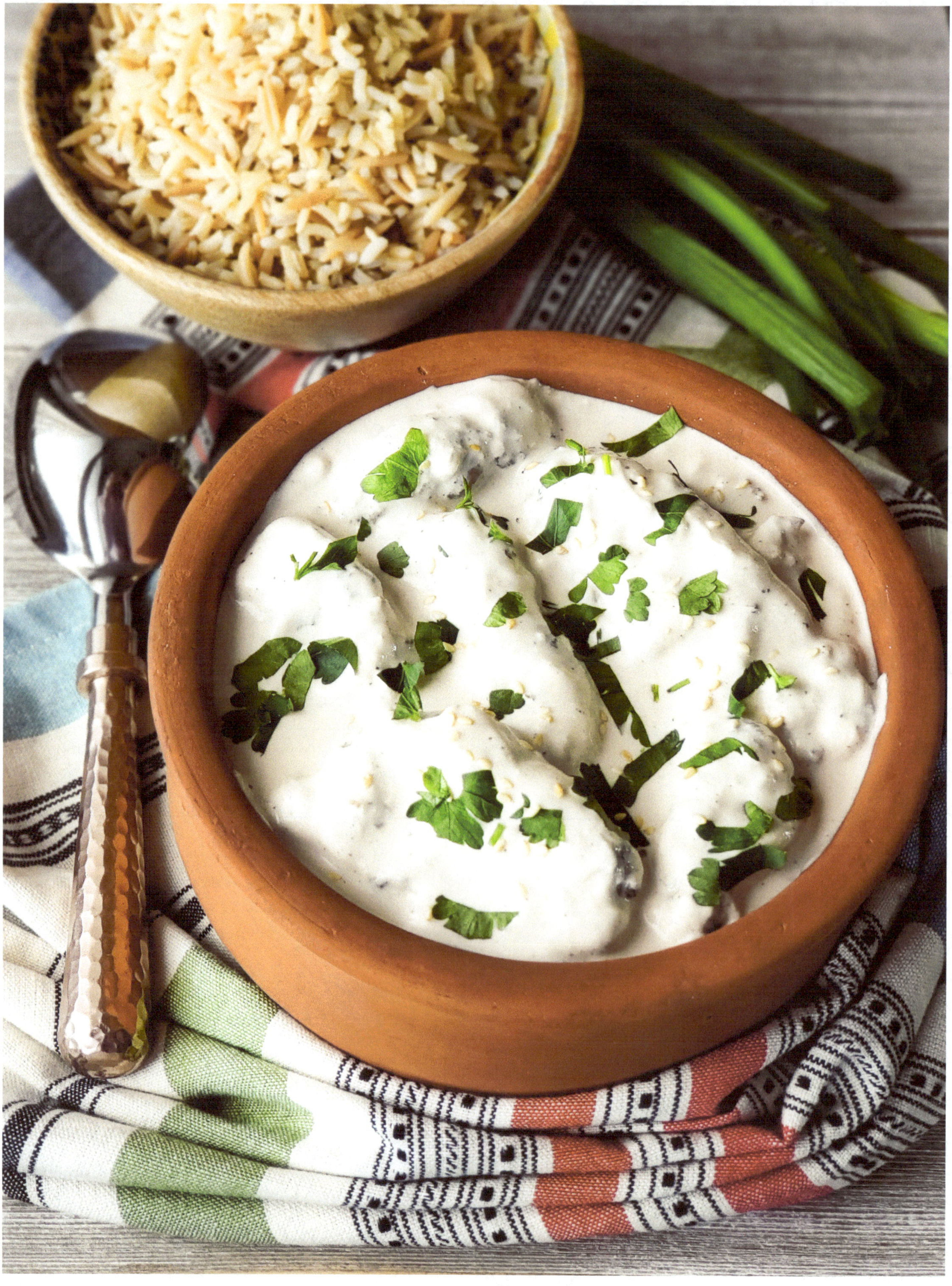

INGREDIENTS

Kafta

Raw extra lean beef, ground (1 kg)
1 large white onion, quartered (320 g)
6 medium green onion stalks, chopped (95 g)
2 bunches Italian Parsley, coarsely chopped (210 g)
1 tbsp olive oil
1 ½ tbsp cinnamon
1 ½ tbsp allspice
1 ½ tbsp 7-spices
2 ½ tsp salt

Sauce

± 3 cups hot water
1 ½ cups tahini
¾ cup lemon juice
1 tbsp garlic, crushed
⅓ tsp cinnamon
⅓ tsp allspice
⅓ tsp 7-spices
⅓ tsp salt

NOTES

- Prepared *kafta* meat is freezer friendly raw or cooked.
- This dish can be sent off to the freezer soon after the prepared ingredients have been layered in the pan and topped with the prepared *tahini* sauce (allow the sauce to cool, though). Thus, instead of placing the ready ingredients in one pan, one can divide them up into 2 smaller pans, and send one off to the freezer (to be baked at a later time).
- Each serving consists of 2 *kafta* patties topped with ~ 2 tbsp sauce.

RECIPE ALTERNATIVE

- One can add a medium russet potato to this dish, sliced up into thin circles, then baked right on the middle rack of a preheated oven at 450 °F for 15 minutes. Lay out the baked potato slices among the *kafta* patties and cover in sauce. When making the sauce, add ~ ½ cup extra water since the potatoes will drink up a bit of the liquid.

INSTRUCTIONS

1. In 2 batches, process the *kafta* vegetables in a large food processor, scraping down the sides as needed, until minced.

2. Place the ground beef in a bowl, then add the *kafta* spices. Pour in the olive oil, add the minced vegetables, then knead until well mixed. Cover, then refrigerate for at least 30 minutes (to decrease stickiness while forming the patties).

3. Form 30 oval *kafta* patties (using a ¼ cup of *kafta* for each), then lay out onto 2 large sheet pans (recommended dimensions: 30 cm x 40 cm or similar). Bake in a preheated oven at 375 °F for 20 minutes.

4. Drain the meat broth (~ ⅔ cup) into a bowl. Add the hot water (adjust the amount of water depending on how much meat broth is obtained, i.e. make sure total liquid equals 3 ⅔ cups), and the rest of the sauce ingredients, then whisk well. Process in 2 batches in a food blender until smooth and homogenous.

5. Using a deep baking pan (recommended dimensions: 25 cm x 35 cm or similar), pour some of the sauce on the bottom of the pan, lay out some of the *kafta* patties, then cover with another layer of sauce. Lay out some more patties, then cover with sauce. Repeat these steps until all the *kafta* patties and sauce have been used up (make sure the last layer of patties is well covered in sauce). Cover with foil, then bake in a preheated oven at 375 °F for 20 minutes.

6. Garnish with fresh parsley and serve with a side of brown rice (recipe on page 129) (some enjoy eating it with pita bread instead of rice), as well as fresh green onions or a salad if desired.

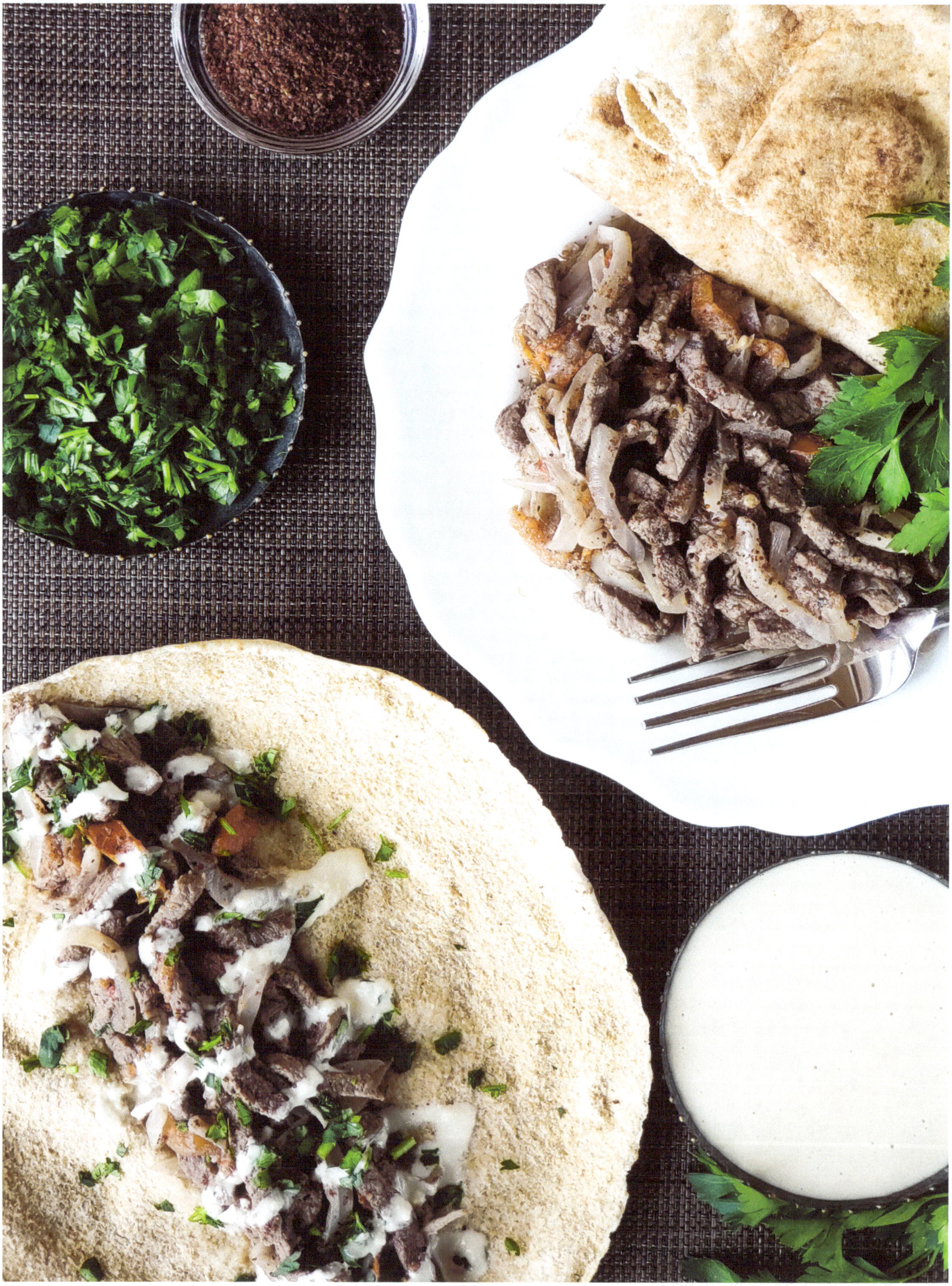

BAKED BEEF SHAWARMA

Shawarma Lahmeh bil Furn شاورما لحمة بالفرن

Shawarma is one of the most famous street foods in Lebanon and other Middle Eastern countries. It is classically made from deeply marinated fatty meat cuts of beef, lamb, or chicken, stacked on a vertical rotating rotisserie to be cooked, then shredded into thin slices and wrapped in pita bread sandwiches with *tahini* sauce. My lighter beef *shawarma* recipe features lean sirloin beef marinated in a light and healthy marinade, then baked in the oven, resulting in the same great flavor of this favorite street dish (my recipe for chicken *shawarma* is on the next page).

RECIPE YIELD 6 cups (12 servings)

DF GF EF FF

INGREDIENTS

Raw lean sirloin beef (no visible fat, no bones), sliced into very thin strips (1 kg)
1 large white onion, sliced into thin strips (320 g)
2 medium tomatoes, sliced into thin crescents (265 g)
4 tbsp apple cider vinegar
1 tbsp olive oil
5 tsp sumac
1 tsp dry mint leaves
1 tsp allspice
1 tsp 7-spices
1 tsp salt
1/8 tsp black pepper
14 whole cardamom pods
4 dry bay leaves

NOTE

- Each serving consists of ½ cup.

INSTRUCTIONS

1. In a large bowl, mix the marinade ingredients (vinegar, olive oil, herbs, spices), then add the cardamom pods and bay leaves.
2. Add the beef and onion slices, then mix well. Cover, then let marinate in the refrigerator for about 8 hours.
3. Place the beef and onions evenly on 2 baking pans (recommended dimensions: 25 cm x 35 cm or similar), then top with the tomato slices.
4. Bake in a preheated oven at 375 °F, uncovered, for about 30 minutes, stirring every 10 minutes, until the meat is cooked.
5. Serve with whole wheat pita bread and *tahini* sauce (recipe on page 139), as well as with chopped parsley if desired.

NUTRITION FACTS PER SERVING

139 Kcal	19 g Protein	5 g Fat	4 g Carbs	1 g Fiber	2 g Sugar

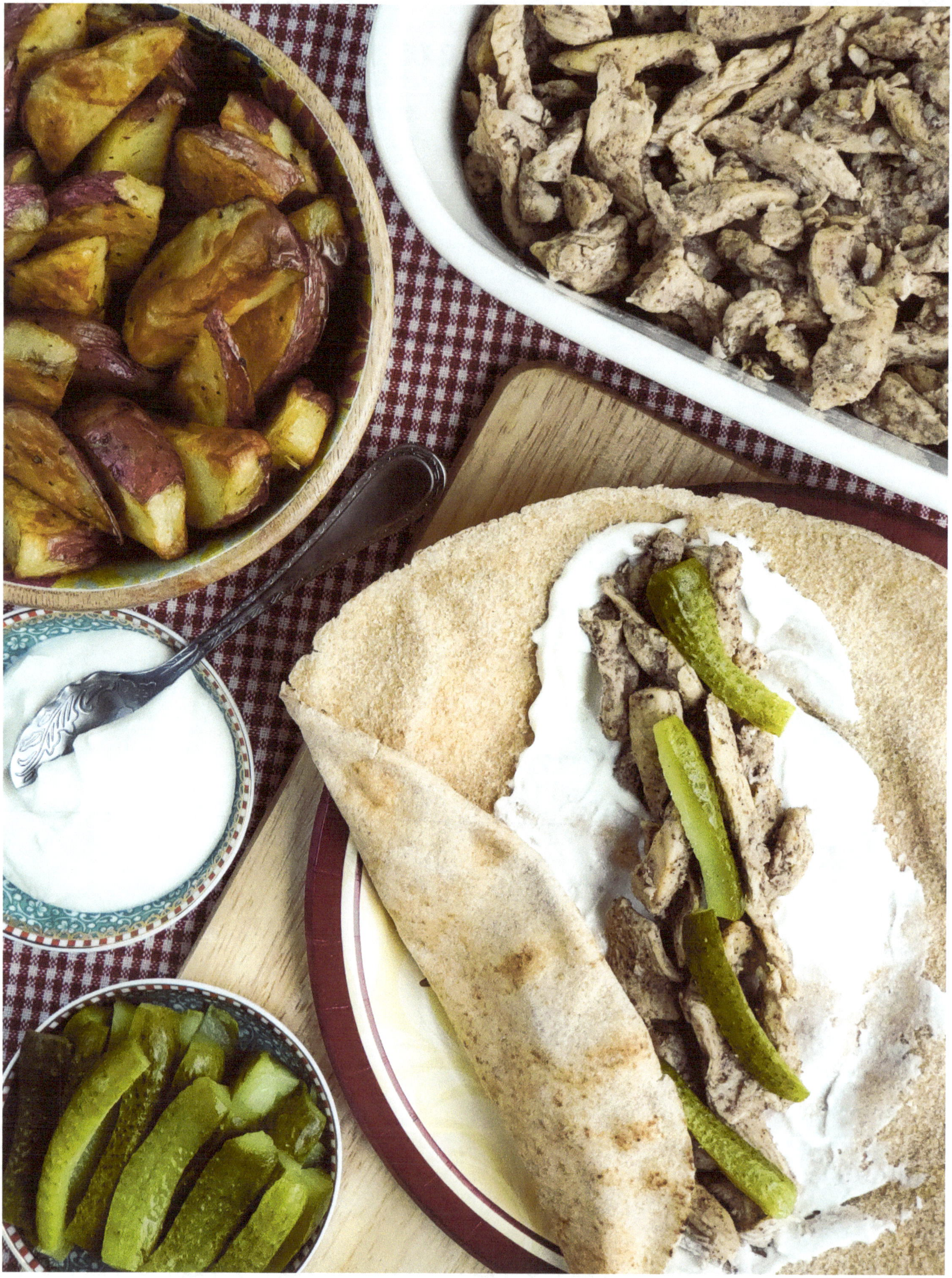

BAKED CHICKEN SHAWARMA

Shawarma Djaij bil Furn شاورما دجاج بالفرن

Beef and chicken *shawarma* are two very famous street foods in the Middle East that classically consist of a fatty meat cut of beef, lamb, or chicken that is deeply marinated then stacked on a vertical rotating rotisserie and cooked. Thinly sliced meat is then eaten on pita bread with traditional *mtawwam* garlic sauce (as described on page 141). My healthier chicken *shawarma* recipe calls for chicken breast in a light marinade baked in the oven and enjoyed with my healthy *mtawwam* garlic sauce.

RECIPE YIELD 5 cups (10 servings)

GF EF FF

INGREDIENTS

2 raw large chicken breasts (no skin, no visible fat, no bones), sliced into thin strips (1 kg)
2 tbsp garlic, crushed
2 tbsp skim yogurt
2 tbsp olive oil
2 tbsp lemon juice
2 tbsp apple cider vinegar
¼ tsp cinnamon
¼ tsp allspice
1 tsp cloves
1 tsp salt
¼ tsp black pepper
12 whole cardamom pods
4 dry bay leaves

NOTES

- The thinner the chicken strips are sliced, the more flavorful the outcome of the *shawarma*. If one wants to cut the strips very thin, cut back on the baking time by 5 minutes.
- Each serving consists of ½ cup.

INSTRUCTIONS

1. In a large bowl, mix the marinade ingredients (garlic, yogurt, olive oil, lemon juice, vinegar, spices), then add the cardamom pods and bay leaves.
2. Add the chicken slices, then mix well. Cover, then let marinate in the refrigerator for about 8 hours.
3. Place the chicken evenly on a baking pan (recommended dimensions: 25 cm x 35 cm or similar), then bake in a preheated oven at 375 °F, uncovered, for about 30 minutes, stirring every 10 minutes, until the chicken is cooked.
4. Serve wrapped in a sandwich with whole wheat pita bread and lots of my healthy garlic sauce (recipe on page 141), as well as with baked potato wedges (recipe on page 137) and pickles if desired.

NUTRITION FACTS PER SERVING

150.5 Kcal	23 g Protein	5.4 g Fat	1 g Carbs	0.2 g Fiber	0.4 g Sugar

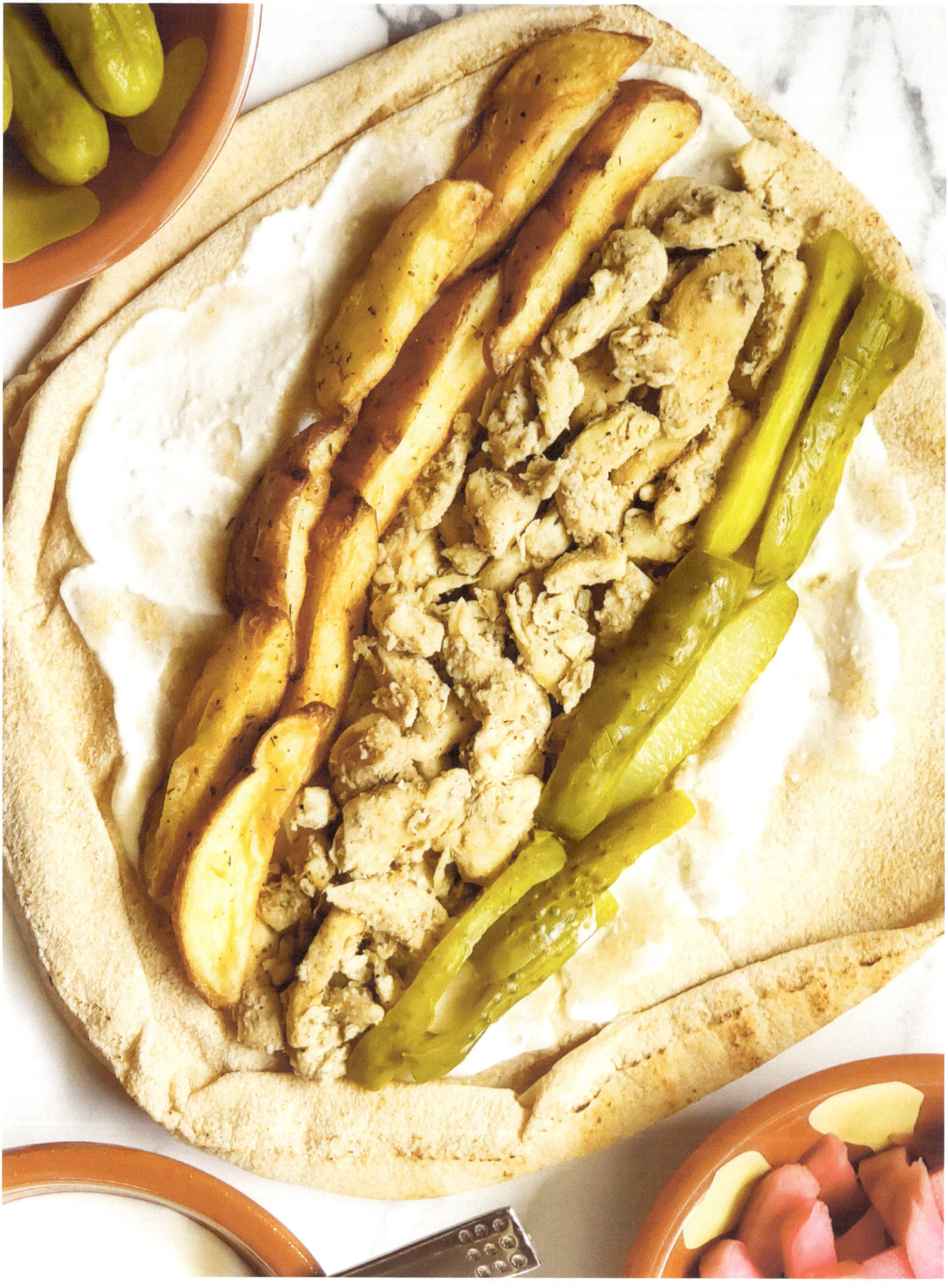

BAKED CHICKEN AND SPICES

This is a recipe I adapted from a traditional Middle Eastern dish (*djaij wa batata*: دجاج و بطاطا) made with chicken (commonly just thighs) and potato slices marinated in a lemony/garlicy sauce and baked in the oven. As I am not fond of chicken thighs or soggy potatoes, my twist for this recipe was inspired by chicken *shawarma* (on the previous page), keeping the potatoes out of the main pan of chicken and marinade, and baking them separately, then eating the dish as a sandwich wrap with my healthy *mtawwam* garlic sauce.

RECIPE YIELD 5 cups (10 servings)

GF EF FF

INGREDIENTS

2 raw large chicken breasts (no skin, no visible fat, no bones), sliced into thin strips (1 kg)
2 tbsp garlic, crushed
2 tbsp skim yogurt
2 tbsp olive oil
5 tbsp lemon juice
2 tsp cumin
1 ½ tsp 7-spices
½ tsp dry coriander leaves
¼ tsp turmeric
1 tsp salt
¼ tsp black pepper
4 dry bay leaves

NOTES

- To imitate the original dish in terms of having more sauce and not eating it as a sandwich, one can add about 1 cup of water to the marinated chicken right before placing in a deep baking pan and covering with foil before baking.
- The thinner the chicken strips are sliced, the more flavorful the outcome of the chicken. If one wants to cut the strips very thin, cut back on the baking time by 5 minutes.
- Each serving consists of ½ cup.

INSTRUCTIONS

1. In a large bowl, mix the marinade ingredients (garlic, yogurt, olive oil, lemon juice, herbs, spices), then add the bay leaves.
2. Add the chicken slices, then mix well. Cover, then let marinate in the refrigerator for about 8 hours.
3. Place the chicken evenly on a baking pan (recommended dimensions: 25 cm x 35 cm or similar), then bake in a preheated oven at 375 °F, uncovered, for about 30 minutes, stirring every 10 minutes, until the chicken is cooked.
4. Serve with whole wheat pita bread and baked potato wedges (recipe on page 137), with lots of my healthy *mtawwam* garlic sauce (recipe on page 141) and pickles if desired.

NUTRITION FACTS PER SERVING

152 Kcal	23 g Protein	5.5 g Fat	2 g Carbs	0.2 g Fiber	0.5 g Sugar

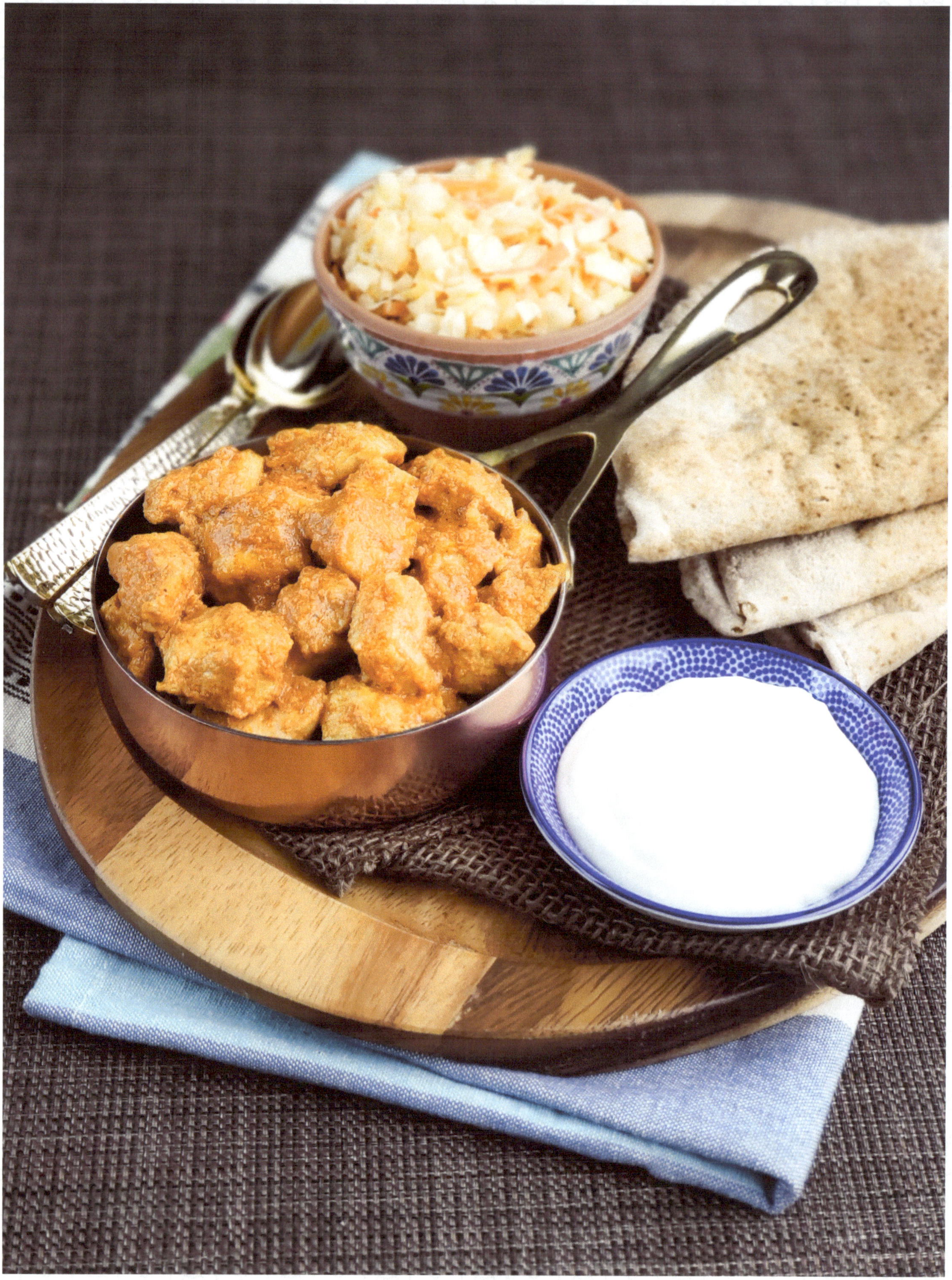

BAKED CHICKEN SHISH TAWOOK

Shish Tawook bil Furn شيش طاووق بالفرن

This traditional dish of 'marinated chicken on skewers' (which is what *shish tawook* means) is very common to Lebanon and other Middle Eastern countries. The marinade of this dish traditionally includes a base of whole yogurt and quite a bit of vegetable oil, to keep the chicken tender and juicy. Variations to the marinade are common, with some including tomato paste and a mixed blend of *shish tawook* spices, while others use ketchup and a couple spices. My recipe features chicken cubes flavored with a light ketchup marinade and baked in the oven with some olive oil. While the grilling of the skewers adds much flavor to the chicken, baking the dish leaves the chicken juicy and just as flavorful. *Shish tawook* is commonly eaten with traditional *mtawwam* garlic sauce (as described on page 141) and wrapped up in a sandwich with pita bread.

RECIPE YIELD 5 cups (10 servings)

GF EF FF

INGREDIENTS

2 raw large chicken breasts (no skin, no visible fat, no bones), cubed (1 kg)
2 tbsp garlic, crushed
½ cup ketchup (130 g)
3 tbsp skim yogurt
1 tbsp mustard
2 tbsp olive oil
1 ½ tsp paprika
½ tsp salt
¼ tsp black pepper

NOTE

- Each serving consists of ½ cup.

INSTRUCTIONS

1. In a large bowl, mix the marinade ingredients (garlic, ketchup, yogurt, mustard, olive oil, spices).
2. Add the chicken cubes, then mix well. Cover, then let marinate in the refrigerator for about 8 hours.
3. Place the chicken evenly on a baking pan (recommended dimensions: 25 cm x 35 cm or similar), then bake in a preheated oven at 375 °F, uncovered, for about 40 minutes, stirring every 10 minutes, until the chicken is cooked.
4. Serve the *shish tawook* wrapped in a sandwich with whole wheat pita bread and lots of my healthy *mtawwam* garlic sauce (recipe on page 141), or serve on a plate with a salad or grilled vegetables as a side if desired (especially good with grilled onions and bell peppers).

NUTRITION FACTS PER SERVING

165 Kcal	23 g Protein	5.5 g Fat	5 g Carbs	0.3 g Fiber	3 g Sugar

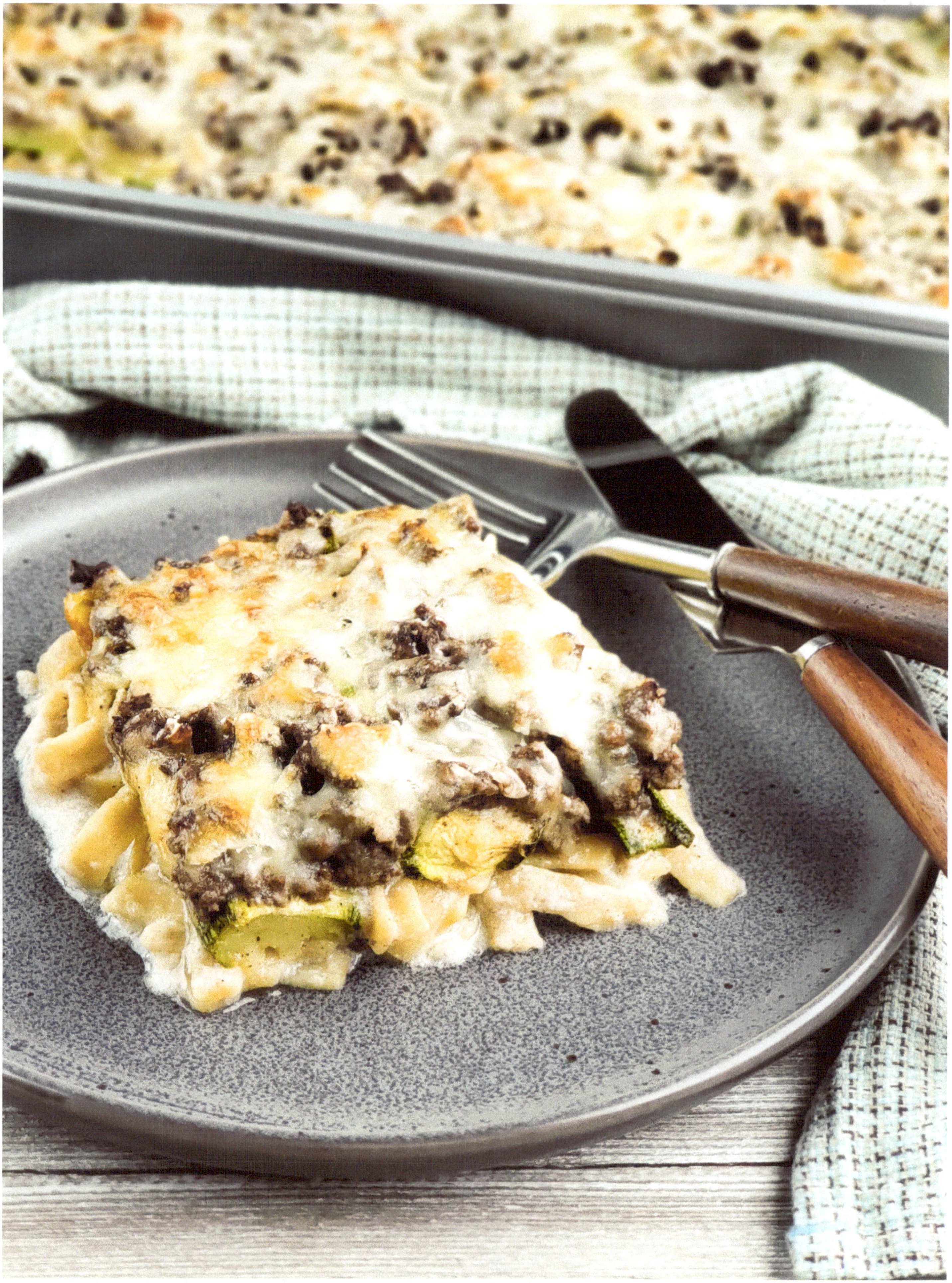

ZUCCHINI BÉCHAMEL CASSEROLE

Kusa bil Béchamel wa Maakarona كوسى بالباشاميل و معكرونة

This recipe combines the features and flavors of two Middle Eastern dishes: an Egyptian dish of zucchini with beef and béchamel sauce, and a Lebanese dish of spaghetti with béchamel sauce. My healthier version of béchamel is unconventional, containing skim milk with no butter, thickened with whole wheat flour, and flavored lightly with warm spices.

RECIPE YIELD 12 slices

EF FF

INGREDIENTS

Raw extra lean beef, ground (500 g)
Dry whole wheat fettuccine (450 g)
9 medium zucchinis, cut into wide lengthwise slices (1 kg)
1 ½ medium yellow onions, sliced into short strips (240 g)
2 cups coarsely grated low-moisture part-skim mozzarella cheese (200 g)
½ cup finely grated parmesan cheese (50 g)
1 tbsp unsalted tomato paste
2 tsp olive oil
8 cups skim milk
6 tbsp whole wheat flour
2 tsp cinnamon
½ tsp allspice
⅓ tsp nutmeg
1 ¾ tsp salt
black pepper, to taste
1 cinnamon stick
2 dry bay leaves

RECIPE ALTERNATIVE

- This dish tastes just as delicious with sautéed/boiled/roasted chicken instead of beef.

INSTRUCTIONS

1. Spread out the zucchini slices on a large sheet pan (recommended dimensions: 30 cm x 40 cm or similar) lined with parchment paper, then bake in a preheated oven at 400 °F for 30 to 40 minutes.
2. In a medium pan or skillet, sauté the meat, stirring frequently until browned. Add the cinnamon stick, bay leaves, onions, tomato paste, and spices (except for the salt), then cook, covered on low heat for 15 minutes, stirring occasionally. Remove the bay leaves and cinnamon stick.
3. In a medium pot, whisk the milk, oil, flour, and salt, then stir on medium-high heat until it just comes to a boil.
4. Stir in the parmesan cheese until well mixed. Remove 2 cups of the béchamel sauce and set aside.
5. Boil the fettuccine in a separate pot with a pinch of salt until an al dente texture. Drain (do not rinse), then return to the pot.
6. Pour the béchamel sauce (minus the 2 cups) over the fettuccine and fold.
7. Pour the fettuccine into a deep baking pan (recommended dimensions: 28 cm x 37 cm or similar), then even out.
8. Lay out the zucchinis over the fettuccine.
9. Add the meat and onions over the zucchinis, then spread out until even.
10. Pour the remaining 2 cups of sauce, then evenly sprinkle the mozzarella cheese over the entire top.
11. Bake, uncovered, in a preheated oven at 375 °F for 25 minutes.
12. Let rest for 10 minutes before serving.

NUTRITION FACTS PER SLICE

361.4 Kcal	26 g Protein	8 g Fat	46 g Carbs	6.4 g Fiber	12.4 g Sugar

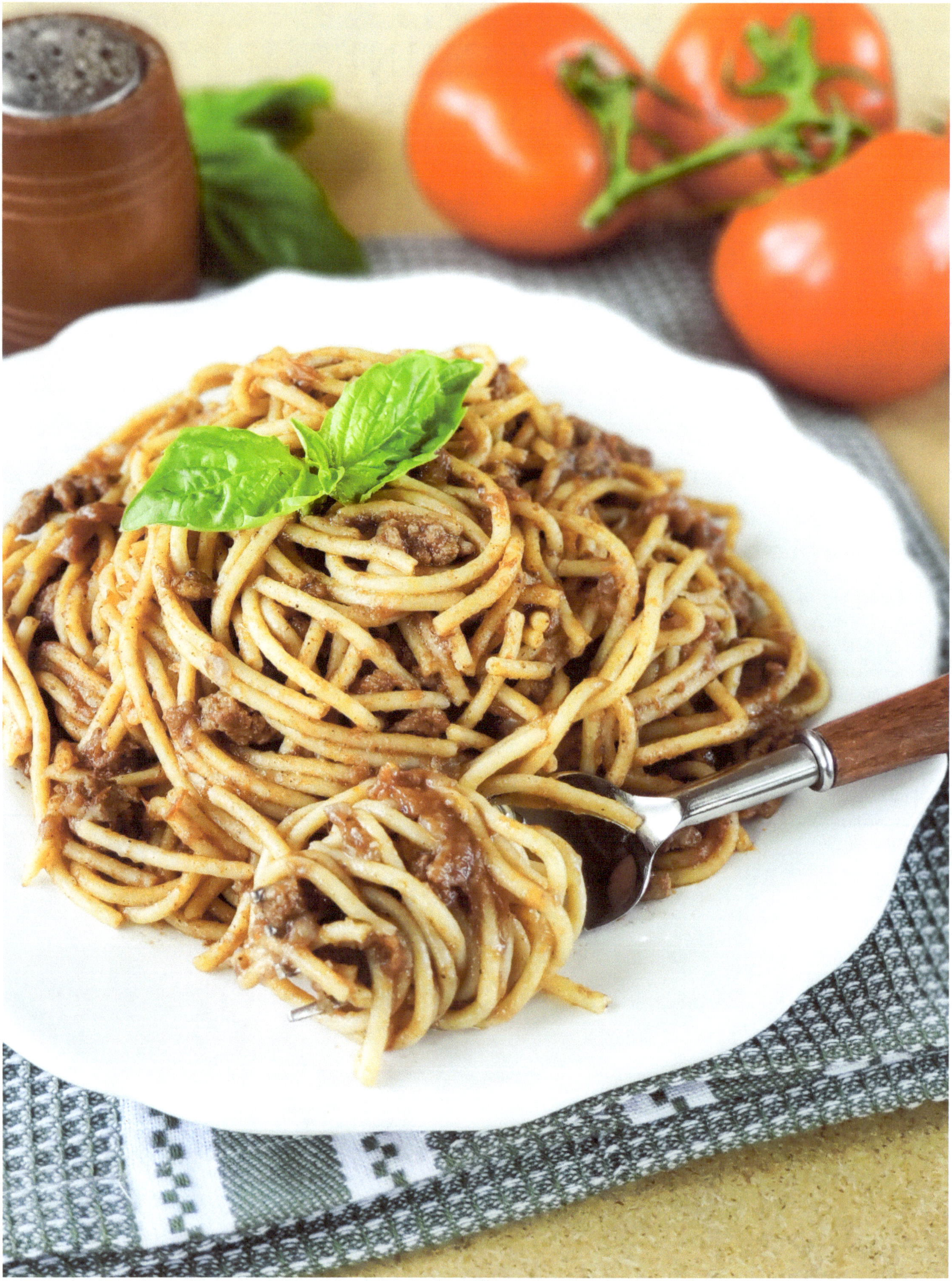

WHOLE WHEAT SPAGHETTI WITH BEEF

This is my basic spaghetti and beef dish with homemade tomato sauce, which I adapted from my mother's recipe. The dish comes close to being a blend between a bolognaise and marinara spaghetti dish, lightly flavored with onions, garlic, warm spices, and herbs, while bursting with the flavor of tomatoes. The dish is hearty, but light, relying on lean beef and heart-healthy olive oil as the fat source.

RECIPE YIELD 17 cups

DF EF FF

INGREDIENTS

Raw extra lean beef, ground (500 g)
Dry whole wheat spaghetti (600 g)
10 medium red tomatoes, quartered (1.3 kg)
2 medium yellow onions, minced (320 g)
2 tsp garlic, crushed
1 cup unsalted tomato paste (240 g)
1 tbsp olive oil
2 cups water
2 tsp cinnamon
2 tsp allspice
2 tsp dry basil leaves
2 $\frac{1}{3}$ tsp salt
black pepper, to taste
1 cinnamon stick
2 dry bay leaves

NOTE

Since all pastas tend to drink up some liquid from the sauce as the dish sits in the refrigerator, always save some of the water from boiling the pasta and use when reheating individual servings as desired.

INSTRUCTIONS

1. In 2 or 3 batches, process the tomatoes in a blender, until well puréed. Pour into a medium pot, then mix in the water, tomato paste, garlic, herbs, and spices. Cover and bring to a boil, then cook, covered, on low heat for 20 minutes, stirring occasionally. Set aside.
2. In a medium pan or skillet, covered, cook the onions with the olive oil, on low heat for 20 minutes (stirring occasionally).
3. Add the meat to the onions, stirring frequently on medium-high heat until browned. Add the cinnamon stick and bay leaves, then cover and cook on low heat for 15 minutes, stirring occasionally. Remove the cinnamon stick and bay leaves. Set aside.
4. In the meantime, boil the spaghetti in a large pot with a pinch of salt to an al dente texture. Drain (but do not rinse), then fold in the meat, onions, and sauce.
5. Let sit for 10 minutes before serving.
6. Serve with fresh basil or a side of salad if desired.

NUTRITION FACTS PER CUP

191.5 Kcal	13 g Protein	3 g Fat	32.4 g Carbs	5 g Fiber	4.4 g Sugar

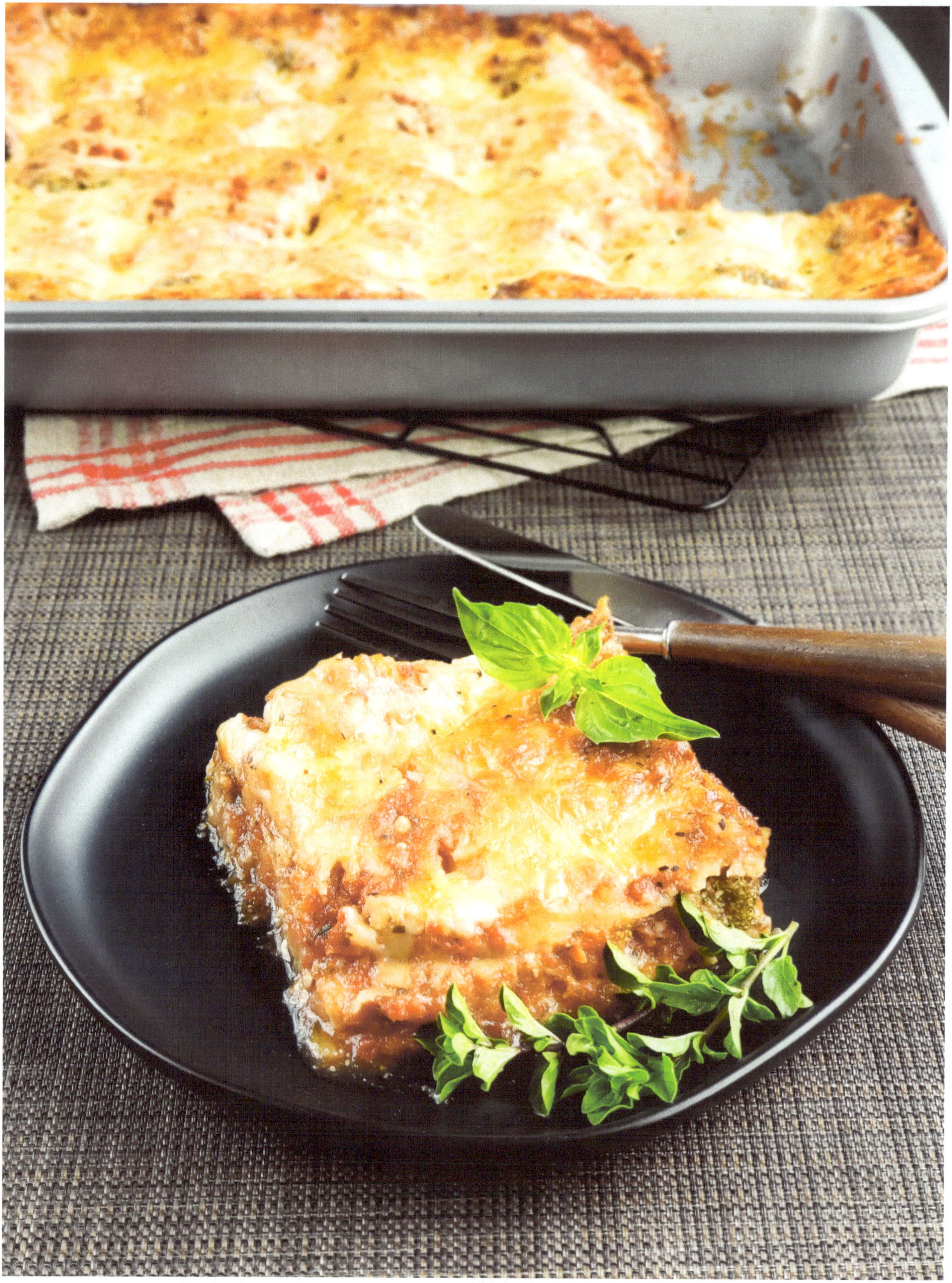

WHOLE WHEAT LASAGNA WITH VEGGIES

This Italian classic is traditionally made with refined white lasagna, and is often high in calories and fat, mostly from all the high fat cheeses that are added to the lasagna layers. My healthy vegetarian lasagna dish is made with whole wheat lasagna pasta and homemade tomato sauce, and calls for low-fat cheeses, as well as less cheese than a traditional lasagna dish would have. It is also loaded with fiber-rich vegetables hiding among the layers of lasagna. This dish is so versatile that any vegetable could be added; peas, fresh spinach, basil, or eggplant would taste good in this dish as well.

RECIPE YIELD 12 slices

EF Vt FF

INGREDIENTS

18 dry whole wheat lasagna sheets (450 g)
15 medium red tomatoes, quartered (2 kg)
1 medium yellow onion, minced (160 g)
1 medium yellow bell pepper, diced (165 g)
1 medium broccoli head (no stems, no stalk), broken into small florets (120 g)
1 medium zucchini, coarsely grated (112 g)
1 medium carrot (no skin), coarsely grated (60 g)
1 tbsp garlic, crushed
3 ½ cups coarsely grated low-moisture part-skim mozzarella cheese (350 g)
1 cup finely grated parmesan cheese (100 g)
1 cup fat-free cottage cheese (230 g)
1 cup part-skim ricotta cheese (230 g)
1 cup unsalted tomato paste (240 g)
2 tbsp maple syrup
2 tbsp olive oil
½ cup water
3 tbsp dry oregano leaves
1 tbsp dry basil leaves
⅓ tsp allspice
2 ¼ tsp salt
¼ tsp black pepper

INSTRUCTIONS

1. Mix the hard cheeses (mozzarella and parmesan) together in a small bowl, then mix the moist cheeses (cottage and ricotta) in a separate bowl. Cover, then set aside in the refrigerator.
2. In 2 or 3 batches, process the tomatoes in a blender, until well puréed. Pour into a medium pot, then mix in the water, olive oil, maple syrup, tomato paste, garlic, herbs, and spices. Cover and bring to a boil, then cook, covered, on low heat for 20 minutes, stirring occasionally.
3. Pour some of the prepared tomato sauce into a deep baking pan (recommended dimensions: 28 cm x 37 cm or similar), covering the bottom completely.
4. Add the prepared vegetables to the pot of sauce, then stir to mix.
5. Lay out 6 lasagna sheets, spread ⅓ of the sauce over the lasagna, then add ½ of the moist cheeses, spreading in an even manner as possible. Sprinkle ¼ of the hard cheeses evenly over the surface.
6. Lay out another 6 lasagna sheets, spread ⅓ of the sauce over the lasagna, then add ½ of the moist cheeses, spreading in an even manner as possible. Sprinkle ¼ of the hard cheeses evenly over the surface.
7. For the final layer, lay out the last 6 lasagna sheets, spread the remaining sauce over the lasagna, then sprinkle the remaining hard cheeses evenly over the surface.

Instructions continued on the next page »

NUTRITION FACTS PER SLICE

373 Kcal	23 g Protein	13 g Fat	46.6 g Carbs	8.6 g Fiber	10.5 g Sugar

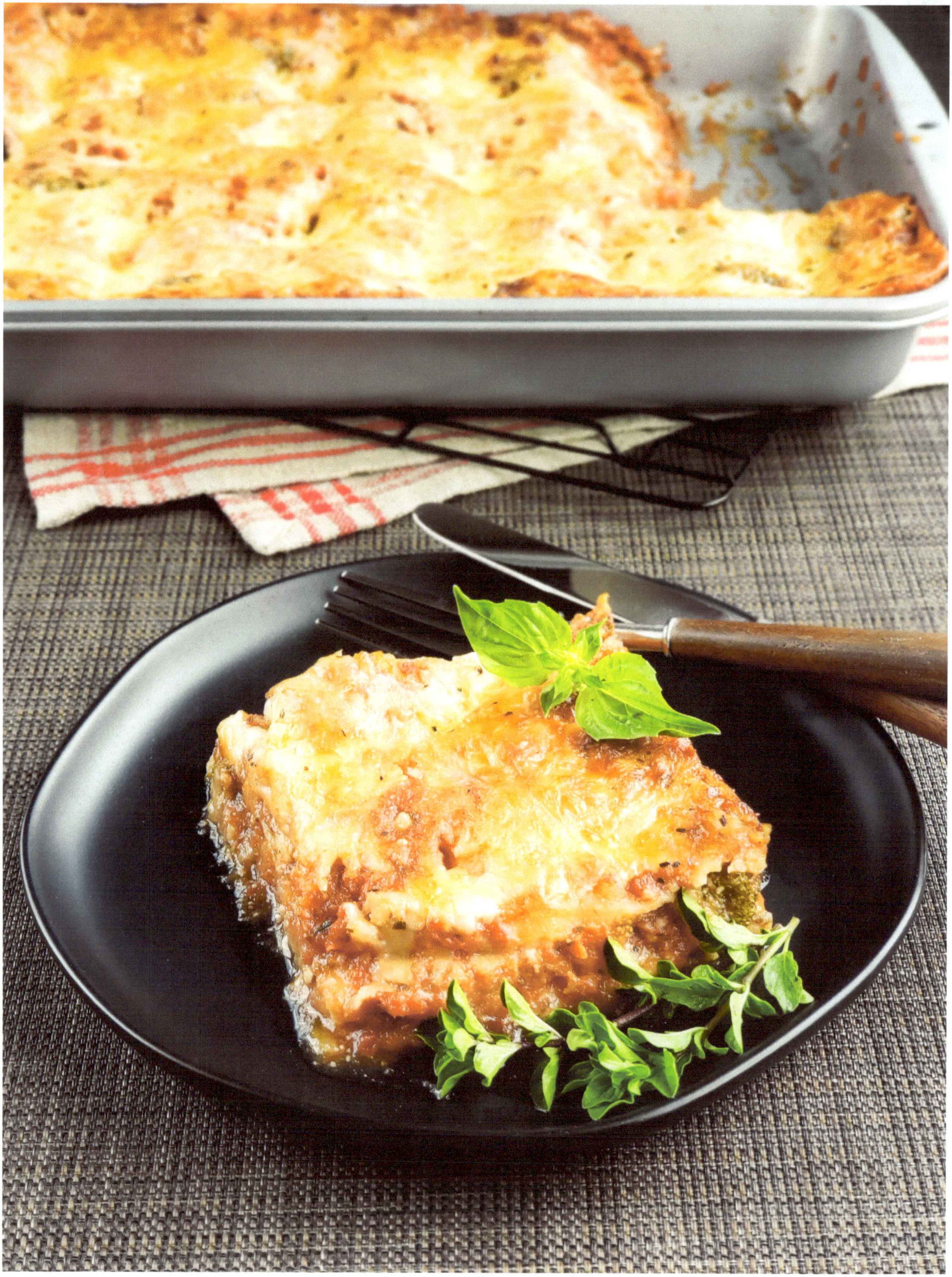

INGREDIENTS

18 dry whole wheat lasagna sheets (450 g)
15 medium red tomatoes, quartered (2 kg)
1 medium yellow onion, minced (160 g)
1 medium yellow bell pepper, diced (165 g)
1 medium broccoli head (no stems, no stalk), broken into small florets (120 g)
1 medium zucchini, coarsely grated (112 g)
1 medium carrot (no skin), coarsely grated (60 g)
1 tbsp garlic, crushed
3 ½ cups coarsely grated low-moisture part-skim mozzarella cheese (350 g)
1 cup finely grated parmesan cheese (100 g)
1 cup fat-free cottage cheese (230 g)
1 cup part-skim ricotta cheese (230 g)
1 cup unsalted tomato paste (240 g)
2 tbsp maple syrup
2 tbsp olive oil
½ cup water
3 tbsp dry oregano leaves
1 tbsp dry basil leaves
⅓ tsp allspice
2 ¼ tsp salt
¼ tsp black pepper

NOTES

❀ I use regular lasagna and not lasagna that has been partially boiled then dried.

❀ Lasagna is best sent off to the freezer prior to baking (this keeps the layers more intact and prevents the lasagna from getting mushy). For future cooking of the frozen lasagna: remove from the freezer 30 minutes before baking. Remove any ice on the under part of the foil as well as any formed ice crystals on the surface of the lasagna. Bake at 375 °F, covered for 1 hour and 15 minutes, then uncover and bake for another 15 to 20 minutes.

INSTRUCTIONS

1. Mix the hard cheeses (mozzarella and parmesan) together in a small bowl, then mix the moist cheeses (cottage and ricotta) in a separate bowl. Cover, then set aside in the refrigerator.

2. In 2 or 3 batches, process the tomatoes in a blender, until well puréed. Pour into a medium pot, then mix in the water, olive oil, maple syrup, tomato paste, garlic, herbs, and spices. Cover and bring to a boil, then cook, covered, on low heat for 20 minutes, stirring occasionally.

3. Pour some of the prepared tomato sauce into a deep baking pan (recommended dimensions: 28 cm x 37 cm or similar), covering the bottom completely.

4. Add the prepared vegetables to the pot of sauce, then stir to mix.

5. Lay out 6 lasagna sheets, spread ⅓ of the sauce over the lasagna, then add ½ of the moist cheeses, spreading in an even manner as possible. Sprinkle ¼ of the hard cheeses evenly over the surface.

6. Lay out another 6 lasagna sheets, spread ⅓ of the sauce over the lasagna, then add ½ of the moist cheeses, spreading in an even manner as possible. Sprinkle ¼ of the hard cheeses evenly over the surface.

7. For the final layer, lay out the last 6 lasagna sheets, spread the remaining sauce over the lasagna, then sprinkle the remaining hard cheeses evenly over the surface.

8. Sprinkle some dry oregano and/or basil if desired, then cover the pan with aluminum foil and bake in a preheated oven at 375 °F for 45 minutes.

9. Uncover, then continue baking for another 10 to 15 minutes.

10. Let sit and cool outside the oven for 15 minutes before slicing and serving.

11. Garnish with fresh basil and/or oregano leaves if desired.

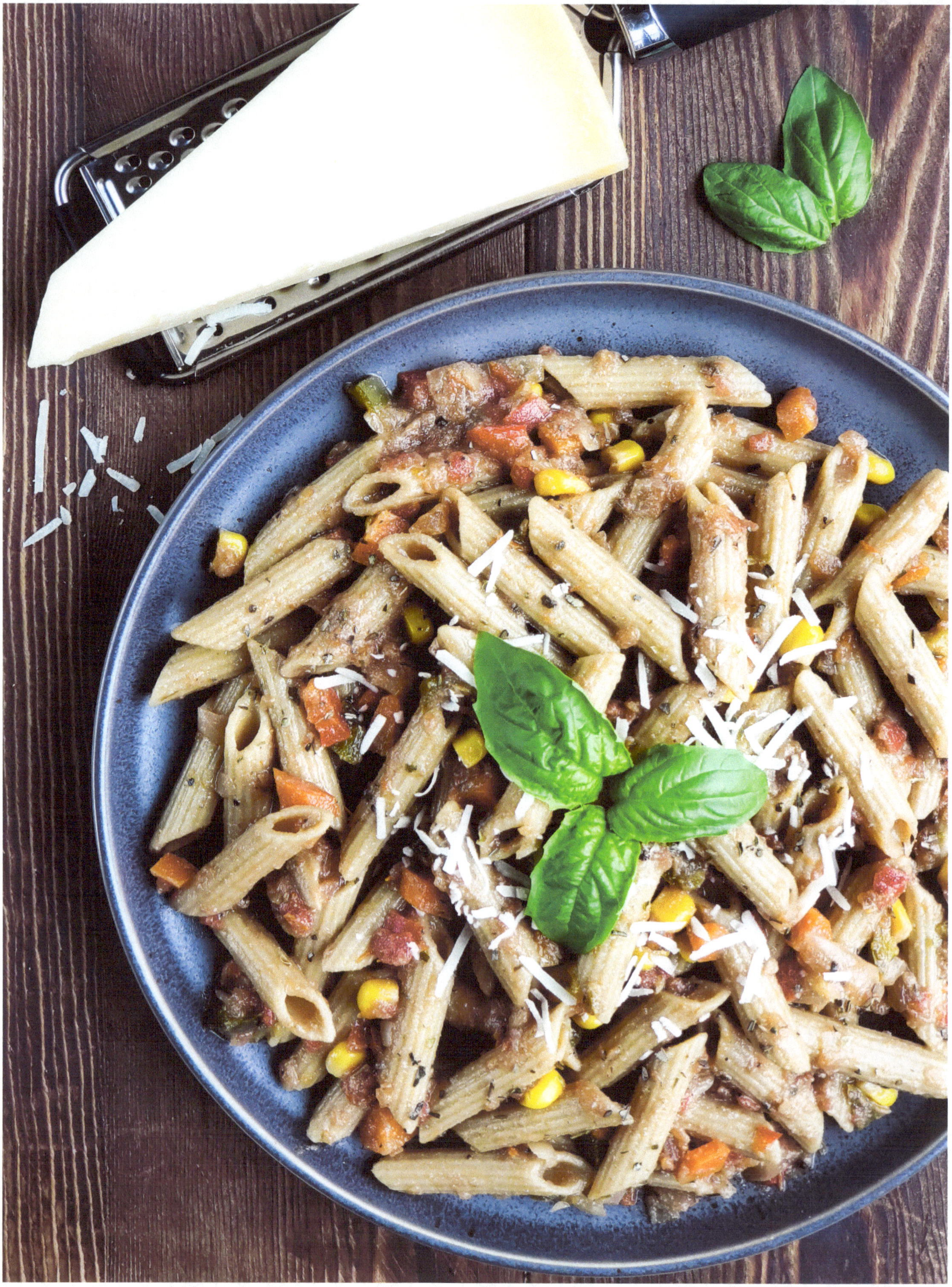

WHOLE WHEAT PENNE WITH VEGGIES

Adapted from a recipe that a cousin of mine and I made up when we were teenagers, this vegetarian pasta is a light, but hearty dish rich in flavor and nutrients. The taste of onions, tomatoes, bell peppers, carrots, and corn come together beautifully with the flavors of cumin, dry oregano, and dry coriander. To pack more fiber and micronutrients into this dish, I use whole wheat penne (but whole wheat rotini pasta or just any other type will do)!

RECIPE YIELD 15 cups

EF Vt FF

INGREDIENTS

Dry whole wheat penne (450 g)
8 medium red tomatoes, quartered (1,065 g)
2 medium bell peppers (1 red, 1 green), diced (330 g)
1 medium yellow onion, diced (160 g)
1 cup sweet corn kernels (160 g)
1 large carrot, diced (100 g)
½ cup part-skim ricotta cheese (115 g)
6 tbsp ketchup
2 tbsp low-salt soy sauce
2 tbsp olive oil
1 cup water
2 tbsp dry oregano leaves
1 tbsp dry coriander leaves
1 tbsp cumin
½ tsp salt

NOTE

Since all pastas tend to drink up some liquid from the sauce as the dish sits in the refrigerator, always save some of the water from boiling the pasta and use when reheating individual servings as desired.

INSTRUCTIONS

1. In 1 or 2 batches, process the tomatoes in a blender, until well puréed. Pour into a medium pot, then whisk in the water, 1 tbsp olive oil, soy sauce, ketchup, ricotta cheese, herbs, and spices. Cover and bring to a boil, then cook, covered, on low heat for 20 minutes, stirring occasionally.
2. In a medium pan or skillet, covered, cook the onions with 1 tbsp olive oil on low heat for 20 minutes, stirring occasionally.
3. Stir in the carrots, cover, then continue cooking on low for 5 minutes.
4. Add the bell peppers, then cook, covered, on low heat for 15 minutes, stirring occasionally
5. Fold in the corn, then place the lid ajar.
6. In the meantime, boil the penne in a large pot with a pinch of salt, to an al dente texture. Drain (but do not rinse), then fold in the vegetables and sauce.
7. Let sit for 10 minutes before serving.
8. Serve with grated parmesan cheese and fresh basil leaves if desired.

NUTRITION FACTS PER CUP

167 Kcal	7 g Protein	4 g Fat	31 g Carbs	6 g Fiber	6.6 g Sugar

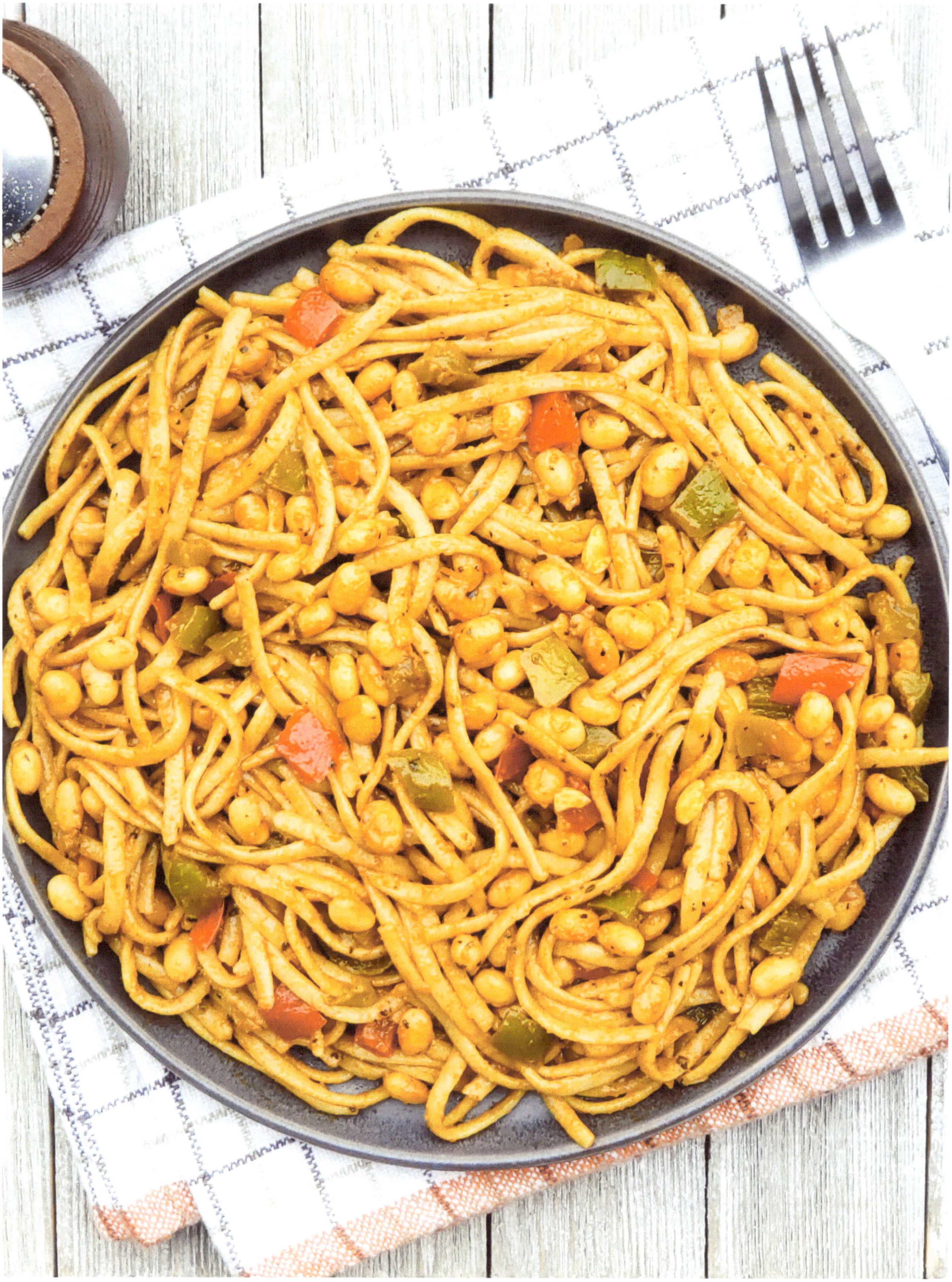

WHOLE WHEAT LINGUINI WITH SOYBEANS

This is my favorite high-protein vegan spaghetti dish of my own creation, loaded with soybeans, vegetables, and whole wheat spaghetti. It offers high-quality protein and heart-healthy fats, while providing a great source of fiber, micronutrients, and antioxidants. Many tend to avoid soy products on the basis that they may cause undesirable health effects such as breast cancer and thyroid problems. Recent research suggests that soy has beneficial and/or neutral effects on various health conditions, and thus, can be safely consumed in moderation (especially when replacing red meat). Soybeans are in fact one of the cheapest richest sources of high-quality protein, ranking as high as the protein quality of meat and dairy (as compared to other beans and plant protein-sources that contain incomplete proteins, i.e. lacking some essential amino acids).

RECIPE YIELD 18 cups

DF EF V FF

INGREDIENTS

2 cups dry soybeans (340 g)
Dry whole wheat linguine (600 g)
5 medium bell peppers (3 green, 2 red), diced (825 g)
1 medium yellow onion, minced (160 g)
2 tsp garlic, crushed
1⅓ cup ketchup (347 g)
1 tbsp mustard
¼ cup low-salt soy sauce
2 tbsp olive oil
1 cup water
1 tbsp mild curry
½ tsp turmeric
2 tsp dry oregano leaves
1 tsp dry basil leaves
1 tsp baking soda
chili pepper powder, optional

NOTE

- Since all pastas tend to drink up some liquid from the sauce as the dish sits in the refrigerator, always save some of the water from boiling the pasta and use when reheating individual servings as desired.

INSTRUCTIONS

1. Soak the soybeans in water with the baking soda for 24 hours (refrigerate). Drain and add fresh water, then soak for another 12 hours.
2. Drain the soybeans, then rinse well. Pick over for bad pieces and for any pieces that don't rehydrate. Place in a pot, cover with water, then bring to a boil. Skim off the white foam that floats to the surface, then cook, covered, on low heat for 3 hours (or until tender). Drain and set aside.
3. In a large pot, covered, cook the onions with the olive oil, on low heat for 20 minutes (stirring occasionally).
4. Add the peppers, then cook, covered, on low heat for another 15 minutes.
5. In a small bowl, mix the water, garlic, ketchup, mustard, soy sauce, herbs, and spices, then pour over the vegetables. Turn up the heat, bring the sauce to a boil, then cook, covered, on low for 5 minutes.
6. Stir in the soybeans.
7. In the meantime, boil the linguini in a separate pot with a pinch of salt to an al dente texture. Drain (but do not rinse), then fold into the vegetables, beans, and sauce.
8. Let sit for 10 minutes before serving.

NUTRITION FACTS PER CUP

238 Kcal	14.6 g Protein	7 g Fat	36.4 g Carbs	7 g Fiber	10 g Sugar

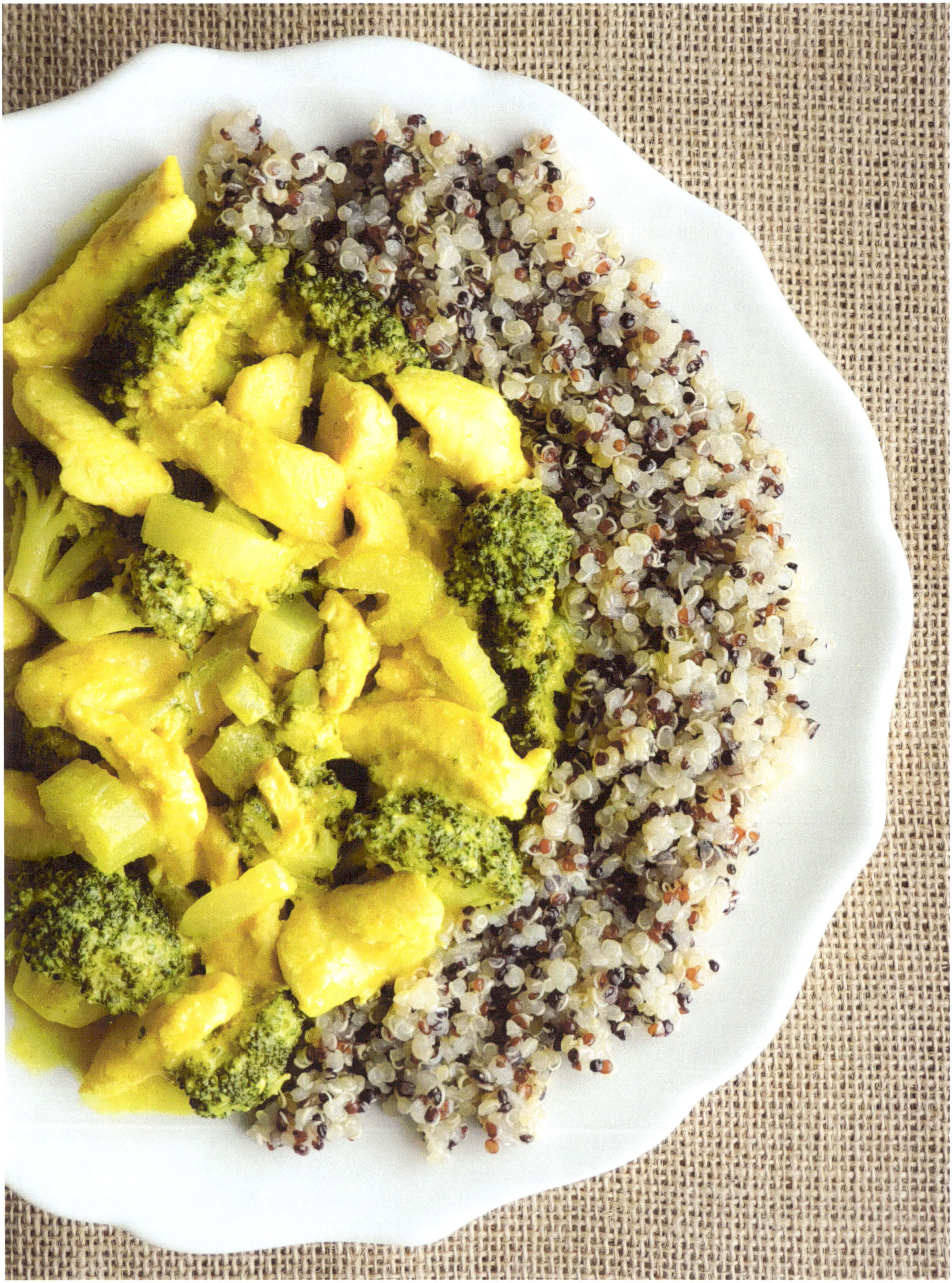

HONEY MUSTARD CHICKEN AND VEGGIES

This dish was adapted from a recipe my mother had developed (which contained quite a bit of mayonnaise as the base for the mustard sauce). I transformed the sauce into a healthier sweet honey mustard sauce made creamy with the addition of skim milk, parmesan cheese, and heart-healthy olive oil. The outcome is light, unique, and very flavorful!

RECIPE YIELD 15 cups

EF FF

INGREDIENTS

2 raw large chicken breasts (no skin, no visible fat, no bones), sliced into strips (1 kg)
4 large broccoli heads (no stalks), broken/chopped into small florets (920 g)
6 large celery stalks (no leaves), chopped (390 g)
1 medium yellow onion, diced (160 g)
½ cup finely grated parmesan cheese (50 g)
¾ cup mustard (180 g)
3 tbsp honey
1 tbsp olive oil
3 cups water
2 cups liquid skim milk
6 tbsp powdered skim milk
6 tbsp whole wheat flour
1 tsp turmeric
1 ½ tsp salt
black pepper, to taste
1 cinnamon stick
2 dry bay leaves

NOTE

If one thinks the pan/skillet they have is not deep enough to fit all the vegetables, use a large pot instead.

INSTRUCTIONS

1. In a large deep pan or skillet, covered, cook the onions with the olive oil on low heat for 5 minutes.
2. Add the celery, then cook, covered, on low for another 10 minutes.
3. Add the broccoli, then cook, covered, on medium-low for another 5 minutes.
4. Place the pan/skillet cover ajar to prevent further cooking of the vegetables.
5. In a medium pan or skillet, sauté the chicken, stirring frequently until the chicken has whitened. Add the cinnamon stick and bay leaves, then cover and cook on low for about 25 minutes, stirring occasionally, until the chicken is cooked. Remove the cinnamon stick and bay leaves.
6. Transfer the chicken to the pan/skillet of cooked vegetables, draining the chicken broth into a large pot.
7. Add the water, mustard, flour, and spices to the broth in the pot, then whisk well. Bring to a boil, then cook, covered, on low for 15 minutes, stirring occasionally.
8. Mix the powdered milk and liquid milk in a small bowl.
9. On medium-high heat, slowly pour in the milk to the sauce, then add the parmesan cheese little by little, stirring well until melted. Stir in the honey.
10. Keep stirring until the sauce just comes to a boil.
11. Add the vegetables and chicken to the sauce, then gently fold. Let sit for 10 minutes before serving.
12. Serve with a side of quinoa (recipe on page 135) or brown rice (recipe on page 129) and add a squeeze of lemon juice if desired.

NUTRITION FACTS PER CUP

194 Kcal	22 g Protein	4 g Fat	18 g Carbs	4 g Fiber	8 g Sugar

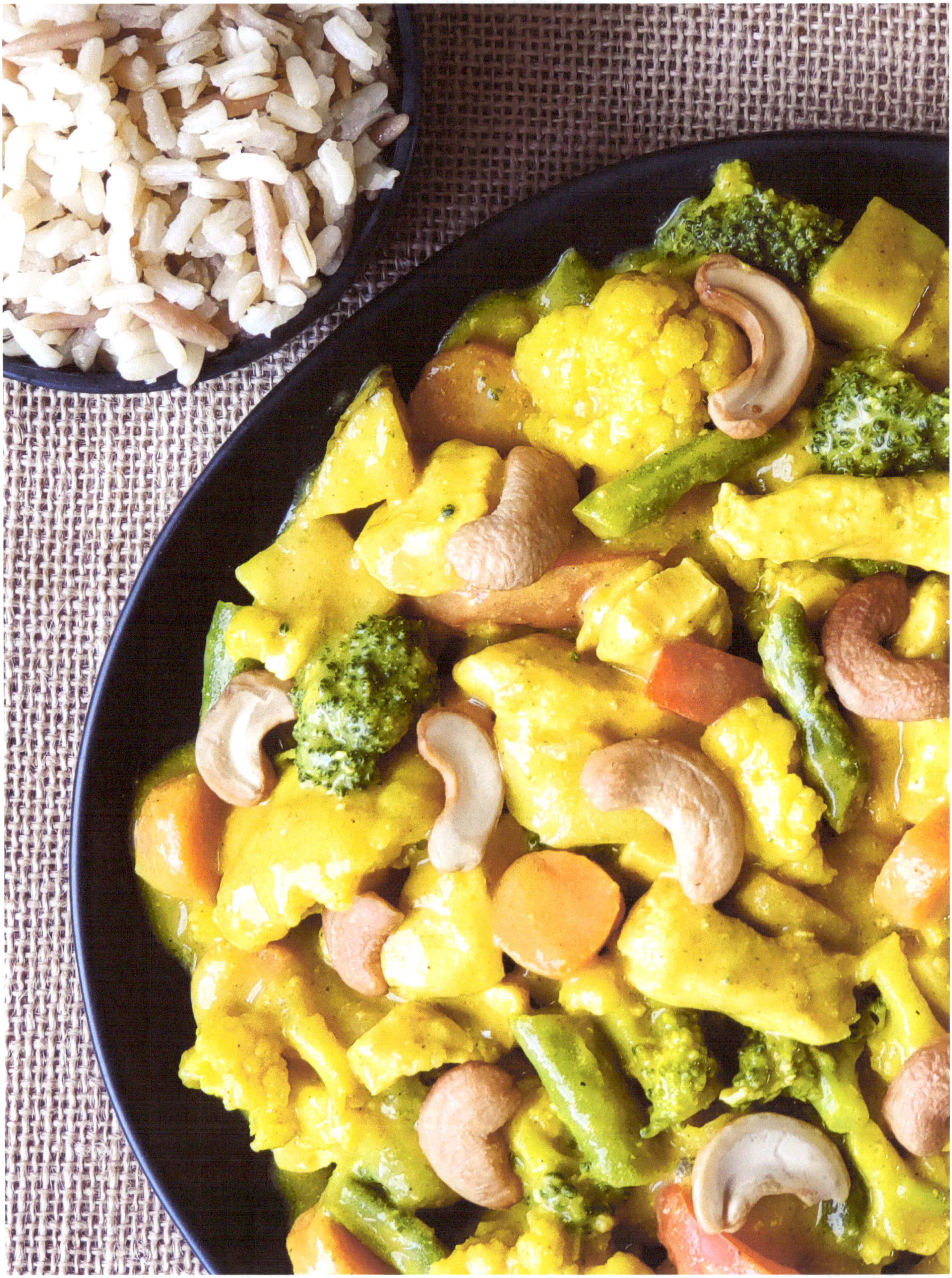

CURRY CHICKEN AND VEGGIES

Adapted from my mother's recipe for Indian curry chicken with vegetables, this dish is a light but flavorful version of the many variations of this simple Indian dish commonly made worldwide. I like to keep my curry sauce dairy-free and light, by using only light coconut milk and no butter, cream, or full-fat milk. Since curry powders vary so much in flavor and strength, I recommend one make this dish with the curry powder one desires. I like flavor, but not hot spice, so I always use mild yellow curry without much red pepper.

RECIPE YIELD 18 cups

DF EF FF

INGREDIENTS

2 raw large chicken breasts (no skin, no visible fat, no bones), sliced into strips (1 kg)
1 small cauliflower head (no stalk), broken/chopped into small florets (700 g)
1 large broccoli head (no stalk), broken/chopped into small florets (230 g)
1 large russet potato (with skin), diced (590 g)
1 ½ large carrots (no skin), sliced into circles (150 g)
1 medium red bell pepper, sliced into short strips (165 g)
1 ½ medium yellow onions, sliced into short strips (240 g)
2 cups frozen cut green beans (230 g), thawed, rinsed, drained well
2 tsp garlic, crushed
2 tbsp olive oil
6 ¾ cups light coconut milk
5 tbsp whole wheat flour
3 tbsp curry
1 tsp turmeric
½ tsp paprika
2 ⅓ tsp salt
1 cinnamon stick
2 dry bay leaves

INSTRUCTIONS

1. Soak the diced potatoes in hot water for 10 minutes, then drain well and pat dry. Toss with a ½ tbsp olive oil, then bake on a sheet pan (recommended dimensions: 25 cm x 35 cm or similar) lined with parchment paper in a preheated oven at 375 °F for 50 minutes. Set aside.
2. In a large deep pan or skillet, covered, cook the onions with 1 tbsp olive oil on low heat for 5 minutes.
3. Add the carrots and sweet peppers, then cook, covered, on medium-low for another 5 minutes.
4. Add the cauliflower and beans, then cook, covered, on medium-low for another 5 minutes.
5. Add the broccoli, then cook, covered, on low for another 5 minutes.
6. Place the pan/skillet cover ajar to prevent further cooking of the vegetables.
7. In a medium pan or skillet, sauté the chicken, stirring frequently until the chicken has whitened. Add the cinnamon stick and bay leaves, then cover and cook on low for about 25 minutes, stirring occasionally, until the chicken is cooked. Remove the cinnamon stick and bay leaves.
8. Transfer the chicken to the pan/skillet of cooked vegetables, draining away the chicken broth into a large pot.

Instructions continued on the next page »

NUTRITION FACTS PER CUP

225.4 Kcal	16 g Protein	9 g Fat	20 g Carbs	4 g Fiber	4 g Sugar

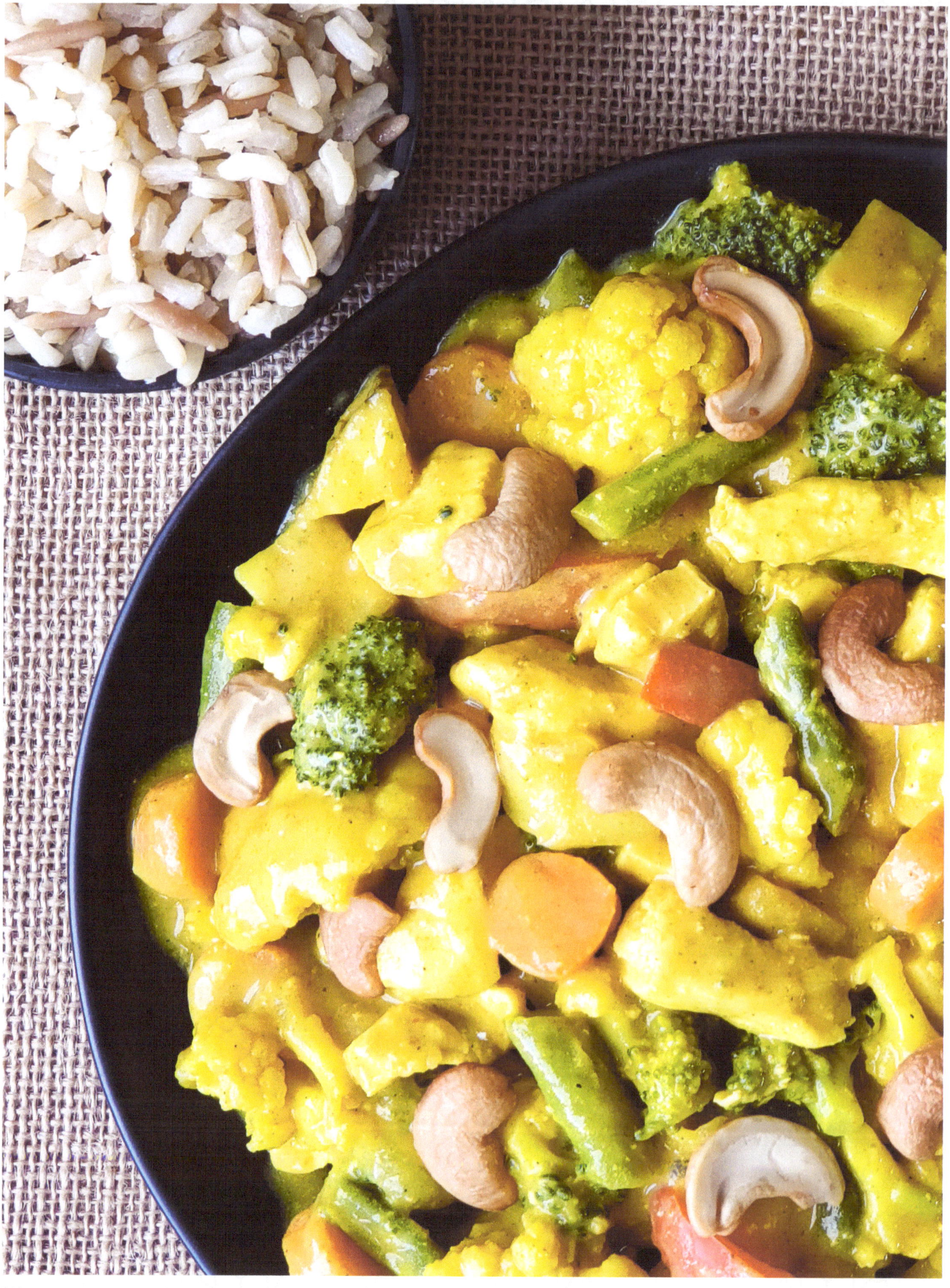

INGREDIENTS

4 halves raw chicken breasts (no skin, no visible fat, no bones), sliced into strips (1 kg)
1 small cauliflower head (no stalk), broken/chopped into small florets (700 g)
1 large broccoli head (no stalk), broken/chopped into small florets (230 g)
1 large russet potato (with skin), diced (590 g)
1 ½ large carrots (no skin), sliced into circles (150 g)
1 medium red bell pepper, sliced into short strips (165 g)
1 ½ medium yellow onions, sliced into short strips (240 g)
2 cups frozen cut green beans (230 g), thawed, rinsed, drained well
2 tsp garlic, crushed
2 tbsp olive oil
6 ¾ cups light coconut milk
5 tbsp whole wheat flour
3 tbsp curry
1 tsp turmeric
½ tsp paprika
2 ⅓ tsp salt
1 cinnamon stick
2 dry bay leaves

NOTES

- If one thinks the pan/skillet they have is not deep enough to fit all the vegetables, use a large pot instead.
- 6 ¾ cup coconut milk is equivalent to 4 (13.5 oz) cans.
- One can add more curry powder to the dish if desired.

INSTRUCTIONS

1. Soak the diced potatoes in hot water for 10 minutes, then drain well and pat dry. Toss with a ½ tbsp olive oil, then bake on a sheet pan (recommended dimensions: 25 cm x 35 cm or similar) lined with parchment paper in a preheated oven at 375 °F for 50 minutes. Set aside.
2. In a large deep pan or skillet, covered, cook the onions with 1 tbsp olive oil on low heat for 5 minutes.
3. Add the carrots and sweet peppers, then cook, covered, on low for another 5 minutes.
4. Add the cauliflower and beans, then cook, covered, on low for another 5 minutes.
5. Add the broccoli, then cook, covered, on low for another 5 minutes.
6. Place the pan/skillet cover ajar to prevent further cooking of the vegetables.
7. In a medium pan or skillet, sauté the chicken, stirring frequently until the chicken has whitened. Add the cinnamon stick and bay leaves, then cover and cook on low for about 25 minutes, stirring occasionally, until the chicken is cooked. Remove the cinnamon stick and bay leaves.
8. Transfer the chicken to the pan/skillet of cooked vegetables, draining away the chicken broth into a large pot.
9. Add the coconut milk, ½ tbsp olive oil, garlic, flour, and spices to the broth in the pot, then whisk well. Bring to a boil, then cook, covered, on low for 15 minutes, stirring occasionally.
10. Add the potatoes, vegetables, and chicken to the sauce, then gently fold. Let sit for 10 minutes before serving.
11. Garnish with dry roasted cashew nuts if desired and serve with a side of brown rice (recipe on page 129).

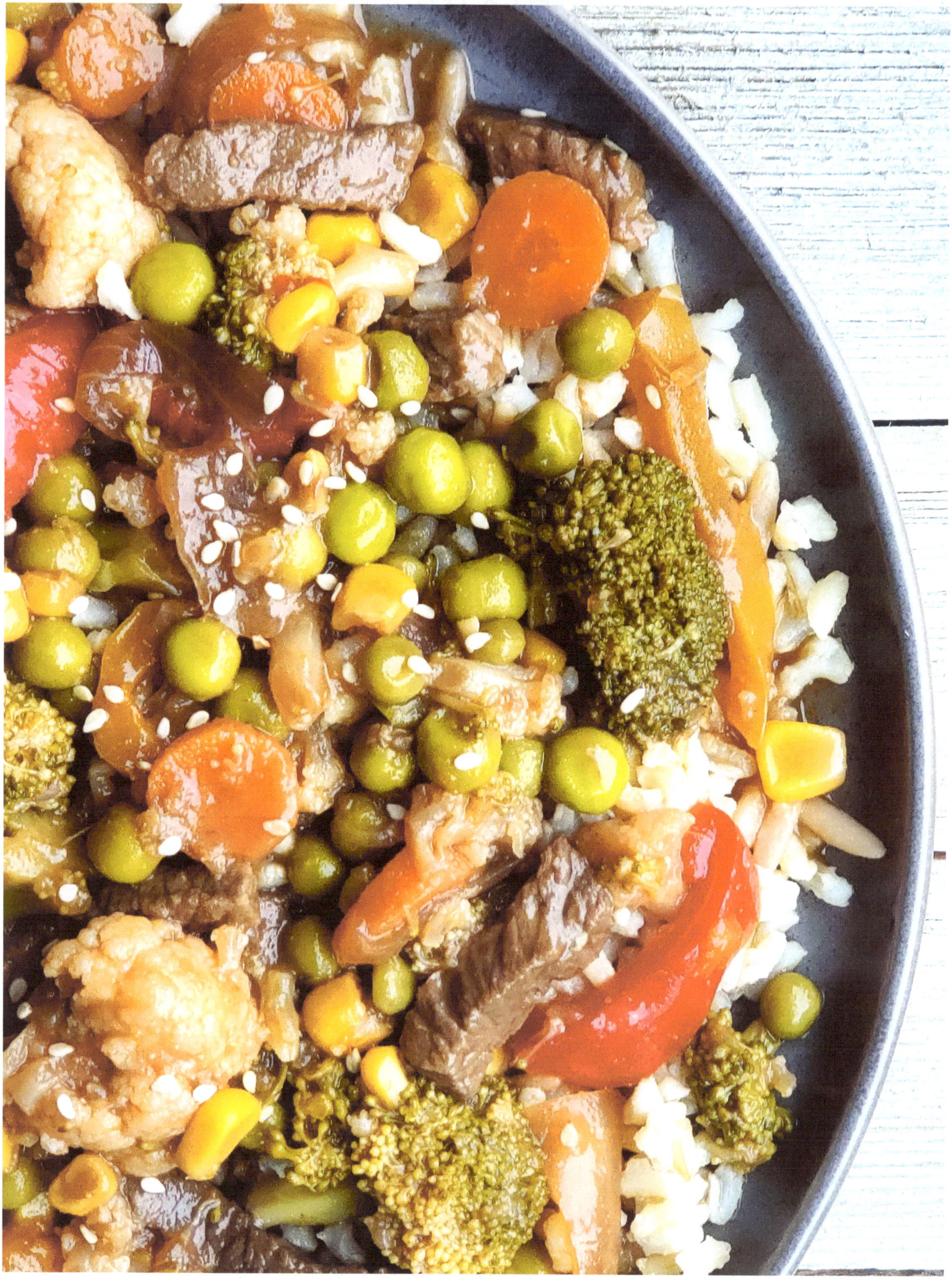

SWEET AND SOUR BEEF AND VEGGIES

Adapted from my mother's recipe for Chinese beef and vegetable stir-fry, this dish offers a blend of the strong flavors of soy sauce and ginger with a subtle sweetness from maple syrup. Though it is typical of a stir-fry dish to call for sautéing the vegetables, I prefer slow cooking over low heat because I prefer a slightly more tender vegetable outcome, and I normally use extra virgin olive oil. Either way, this dish is sure to please your sweet and sour tastes with an array of colorful vegetables and tender lean beef.

RECIPE YIELD 16 cups

DF EF FF

INGREDIENTS

Raw lean sirloin beef (no visible fat), sliced into thin strips (750 g)
1 small cauliflower head (no stalk), broken/chopped into small florets (700 g)
3 large broccoli heads (no stalks), broken/chopped into small florets (690 g)
2 medium bell peppers (1 red, 1 yellow), sliced into short strips (330 g)
1 ½ medium yellow onions, sliced into short strips (240 g)
2 large carrots (no skin), sliced into circles (200 g)
2 cups frozen peas (250 g), thawed, rinsed, drained
1 ½ cups sweet corn kernels (240 g)
2 tbsp garlic, crushed
1 tbsp ginger root, finely grated
⅔ cup ketchup (173 g)
¾ cup low-salt soy sauce
3 tbsp maple syrup
6 tbsp lemon juice
2 tsp olive oil
2 cups water
4 tbsp whole wheat flour
1 tsp ginger

NOTE

If one thinks the skillet they have is not deep enough to fit all the vegetables, use a large pot instead.

INSTRUCTIONS

1. In a large bowl, mix the marinade ingredients (garlic, ginger root, ketchup, soy sauce, maple syrup, lemon juice, ginger). Add the beef, then mix well. Cover, then let marinate for 4 hours.
2. In a large deep pan or skillet, covered, cook the onions with the olive oil on low heat for 5 minutes.
3. Add the carrots and sweet peppers, then cook, covered, on low for another 5 minutes.
4. Add the cauliflower, then cook, covered, on medium-low for another 5 minutes.
5. Add the broccoli, peas, and corn, then cook, covered, on medium-low for another 5 minutes.
6. Place the pan/skillet cover ajar to prevent further cooking of the vegetables.
7. Drain the beef from the marinade, pouring the marinade into a large pot. Put the drained meat in a medium pan or skillet, then on high heat, sauté the meat stirring frequently until browned. Cover, then cook on low for about 25 minutes, stirring occasionally, until the meat is cooked.
8. Transfer the meat to the pan/skillet of cooked vegetables, draining the broth into the pot of marinade.
9. Add the water and flour to the marinade, then whisk well. On high heat, bring to a boil while stirring frequently. Cook, covered, on low for 15 minutes, stirring occasionally.
10. Add the vegetables and beef to the marinade, then gently fold. Let sit for 10 minutes before serving.
11. Garnish with toasted sesame seeds if desired and serve with a side of brown rice (recipe on page 129).

NUTRITION FACTS PER CUP

186 Kcal	16 g Protein	3 g Fat	25.5 g Carbs	5 g Fiber	12.6 g Sugar

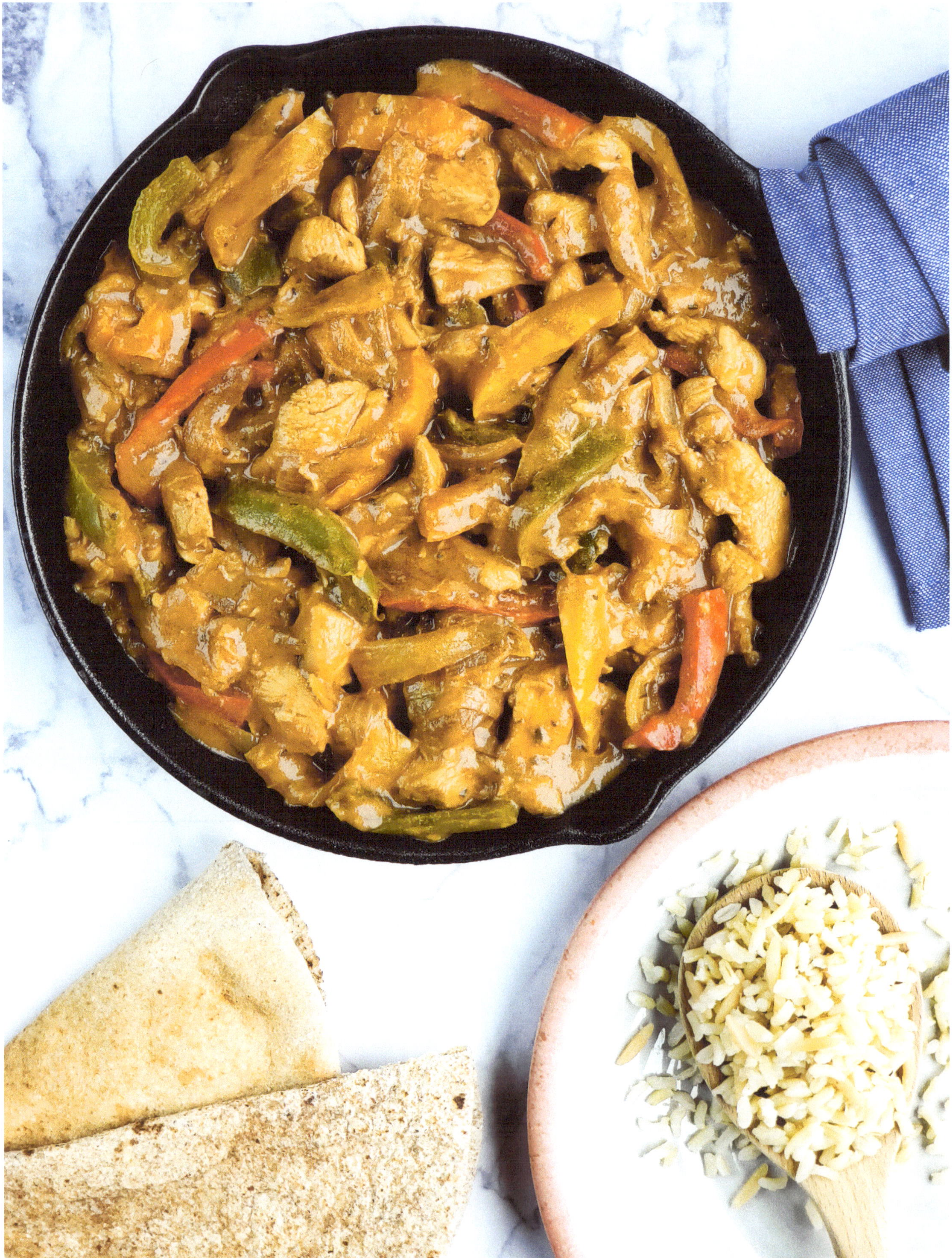

FAJITA CHICKEN AND VEGGIES

Traditional fajita dishes are often complemented with a side of guacamole, salsa, sour cream, or cheese. My recipe, adapted from my mother's recipe for Mexican fajita chicken with vegetables, is super flavorful on its own, not necessitating any additions. I enjoy my fajita with a side of brown rice, and thus bump up the marinade a bit to make it juicier. Since I am fond of flavor but not hot spice, I avoid adding any hot peppers, but one can spice up their fajita as they wish. Fajitas can be prepared in many ways, and I like doing the vegetables in the oven while the chicken and sauce are cooking on the stove.

RECIPE YIELD 12 cups

DF EF FF

INGREDIENTS

3 raw large chicken breasts (no skin, no visible fat, no bones), sliced into strips (1.5 kg)
5 medium bell peppers (2 green, 1 red, 1 orange, 1 yellow), sliced into short strips (825 g)
2 large white onions, sliced into short strips (640 g)
1 tbsp garlic, crushed
2 tsp ginger root, finely grated
⅔ cup ketchup (173 g)
2 tbsp mustard
½ cup low-salt soy sauce
2 tbsp olive oil
½ cup water
2 tbsp whole wheat flour
1 tbsp dry oregano leaves
2 ½ tsp cumin
1 tsp ginger
1 tsp paprika
⅛ tsp black pepper
1 cinnamon stick
2 dry bay leaves

NOTE

❀ For those who wish to eat this dish rolled up in sandwiches using tortillas or even Arabic bread, do not add the ½ cup water called for in the recipe.

INSTRUCTIONS

1. In a large bowl, mix the marinade ingredients (garlic, ginger root, ketchup, mustard, soy sauce, 1 tbsp olive oil, flour, herbs, spices). Add the chicken, then mix well. Cover, then let marinate for 4 hours.
2. Toss the onions and sweet peppers into another large bowl with the remaining 1 tbsp of oil, then spread on 2 sheet pans (recommended dimensions: 25 cm x 35 cm or similar) lined with parchment paper. Bake in a preheated oven at 375 °F for 20 minutes (give the pans a light shake 10 minutes into cooking).
3. In the meantime, sauté the chicken in the marinade in a large pot, stirring frequently until the chicken has whitened. Add the water, cinnamon stick, and bay leaves, then bring to a boil. Cover and cook on low for about 25 minutes, stirring occasionally, until the chicken is cooked. Remove the cinnamon stick and bay leaves.
4. Add the cooked vegetables over the chicken, then gently fold. Let sit for 10 minutes before serving.
5. Serve with a side of brown rice (recipe on page 129).

NUTRITION FACTS PER CUP

252 Kcal	31 g Protein	6 g Fat	18.5 g Carbs	3 g Fiber	10.5 g Sugar

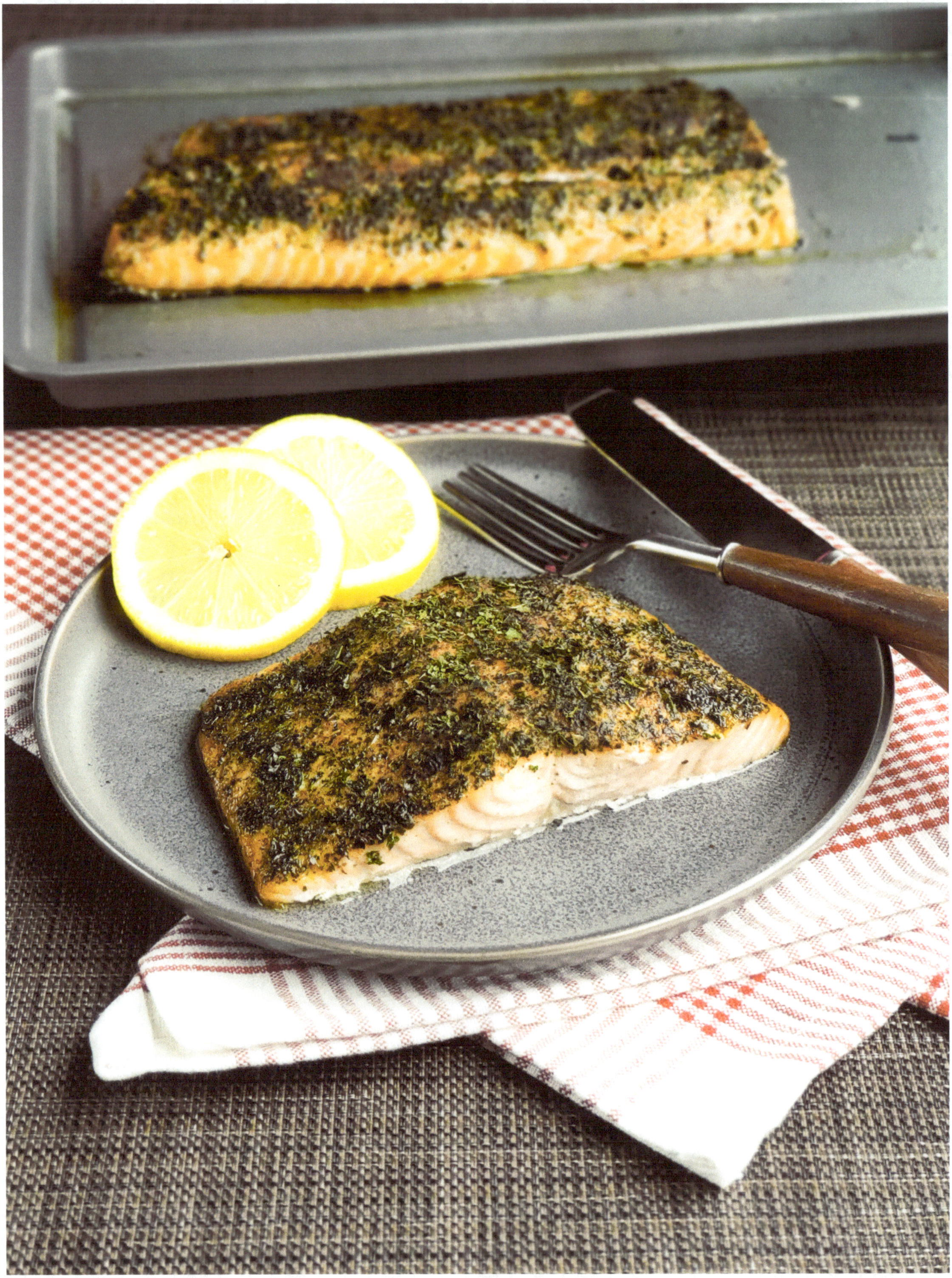

BAKED SALMON

This is my super simple, fast, flavorful, and healthy recipe for baked salmon. It is adapted from a recipe handed down to my father from my maternal grandfather - who loved salmon! My father ended up falling in love with this recipe, and it wasn't long before salmon became a biweekly meal in our household while I was growing up!

RECIPE YIELD 4 slices

DF GF EF FF

INGREDIENTS

Raw salmon fillet (with skin, no bones) (950 g)
1 tsp olive oil
1 tbsp dry basil leaves
¼ tsp paprika
⅔ tsp garlic salt
¼ tsp black pepper

NOTES

- One can substitute the garlic salt with fresh garlic if desired. Mix 1 tsp crushed garlic with ½ tsp salt (until a paste is formed), then spread onto the oiled fish before sprinkling on the rest of the spices/herbs.
- Adding onion powder to the spice mix adds a nice flavor as well.
- If one is using refined olive oil, one can bake the salmon in a hotter oven, at a broil setting of 450 °F for 12 to 15 minutes, on one level higher than the middle oven rack (thinner sections of the fillet will take about 7 to 10 minutes only).

INSTRUCTIONS

1. Mix the spices (paprika, garlic salt, pepper) together in a small bowl.
2. Place the salmon fillet (skin down) on a lightly greased sheet pan (recommended dimensions: 25 cm x 35 cm or similar).
3. Brush the fillet with olive oil, then evenly sprinkle on the spice mix.
4. Evenly sprinkle on the dry basil, covering the surface of the fish.
5. Bake, uncovered, in a preheated oven at 375 °F for about 20 minutes (if the fillet is not of uniform thickness, make sure to bake the thinner sections for 12 to 15 minutes only, then cut off, set aside, and keep warm while the thicker piece continues to bake).
6. Squeeze on some lemon juice and serve with a side of baked vegetables or a salad if desired. For a Middle Eastern twist, serve with my *tahini* sauce (recipe on page 139).

NUTRITION FACTS PER SLICE

368.4 Kcal	50 g Protein	17 g Fat	0.6 g Carbs	0.5 g Fiber	0.05 g Sugar

DESSERTS

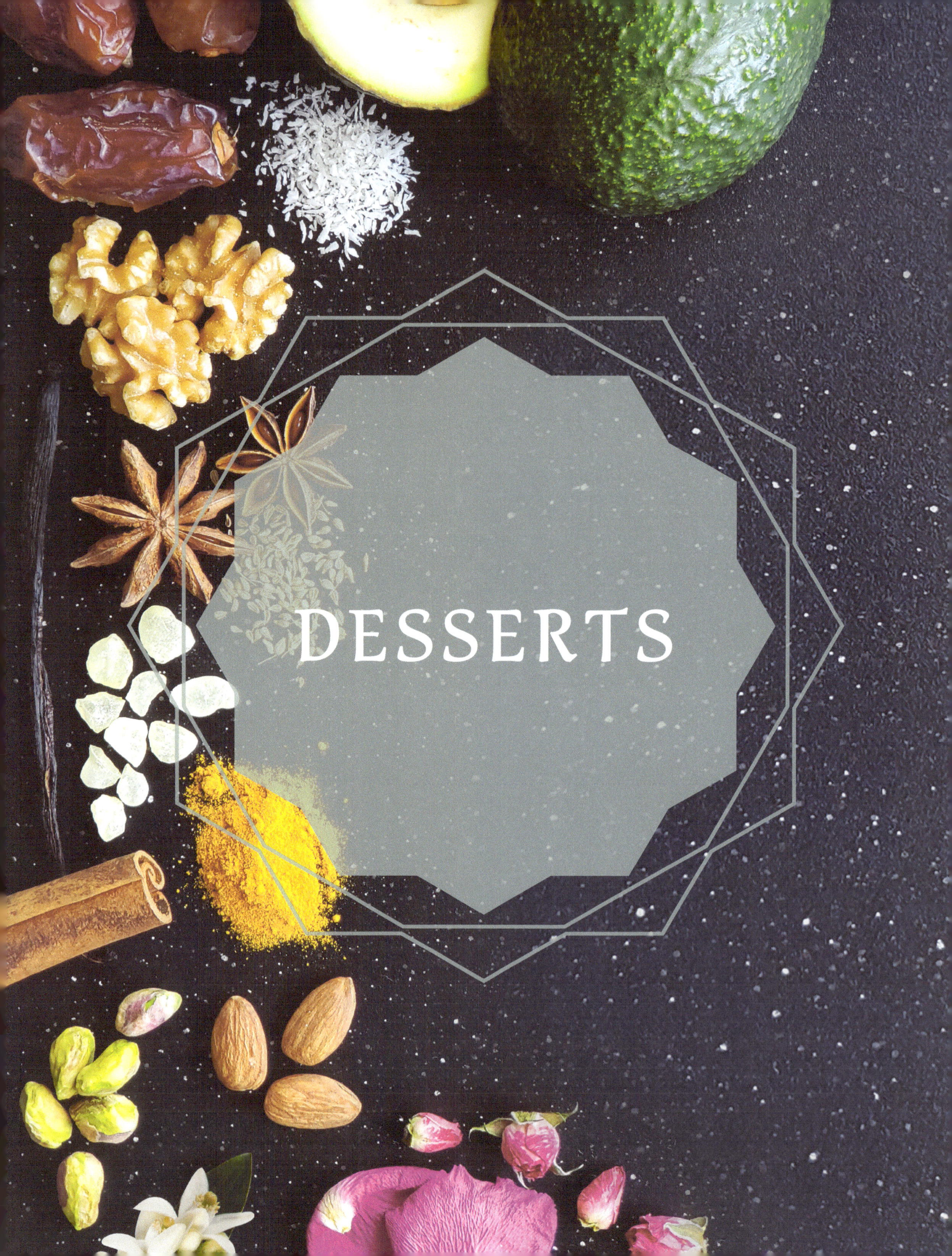

Lebanese desserts are famous for their variety in ingredients and their richness in flavor and sweetness. Many desserts common to the Lebanese cuisine are also commonly made in other Middle Eastern countries, with possible slight variations in nomenclature, ingredients, and methods. Lebanese desserts presented in this section are named with the traditional Arabic name of the dessert, along with an English transliteration of the Arabic. Desserts without an Arabic name are not Lebanese/Middle Eastern. They are either recipes of my own creation or are ones adapted from recipes handed down to me by my mother.

SOME GENERAL REMARKS AND RECOMMENDATIONS

- Since I use honey in many of my desserts, vegans who prefer avoiding honey in their diet may shy away from trying these recipes. Instead of doing so, opt for trying maple syrup, carob molasses, or agave nectar instead of the called for honey (in equal substitutions).

- All nuts and seeds called for in the dessert recipes are shelled, raw, and unsalted (unless otherwise specified). Nuts and seeds not indicated as chopped or ground are intended to be added whole.

- Make sure to measure the called for amounts of fruit and vegetables using dry measuring cups.

- Make sure to measure the called for amounts of yogurt and *tahini* using dry measuring cups.

- Make sure to measure the called for amounts of sweetener and oil using liquid measuring cups.

- Sifting dry ingredients allows for better mixing of the ingredients together and adds fluffiness to the final product. Since my desserts call for either regular whole wheat flour or whole wheat pastry flour, do not discard any bran pieces that are caught in the sifter, but instead just pour them back into the mixing bowl containing the batter.

- One of the trickiest aspects in baking is oven heat variability. No oven is perfect, and no oven bakes in the same way as another oven. Get to know your oven, and how 'hot' it is - how much time it takes to bake your goods and at what temperature. Using an inexpensive oven thermometer may be a good way to give you a sense of how your oven functions, allowing you to set your oven thermostat higher or lower depending on whether your oven tends to run cool or hot.

- Start preheating your oven at least 5 minutes before getting ready to place the dessert in the oven. My rule of thumb: set your oven at the desired temperature, then grease the baking pan, mix the wet and dry ingredients together, and then pour the batter into the pan and place immediately in the oven.

- I prefer baking my desserts at temperatures not higher than 325 °F (165 °C) since they contain honey, which is darker to start with than refined sugar and tends to brown the baked product even more during baking. Also, because of the presence of whole wheat flour in these recipes, the baked product will look browner than if baked with refined white flour.

- Bake desserts on the middle rack of the oven, unless otherwise specified.

- There is quite a variability between different brands of baking powder in the market, unlike baking soda. And this variability is often enough to cause a difference in outcomes of baked goods (sometimes more pronounced than others depending on the baking powder ingredients as well as the recipe itself). The baking powder I use for my desserts is a double-acting one containing the following ingredients in this order: cornstarch, sodium bicarbonate, sodium aluminum sulfate, and monocalcium phosphate.

- Although some of my baked desserts are somewhat freezer friendly, others are not, primarily because they are very dense and moist due to the presence of whole wheat flour and liquid sweeteners. As such, I prefer keeping my baked goods in the refrigerator and consuming within a week.

- If one does not have the called for type of wheat flour for a given recipe, below is a simple estimated flour-substitution guide that I have devised (this substitution may work better for some recipes than for others):

  - If needing to use white whole wheat flour instead of whole wheat pastry flour, decrease the amount of flour by 2 tbsp for each cup of flour.

  - If needing to use regular whole wheat flour instead of whole wheat pastry flour, decrease the amount of flour by 3 tbsp for each cup of flour. However, if a recipe calls for a total of 2 or more cups of flour, one may need to slightly adjust (decrease) the liquid/semi liquid ingredients (either water, milk, or yogurt) in the recipe.

  - If needing to use refined white flour instead of whole wheat pastry flour, increase the amount of flour by 1 tbsp for each cup of flour.

  - If needing to use white whole wheat flour instead of regular whole wheat flour, increase the amount of flour by 1 tbsp for each cup of flour.

  - If needing to use refined white flour instead of regular whole wheat flour in a recipe, increase the amount of flour by 4 tbsp for each cup of flour. However, if a recipe calls for a total of 2 or more cups of flour, one may need to slightly adjust (increase) the liquid/semi liquid ingredients (either water, milk, or yogurt) in the recipe.

- The 'sugar' value in the nutrition facts of recipes refers to the total amount of sugar (both simple and complex) that is naturally occurring in the various ingredients.

- I grease my baking pans with coconut oil, unless otherwise specified.

- The fat source called for greasing baking pans is NOT included in the nutrition facts. Reasons include the fact that different desserts absorb the pan grease differently, and some people may opt for covering all their pans with parchment paper before pouring in the dessert batter.

- Food items suggested as garnish are NOT included in the nutrition facts.

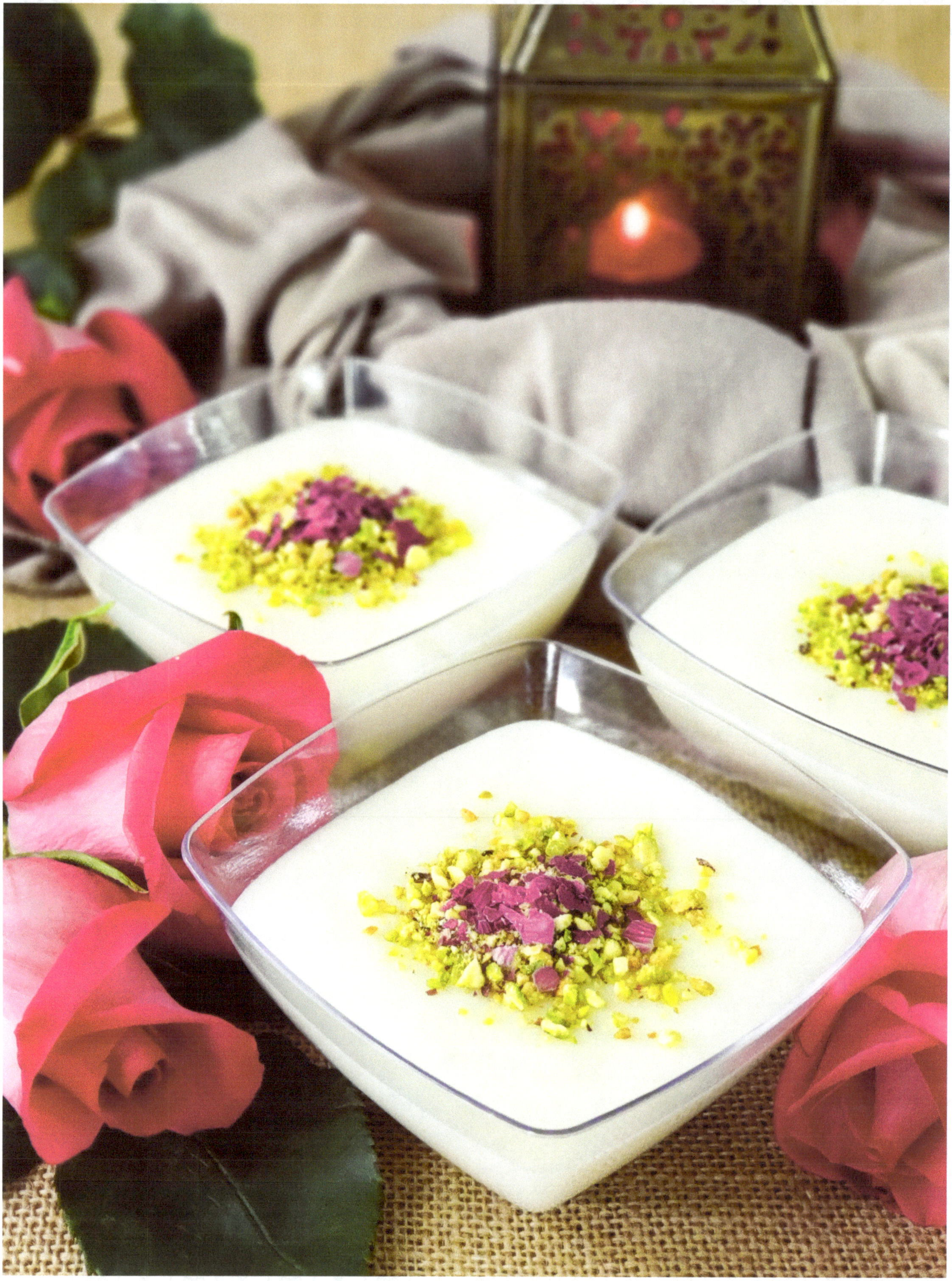

PLAIN MILK PUDDING

Mhalbiyyeh مهلبيّة

This smooth and creamy rose water-infused Lebanese pudding is light and refreshing, made with only a handful of simple ingredients. Traditionally made with full-fat milk, refined white sugar, and a lot of cornstarch, my healthier and more whole version calls for skim milk thickened with powdered milk, honey, and equal parts brown rice flour and cornstarch.

RECIPE YIELD 10 cups

GF EF OF Vt

INGREDIENTS

Dry Ingredients

½ cup + 1 ½ tbsp brown rice flour (80 g)
½ cup + 1 ½ tbsp cornstarch (80 g)
⅔ cup skim powdered milk (60 g)

Wet Ingredients

10 cups skim liquid milk
⅓ cup honey
6 tbsp rose water

NOTE

- To prevent scorching, it is recommended to add an extra burner grate on the stove top underneath the pot during cooking.

RECIPE ALTERNATIVE

- One could make this pudding with only brown rice flour (i.e. without any cornstarch), but the texture of the pudding will be 'grainy', and the appearance will look dull (as cornstarch gives the pudding a shiny appearance).

INSTRUCTIONS

1. In a large pot, mix the dry ingredients, then pour in the liquid milk, whisking well. Let sit in the refrigerator for 30 minutes.
2. Over medium-high heat, stir the pudding frequently until slightly thickened.
3. Add the honey, then continue stirring well until it comes to a boil.
4. Cook, uncovered, on medium-low heat for 5 minutes, stirring well to prevent scorching.
5. Add the rose water, then stir to mix.
6. Pour into 10 bowls (1 cup per bowl). Let cool to room temperature.
7. Refrigerate for at least 2 hours before serving.
8. I enjoy this pudding plain with no toppings, but one can garnish with ground pistachios and crushed dry rose petals if desired.
9. Store, covered, in the refrigerator.

NUTRITION FACTS PER CUP

194 Kcal	11 g Protein	0.4 g Fat	38 g Carbs	0.5 g Fiber	24 g Sugar

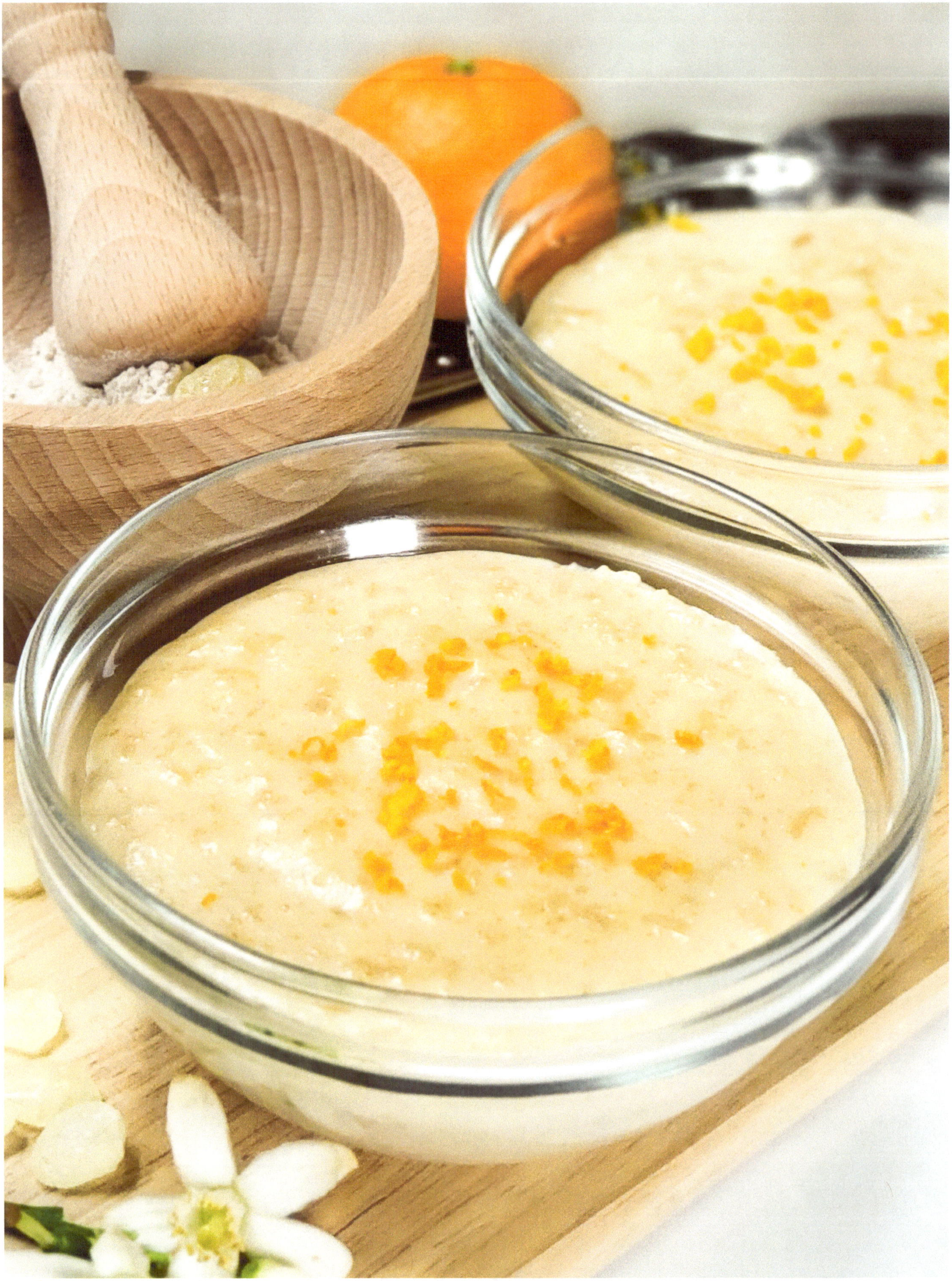

RICE MILK PUDDING

Riz bi Haleeb رز بحليب

This 'rice in milk' pudding is a traditional Lebanese dessert flavored with orange blossom water and mastic. While traditionally made with white rice, full-fat milk, refined white sugar, and quite a bit of corn starch, my healthy modified version contains parboiled brown rice and some oatmeal, skim milk, honey, and brown rice flour. Another healthy traditional version of this pudding calls for the use of whole wheat kernels instead of rice. This pudding is sure to satisfy a sweet craving and makes for a healthy breakfast as well!

RECIPE YIELD 8 cups

GF EF OF Vt

INGREDIENTS

Dry Ingredients

- ⅔ cup dry parboiled brown rice (121 g)
- ¼ cup dry quick oats (22 g)
- 6 tbsp skim powdered milk
- 2 tbsp brown rice flour
- 2 tbsp cornstarch
- 1 small or medium piece of mastic

Wet Ingredients

- 10 cups skim liquid milk
- ⅓ cup honey
- 1 tsp orange blossom water

NOTES

- To prevent scorching, it is recommended to add an extra burner grate on the stove top underneath the pot during cooking.
- I enjoy this pudding plain with no toppings, but one can garnish with some orange zest if desired.

INSTRUCTIONS

1. Measure out the brown rice flour into a small bowl. Remove 1 tsp of the flour and add to the mastic in a pounder. Pound the mastic until well ground and non-sticky. Set aside.
2. Pick over the rice, removing any bad pieces. Rinse well, then drain.
3. In a large pot, mix the dry ingredients (except for the cornstarch and mastic), then pour in the liquid milk, whisking well. Let sit in the refrigerator for 2 hours.
4. Over medium-high heat, stir the pudding frequently until it comes to a boil.
5. Cook, covered, on medium-low heat for 35 minutes, stirring occasionally to prevent scorching.
6. Measure out the honey into a small bowl. Remove some of the pudding and add to the honey, then whisk in the cornstarch. Return slowly to the pot of pudding and stir to mix.
7. Bring back to a boil, then cook, uncovered, on medium-high heat for 15 minutes, stirring well to prevent scorching.
8. Stir in the ground mastic, then continue cooking for another 10 minutes.
9. Add the orange blossom water, then stir to mix.
10. Pour into 8 bowls (1 cup per bowl). Let cool to room temperature.
11. Refrigerate for at least 2 hours before serving.
12. Store, covered, in the refrigerator.

NUTRITION FACTS PER CUP

239 Kcal	13 g Protein	1 g Fat	45 g Carbs	1 g Fiber	28.6 g Sugar

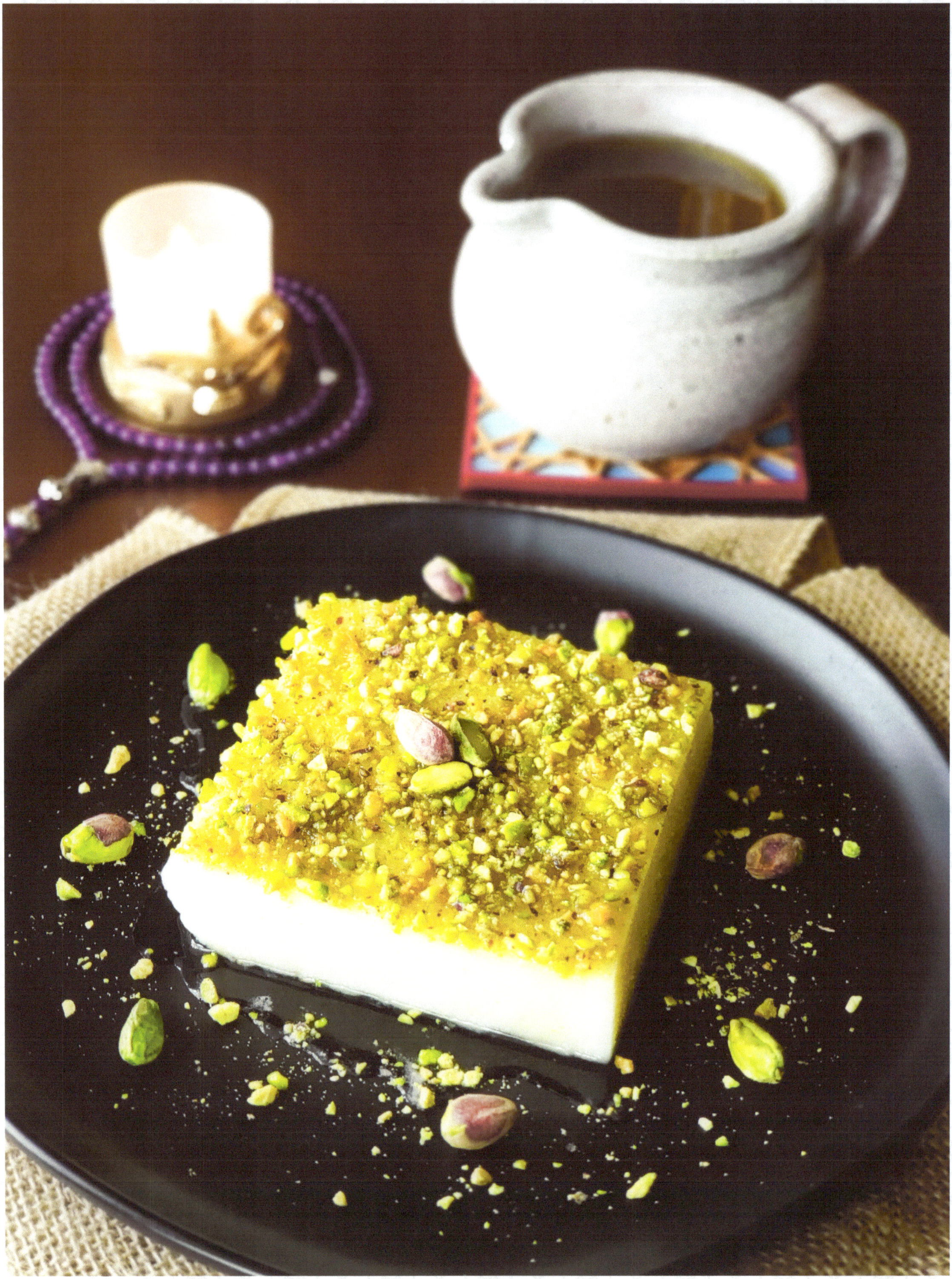

LEBANESE NIGHTS PUDDING

Layali Lubnan ليالي لبنان

This pudding makes me very nostalgic of Lebanon and its beautiful clear night skies with shining stars, bringing back many cherished memories every time I prepare it. While very easy to make, this pudding is traditionally very rich, made with full-fat milk, topped with a layer of a rich Middle Eastern clotted cream (known as *qashta*), as well as a layer of sweet whipping cream, then covered with a rich floral-infused sugar syrup (known as *qatir*). My healthy version is just as flavorful but much simpler and lighter, using skim milk thickened with powdered milk, skipping both the heavy cream and sweet whipping cream, while simply substituting traditional *qatir* with honey infused with floral waters.

RECIPE YIELD 18 slices

EF OF Vt

INGREDIENTS

Dry Ingredients

2 cups fine semolina flour (300 g)
½ cup skim powdered milk (45 g)
1 cup ground pistachios (140 g)

Wet Ingredients

10 cups skim liquid milk
1 tsp liquid vanilla extract
1 tbsp rose water
1 tbsp orange blossom water

Honey Syrup

1 cup honey
2 tsp rose water
2 tsp orange blossom water

NOTES

- To prevent scorching, it is recommended to add an extra burner grate on the stove top underneath the pot during cooking.
- The pudding could be poured into individual bowls if desired (top with pistachios and syrup just before serving).
- The nutrition facts do not include the honey syrup. 1 tbsp of pure honey contains 64 kcal; thus, 1 tbsp of my diluted honey syrup contains a bit less.

INSTRUCTIONS

1. In a large pot, mix the flour and powdered milk, then pour in the liquid milk and vanilla, whisking well. Let sit in the refrigerator for 30 minutes.
2. Over medium-high heat, bring to a light boil, stirring frequently.
3. Turn the heat down to medium-low, then cook, uncovered, for 5 minutes, stirring well to prevent scorching.
4. Add the floral waters, then stir to mix.
5. Pour into 2 deep glass or stoneware serving dishes (I use a large and a medium pan to accommodate the pudding; recommended dimensions: 23.5 cm x 33.5 cm and 20 cm x 28 cm or similar. Regardless of the number and dimensions of the pans used, pour the pudding in a way that the thickness of the pudding is not more than 2 to 3 cm high). Let cool to room temperature.
6. Refrigerate for at least 2 hours before serving.
7. Whisk the honey and floral waters in a small bowl.
8. Top the pudding surface with ground pistachios (⅔ cup for the large pan and ⅓ cup for the medium pan) before slicing, then drizzle each slice with honey syrup (~ 1 tbsp) just before serving.
9. Store, covered, in the refrigerator.

NUTRITION FACTS PER SLICE

156.5 Kcal	9 g Protein	4 g Fat	22 g Carbs	1 g Fiber	8.4 g Sugar

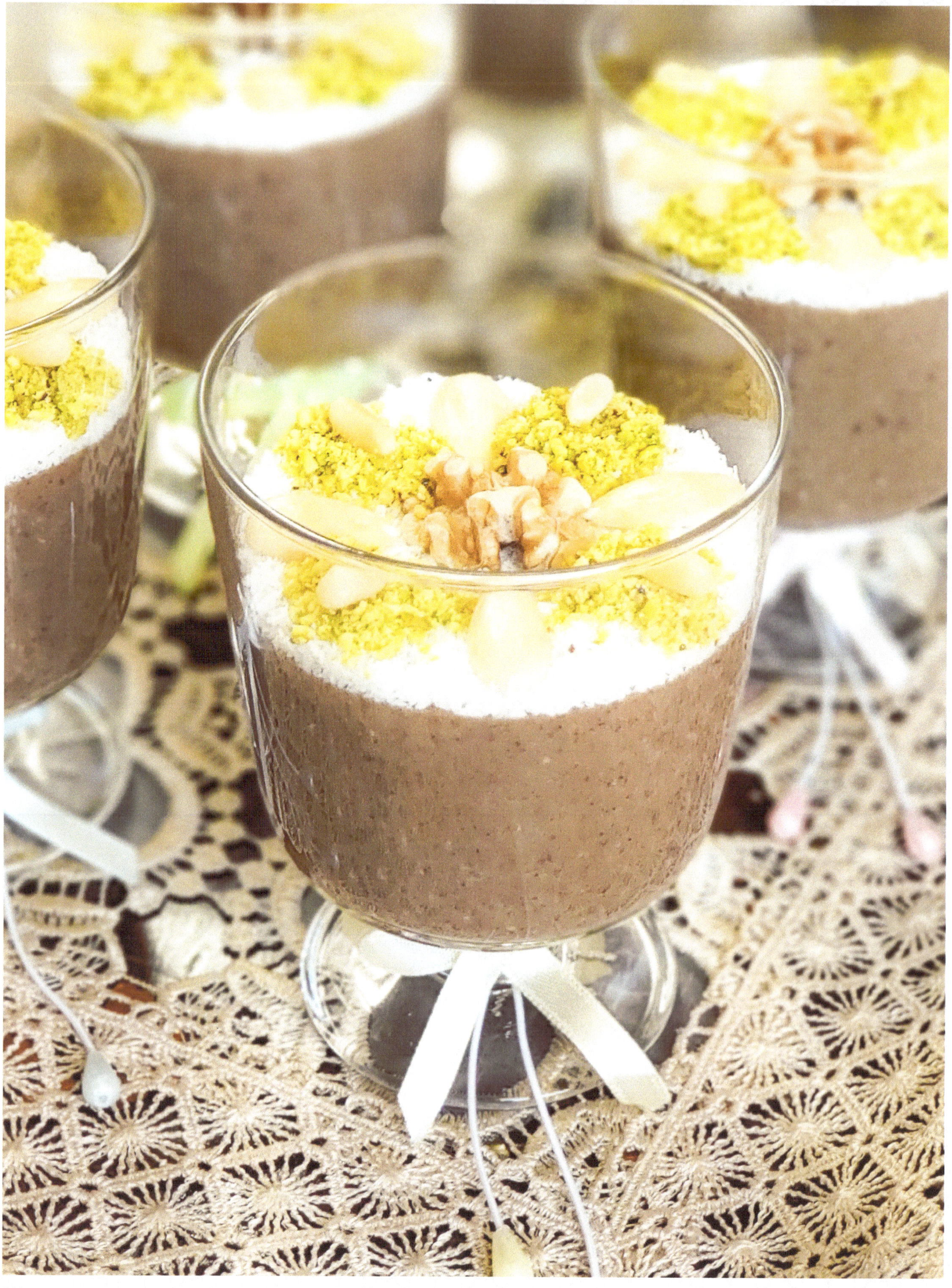

SPICY RICE PUDDING

Moghleh مغلي

This flavorful rice pudding is traditionally made and served in countries of the Middle East to celebrate the joy of the birth of a baby. It is a simple pudding spiced up with lots of caraway and cinnamon, with a little anise sometimes, and traditionally prepared with refined rice flour and white sugar. It is usually topped with shredded coconut, ground pistachios and other nuts such as walnuts, almonds, and pine nuts. My healthier take on this delicious pudding is made with whole brown rice flour and is sweetened with honey and dates.

RECIPE YIELD 11 cups

DF GF EF OF V

INGREDIENTS

Dry Ingredients

2 ½ cups brown rice flour (325 g)
2 tbsp caraway
2 tbsp cinnamon
2 tbsp anise seeds
¼ tsp salt

Wet Ingredients

16 large soft pitted medjool dates (305 g)
11 ½ cups water
1 ½ cups hot water
½ cup honey

Toppings

11 tbsp finely shredded unsweetened coconut flakes
11 tsp ground pistachios
11 walnut halves
44 blanched almond halves
44 pine nuts

NOTES

- To prevent scorching, it is recommended to add an extra burner grate on the stove top underneath the pot during cooking.
- It is best to add the toppings to each bowl just before serving to keep the coconut from absorbing moisture from the pudding.

INSTRUCTIONS

1. Pour the 11 ½ cups water into a pot, then whisk in the rice flour and spices. Cover, then let sit for 1 hour.
2. Rinse the walnuts, almonds, and pine nuts, then soak each one separately in a small bowl of cold water.
3. Sort through the anise seeds and remove any impurities. Place in a small bowl, then add ½ cup hot water. Let sit.
4. Place the dates and the remaining 1 cup hot water in a small food processor and blend very well.
5. Transfer the pot of water, flour, and spices to the stove. Over medium-high heat, bring to a boil, stirring frequently.
6. Cook, uncovered, on medium-low heat for 30 minutes, stirring occasionally to prevent scorching.
7. Pour in the honey and add the date paste as well as the anise water (discard the seeds), then whisk well to mix. On medium-high heat, continue stirring until the pudding returns to a rapid boil.
8. Turn back down to medium-low and cook for another 30 minutes, stirring occasionally.
9. Pour into 11 bowls (1 cup per bowl). Let cool to room temperature.
10. Store, covered, in the refrigerator.
11. Top each bowl with 1 tbsp of shredded coconut, 1 tsp ground pistachios, 4 almond halves, 1 walnut half, and 4 pine nuts (as shown in the picture, if desired).

NUTRITION FACTS PER CUP

327 Kcal	5 g Protein	9.4 g Fat	62 g Carbs	6 g Fiber	32 g Sugar

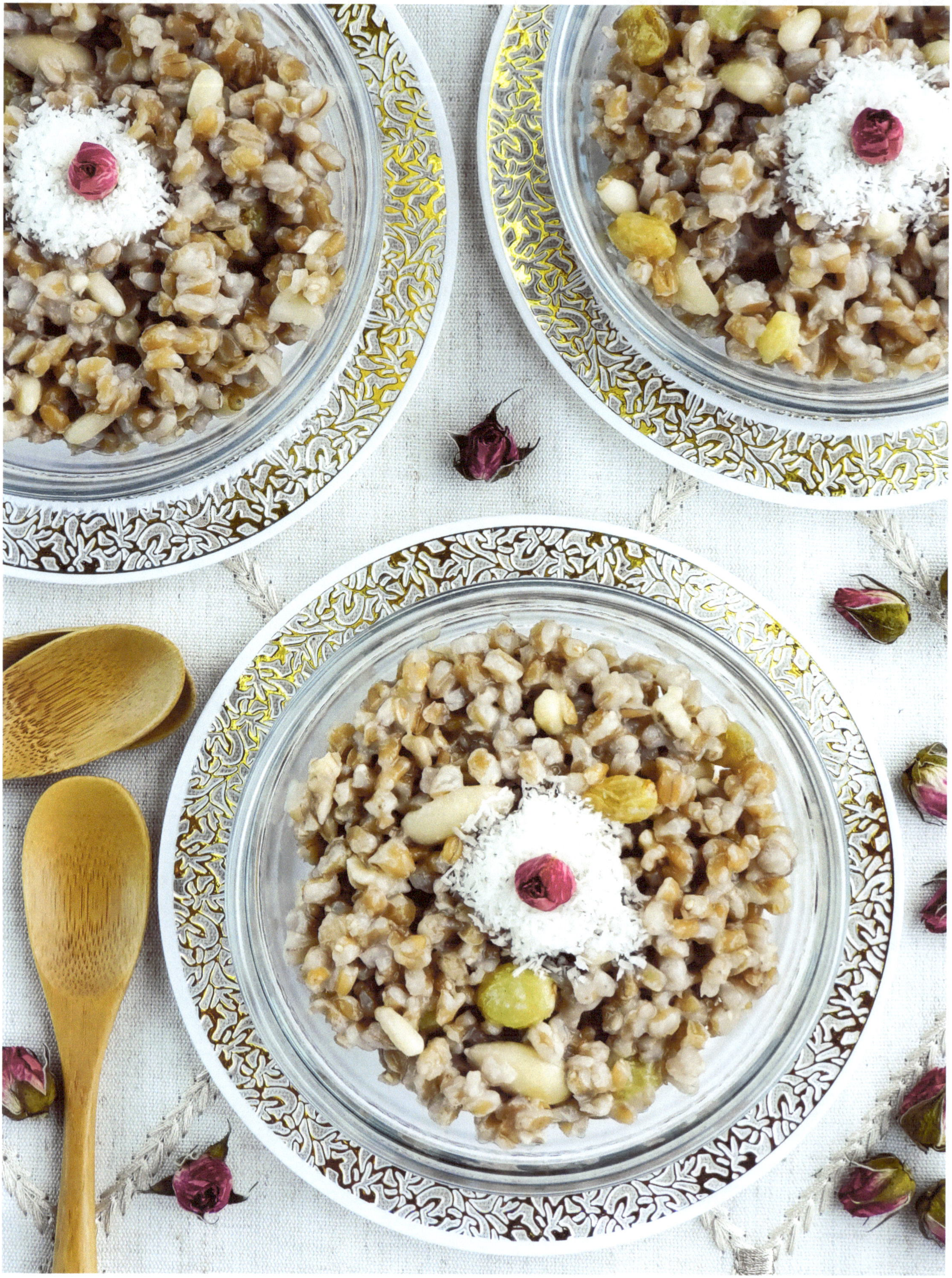

WHEAT AND NUTS PUDDING

Qamhiyyeh قمحيّة

This Middle Eastern dessert is traditionally made to celebrate the cutting through of a baby's first tooth! Cooked wheat berries are mixed with a variety of nuts, beautifully flavored with floral waters (orange blossom and rose), sweetened with sugar (and sometimes raisins, too), then topped with shredded coconut. I prefer sweetening this simple "pudding" with honey as well as raisins, while loading it with heart-healthy nuts. Though some make this pudding with milk, I prefer the vegan version and cook the wheat in just water. I like enjoying this hearty dessert as a healthy breakfast or light dinner as well.

RECIPE YIELD 12 cups

DF EF OF V FF

INGREDIENTS

Dry Ingredients

4 cups dry whole wheat farro berries (680 g)
⅓ cup coarsely chopped walnuts (40 g)
⅓ cup blanched almond halves (40 g)
⅓ cup pine nuts (45 g)
½ cup yellow seedless raisins (68 g)
2 tbsp finely shredded unsweetened coconut flakes

Wet Ingredients

6 cups water
⅓ cup honey
⅔ cup rose water
⅓ cup orange blossom water

NOTE

Wheat berries commonly used for this dessert in Middle Eastern countries are the softer and longer wheat kernels (including farro and kamut), which are similar in their nutty flavor and chewy texture. In the US, hard red and hard white wheat berries are more commonly available in the market (these are more chewy and shorter). Depending on what wheat kernel is used to make this dessert, cooking time and how much water is required may vary, as well as the recipe yield differing slightly as well.

INSTRUCTIONS

1. Rinse the three types of nuts, then place together in a small bowl and soak in cold water for 15 minutes. Drain, then rinse. Set aside.
2. Rinse the wheat well, then drain.
3. Place the wheat and water in a large pot. Cover, then bring to a boil.
4. Cook, covered, on low heat for 20 to 30 minutes (or until the wheat is soft), stirring occasionally (do not drain away any water once done).
5. Add the honey, floral waters, raisins, and nuts, then stir to mix.
6. Serve warm in individual bowls (1 cup per bowl) and top each bowl with ½ tsp of coconut just before serving.
7. Store, covered, in the refrigerator.

NUTRITION FACTS PER CUP

321 Kcal	8.4 g Protein	8 g Fat	56 g Carbs	8 g Fiber	12 g Sugar

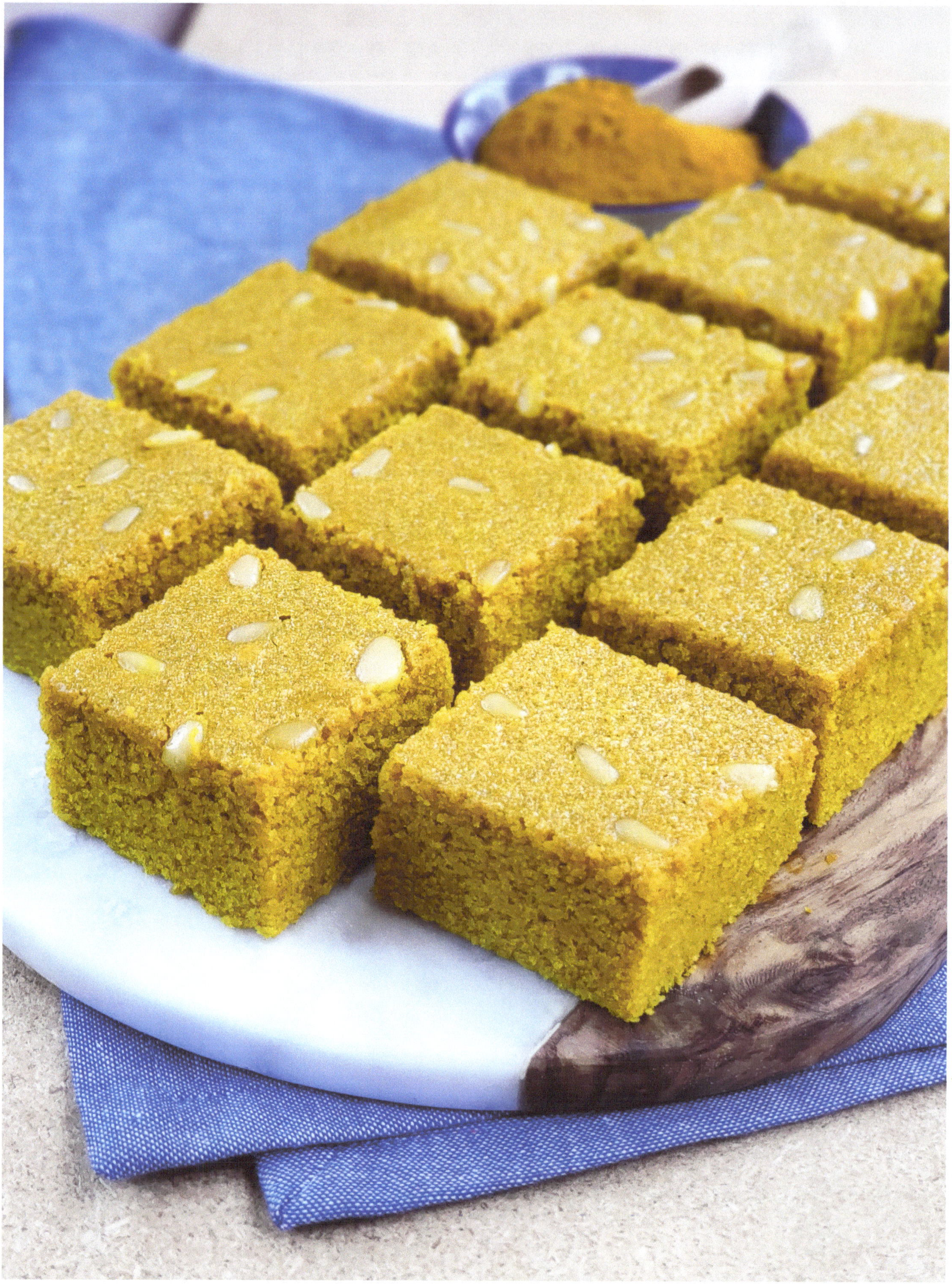

TURMERIC CAKE

Sfoof صفوف

With a distinct yellow color and a funny-sounding name, this Lebanese dessert is quite unique and nutritious. Traditionally made with equal parts of refined white flour and fine semolina flour, *sfoof* is soft and cake-like, with refined white sugar or carob molasses as the source of sweetness. I prefer using honey over molasses to maintain the yellow color and flavor imparted by all the turmeric present. *Sfoof* is traditionally made with refined vegetable oils, or a mix of butter and oil, but I have found that making it with extra-virgin olive oil produces a wonderfully moist product! This turmeric cake is often made vegan with only water and no cow milk, however, I like the fuller and richer flavor of milk. Since *sfoof* is not super sweet, I normally enjoy eating it for breakfast or for a light snack.

RECIPE YIELD 35 slices

EF Vt

INGREDIENTS

Dry Ingredients

3 cups whole wheat pastry flour (360 g)
1 cup fine semolina flour (150 g)
6 tbsp skim powdered milk
5 tsp baking powder
4 tbsp turmeric
½ tsp salt
1 ½ tbsp pine nuts

Wet Ingredients

2 ⅔ cups skim liquid milk
⅔ cup olive oil
1 ⅓ cups honey
2 tbsp liquid vanilla extract

NOTES

- *Tahini* is traditionally used to grease the pan when making turmeric cake, imparting a slight *tahini* flavor to the end product.
- After baking, the surface of this cake will develop a lighter yellow color and will have the appearance of some tiny bubbles, both of which will fade away and look more homogenous once the cake has completely cooled.

INSTRUCTIONS

1. Measure out the dry ingredients (except for the powdered milk and the nuts) into a bowl. Mix gently and set aside.
2. In a separate bowl, mix the oil and honey, then add the vanilla.
3. Mix the powdered milk and liquid milk in a separate bowl, then add to the oil and honey, stirring well to mix.
4. Preheat the oven to 325 °F.
5. Grease a baking pan (recommended dimensions: 29 cm x 35 cm or similar).
6. In 3 batches, add the wet ingredients to the dry ingredients, mixing gently, while making sure no lumps are formed.
7. Pour the batter into the pan then sprinkle the pine nuts evenly over the top.
8. Bake for 30 minutes.
9. Let cool for at least an hour before slicing and serving.
10. Store, covered, at room temperature or in the refrigerator.

NUTRITION FACTS PER SLICE

146 Kcal	3 g Protein	5 g Fat	24 g Carbs	1.4 g Fiber	12 g Sugar

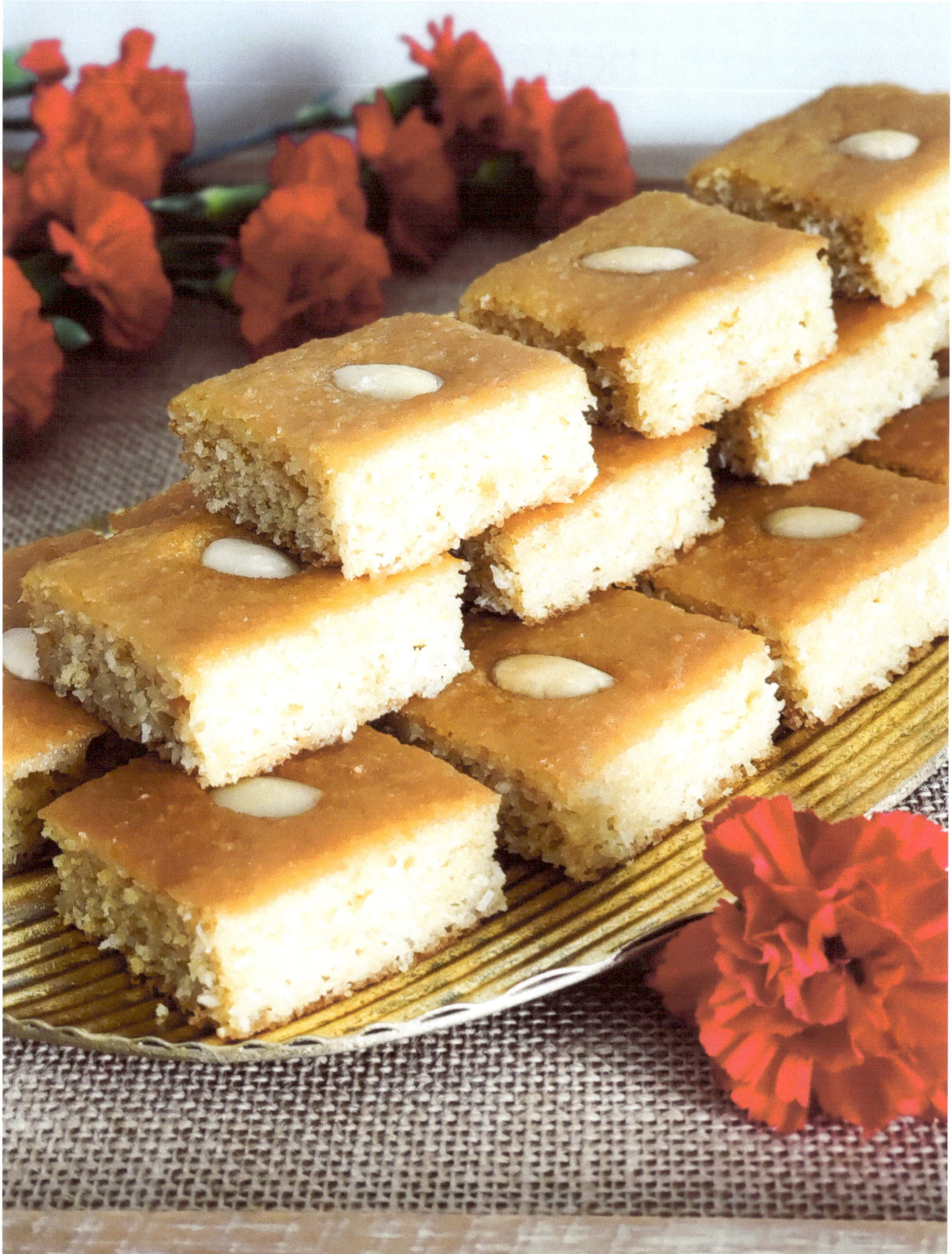

SEMOLINA COCONUT CAKE

Nammoura نمّورة

This simple Middle Eastern classic dessert comes with many names and variations between countries. In Lebanon, it is known as *nammoura* and is traditionally made with coarse semolina flour, butter or ghee, and full-fat yogurt or milk, with some liking to make it with coconut, while others leaving it plain. This dessert is then traditionally soaked with a rich floral-infused sugar syrup (known as *qatir*), for a shiny, dense, and moist end result! My healthy take on this classic recipe calls for using part semolina flour, part whole wheat flour, using skim yogurt and olive oil, and covering the finished surface with my simple honey syrup scented with floral waters.

RECIPE YIELD 48 slices

EF Vt

INGREDIENTS

Dry Ingredients

1 cup whole wheat flour (130 g)
2 cups coarse semolina flour (310 g)
1 ½ cups finely shredded unsweetened coconut flakes (126 g)
2 tsp baking soda
½ tsp salt
48 blanched almond halves

Wet Ingredients

3 cups skim yogurt (705 g)
¾ cup olive oil
⅓ cup honey
1 tsp orange blossom water
1 tsp rose water

Honey Syrup

1 cup honey
1 ½ tbsp orange blossom water
1 ½ tbsp rose water

INSTRUCTIONS

1. Measure out the dry ingredients (except for the almonds) into a bowl. Mix gently and set aside.
2. In a separate bowl, mix the oil and honey, then add the yogurt and floral waters, stirring well to mix.
3. Add the dry ingredients over the wet ingredients, then mix well.
4. Preheat the oven to 325 °F.
5. Grease a large sheet pan (recommended dimensions: 30 cm x 40 cm or similar).
6. Pour the batter into the pan, spreading it out evenly.
7. Lightly score the surface with a sharp knife to define the 48 slices, then place one almond half in the middle of each piece.
8. Bake for 25 to 30 minutes (depending on how golden brown one wants the surface to turn).
9. In the meantime, whisk the honey syrup ingredients together then set aside in the refrigerator to chill up a bit.
10. As soon as the cake comes out of the oven, pour the honey syrup slowly over the entire surface, spreading it out evenly until it gets soaked up by the cake. Return the pan to the turned off oven for 5 minutes.
11. Let cool for at least an hour before slicing and serving.
12. Store, covered, at room temperature or in the refrigerator.

See next page for notes »

NUTRITION FACTS PER SLICE

120 Kcal	2.5 g Protein	5.6 g Fat	16 g Carbs	1 g Fiber	9 g Sugar

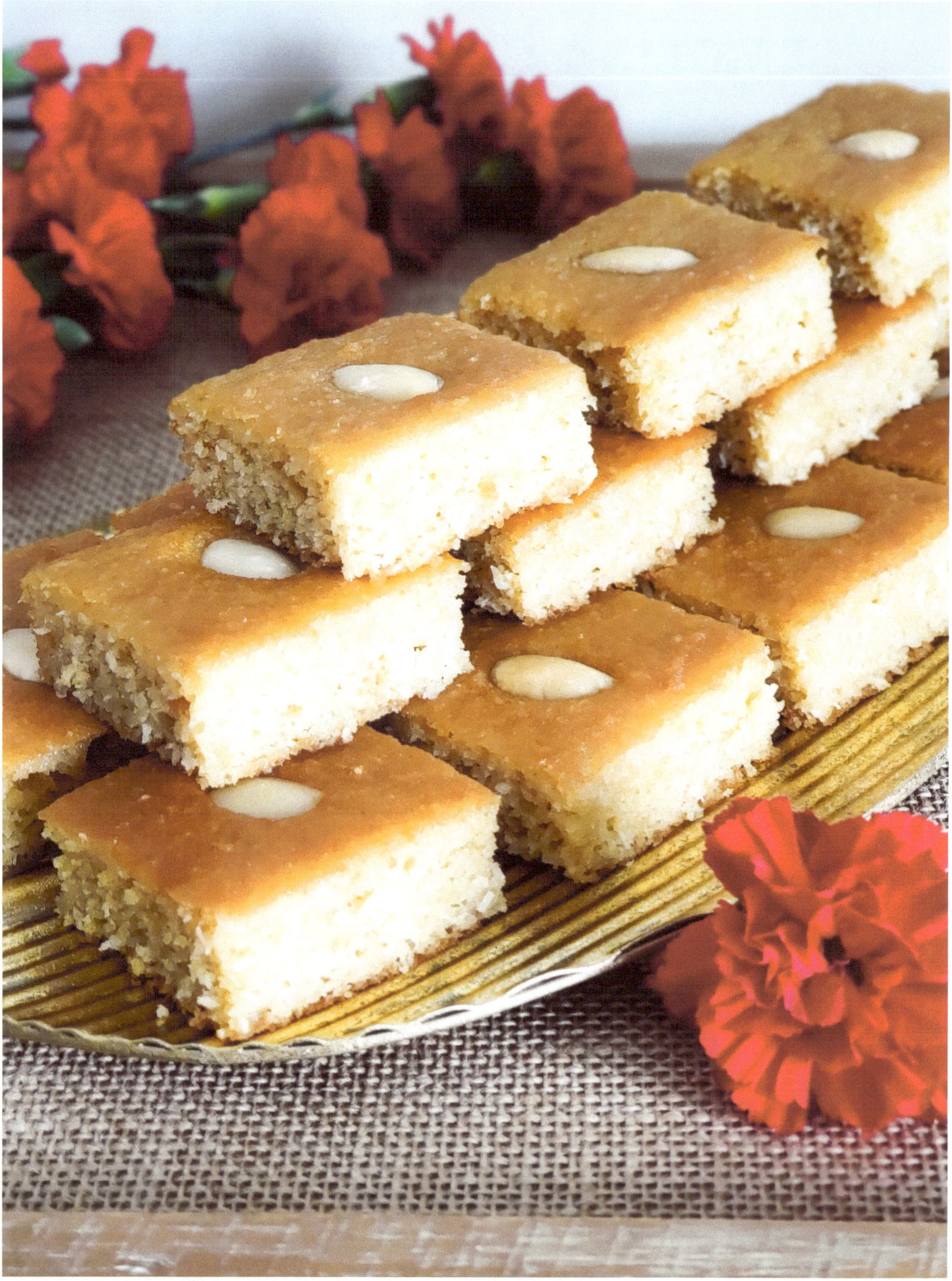

INGREDIENTS

Dry Ingredients

1 cup whole wheat flour (130 g)

2 cups coarse semolina flour (310 g)

1 ½ cups finely shredded unsweetened coconut flakes (126 g)

2 tsp baking soda

½ tsp salt

48 blanched almond halves

Wet Ingredients

3 cups skim yogurt (705 g)

¾ cup olive oil

⅓ cup honey

1 tsp orange blossom water

1 tsp rose water

Honey Syrup

1 cup honey

1 ½ tbsp orange blossom water

1 ½ tbsp rose water

NOTES

- Fine semolina flour can be used for this dessert, but the texture will obviously be finer and smoother than the traditional grainy feel imparted by coarse semolina flour.
- *Tahini* is traditionally used to grease the pan when making this semolina cake, imparting a slight *tahini* flavor to the end product.
- Many make this desert on the thinner side and tend to dry it out a bit in the oven before soaking it in the syrup. I like my semolina cake on the thicker and more moist side.

INSTRUCTIONS

1. Measure out the dry ingredients (except for the almonds) into a bowl. Mix gently and set aside.
2. In a separate bowl, mix the oil and honey, then add the yogurt and floral waters, stirring well to mix.
3. Add the dry ingredients over the wet ingredients, then mix well.
4. Preheat the oven to 325 °F.
5. Grease a rectangular pan (recommended dimensions: 30 cm x 40 cm or similar).
6. Pour the batter into the pan, spreading it out evenly.
7. Lightly score the surface with a sharp knife to define the 48 slices, then place one almond half in the middle of each piece.
8. Bake for 25 to 30 minutes (depending on how golden brown one wants the surface to turn).
9. In the meantime, whisk the honey syrup ingredients together then set aside in the refrigerator to chill up a bit.
10. As soon as the cake comes out of the oven, pour the honey syrup slowly over the entire surface, spreading it out evenly until it gets soaked up by the cake. Return the pan to the turned off oven for 5 minutes.
11. Let cool for at least an hour before slicing and serving.
12. Store, covered, at room temperature or in the refrigerator.

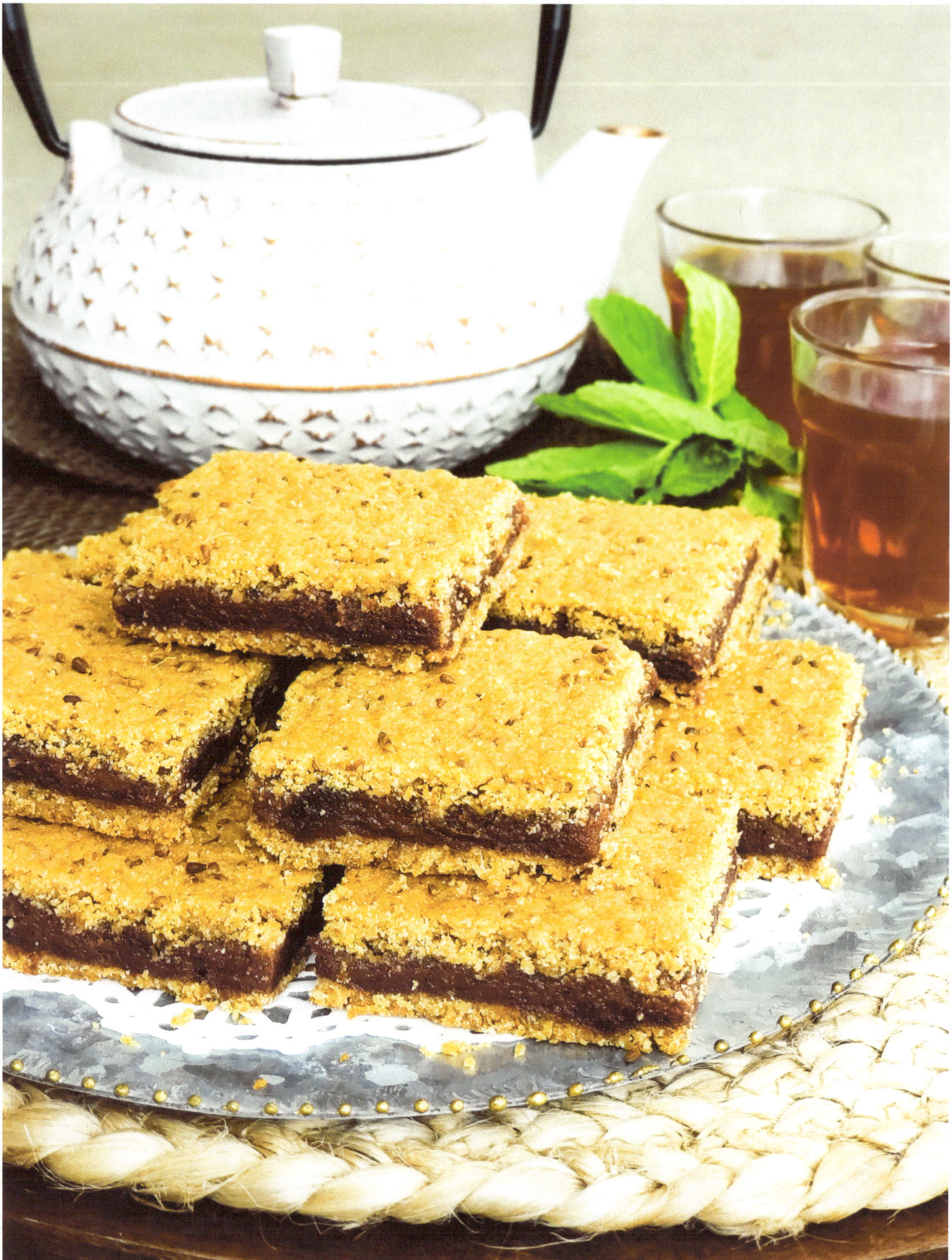

DATE ANISE BARS

Maamoul Madd bi Tamir wa Yansoon معمول مد بتمر و يانسون

These delicious and healthy anise-flavored date-filled bars were inspired by two different Lebanese sweets: anise *maakaroun* (which are semolina fingers traditionally deep fried then soaked in syrup) and *maamoul madd* (the pan-pressed version of *maamoul*, which are decorative, stuffed cookies traditionally made with refined flour, semolina, sugar, and butter). First adapted from an uncle's recipe of baked anise *maakaroun* filled with date paste, I modified it to include only heart-healthy oils and whole ingredients (whole wheat flour and honey instead of refined flour and sugar). To add convenience to this recipe, I found myself rolling out the dough and layering the date paste to resemble *maamoul madd* baked in the oven.

RECIPE YIELD 48 slices

DF EF V FF

INGREDIENTS

Crust Dough

4 cups whole wheat flour (520 g)
¼ cup anise seeds (25 g)
1 tbsp baking powder
2 tsp mahlab
⅓ tsp salt
¾ cup hot water
½ cup olive oil
½ cup avocado oil
⅓ cup honey

Filling

37 large soft pitted medjool dates (705 g)
2 tbsp orange blossom water

INSTRUCTIONS

1. For the dough, start with sorting through the anise seeds and removing any impurities. Place in a small bowl, then add the water and stir to mix. Let sit to cool.

2. Measure out the flour, baking powder, mahlab, and salt into a bowl. Mix gently and set aside.

3. In a separate bowl, mix the oils and honey, then pour over the dry ingredients. Add the anise seeds with the water, then mix well until a uniform dough is formed. Knead the dough for a few minutes, then cover the bowl with a plate or towel and let rest for an hour.

4. For the date filling, place the dates and orange blossom water in a large food processor and blend, scraping down the sides as needed (no need to make the date paste super smooth; some small chunks of dates add a nice texture to the bars).

5. Grease a large sheet pan (recommended dimensions: 30 cm x 40 cm or similar) with some olive oil, then divide the dough in half.

6. Using a coarse cheese grater, grate one half of the dough onto the pan. Press down with one's hands to flatten the surface and bind the grated dough together until the surface is even and the base of the pan is completely covered (this process takes some time and patience).

Instructions continued on the next page »

NUTRITION FACTS PER SLICE

131 Kcal	2.4 g Protein	5 g Fat	21 g Carbs	3 g Fiber	12 g Sugar

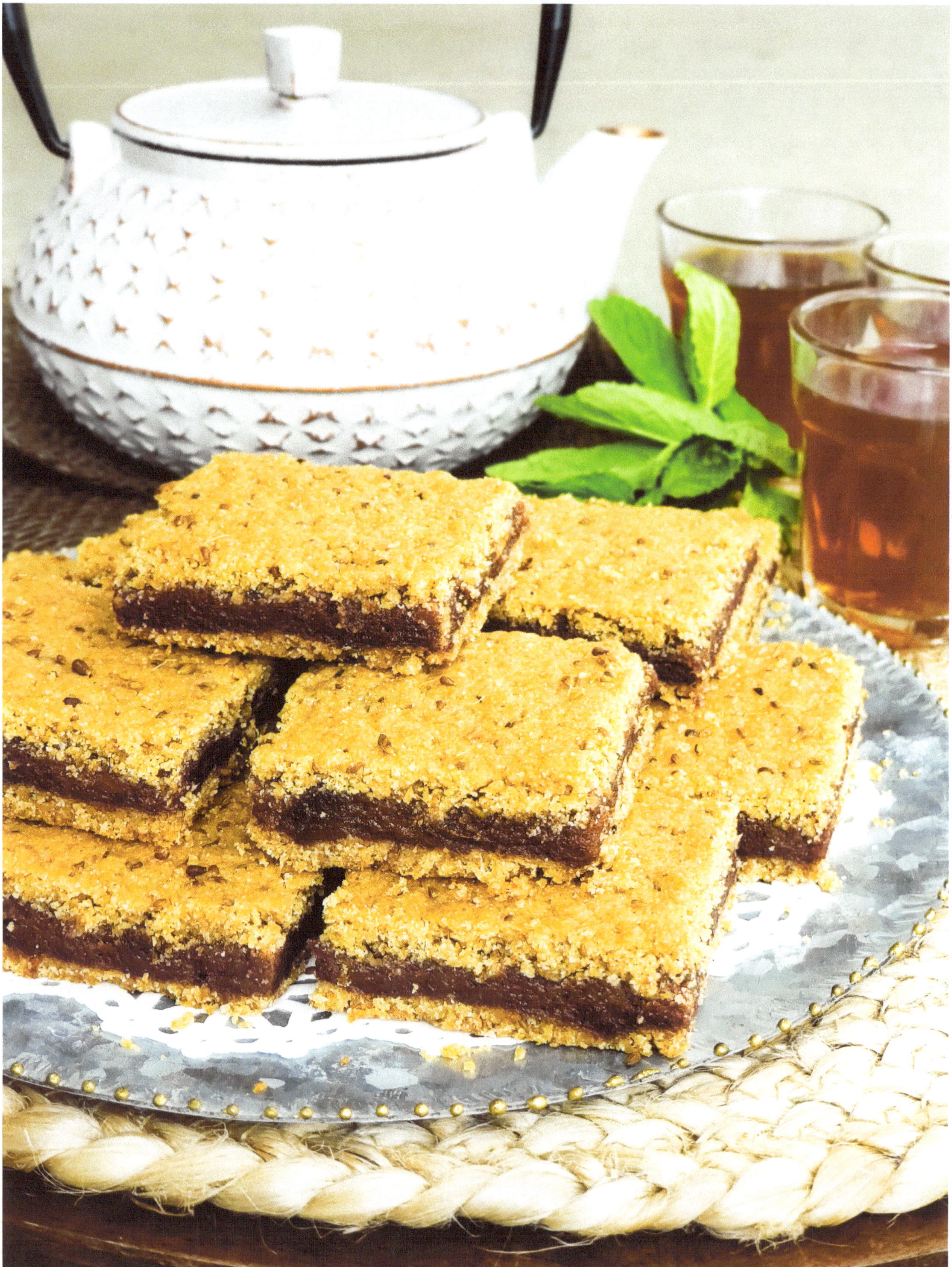

INGREDIENTS

Crust Dough

4 cups whole wheat flour (520 g)

¼ cup anise seeds (25 g)

1 tbsp baking powder

2 tsp mahlab

⅓ tsp salt

¾ cup hot water

½ cup olive oil

½ cup avocado oil

⅓ cup honey

Filling

37 large soft pitted medjool dates (705 g)

2 tbsp orange blossom water

NOTES

- Since the date paste is quite sticky, it is best to dip one's hands in water or oil to help spread the paste over the dough layer.
- If a smoother look to the baked crust is desired, one can, in steps 6 and 9, avoid using a cheese grater, and instead, flatten small patches of the dough between the hands and lay out onto the pan or over the filling. Join the patches and mold them together with one's hands, patting down gently, until a uniform surface is formed. One can also use a small roller to smoothen out the look of the surface if desired.

RECIPE ALTERNATIVE

- To make fig anise bars, make the following changes to the wet ingredients: substitute the dates with 850 g of fresh figs (no skin), omit the orange blossom water, and add 1 tbsp lemon juice. Mash up the figs, then cook in a saucepan, covered, on low heat for 1 hour, stirring occasionally. Mix in an additional 2 teaspoons of anise seeds, then set aside to cool, before spreading out onto the first layer of dough. Continue with the rest of the steps just as above.

INSTRUCTIONS

1. For the dough, start with sorting through the anise seeds and removing any impurities. Place in a small bowl, then add the water and stir to mix. Let sit to cool.
2. Measure out the flour, baking powder, mahlab, and salt into a bowl. Mix gently and set aside.
3. In a separate bowl, mix the oils and honey, then pour over the dry ingredients. Add the anise seeds with the water, then mix well until a uniform dough is formed. Knead the dough for a few minutes, then cover the bowl with a plate or towel and let rest for an hour.
4. For the date filling, place the dates and orange blossom water in a large food processor and blend, scraping down the sides as needed (no need to make the date paste super smooth; some small chunks of dates add a nice texture to the bars).
5. Grease a large sheet pan (recommended dimensions: 30 cm x 40 cm or similar) with some olive oil, then divide the dough in half.
6. Using a coarse cheese grater, grate one half of the dough onto the pan. Press down with one's hands to flatten the surface and bind the grated dough together until the surface is even and the base of the pan is completely covered (this process takes some time and patience).
7. Drop the date paste onto the dough in small batches. Using one's hands, spread the date paste over the dough, patting down well until the whole surface is covered.
8. Preheat the oven to 325 °F.
9. Grate the remainder half of the dough over the date layer. Press down with one's hands to flatten the surface and bind the grated dough together until the surface is even and the date paste is completely covered.
10. Score the top layer with a sharp knife to define the 48 slices.
11. Bake for 40 minutes (one can then broil the surface until light brown and crisp if desired).
12. Let cool for at least an hour before slicing and serving.
13. Store, covered, at room temperature or in the refrigerator.

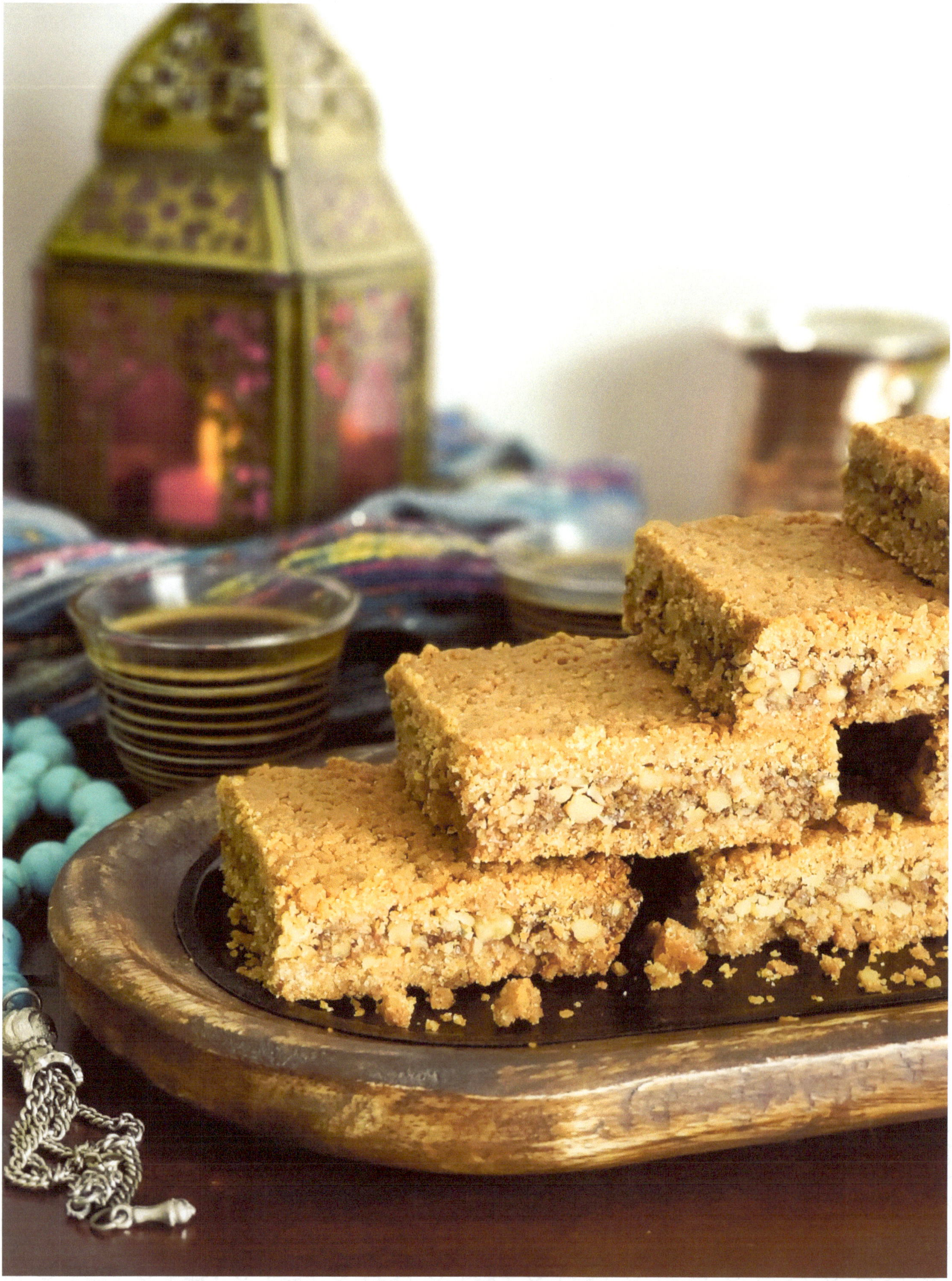

WALNUT BARS

Maamoul Madd bi Joze معمول مد بجوز

Maamoul madd is the pan-pressed version of *maamoul*, which is a traditional Middle Eastern decorative cookie stuffed with ground dates, pistachios, or walnuts. Traditionally made with refined white flour, semolina, butter, and sugar, my healthy and whole modified *maamoul madd* includes whole wheat flour and heart-healthy oils and is lightly sweetened with honey and freshly squeezed orange juice! Pictured is my *maamoul madd bi joze*, made with ground walnuts and flavored with cinnamon and orange blossom water. To pack more omega-3 fats into this dessert, I like adding flax seeds along with the walnuts!

RECIPE YIELD 30 slices

DF EF Vt FF

INGREDIENTS

Crust Dough

4 cups whole wheat flour (520 g)
1 tbsp baking powder
2 tsp mahlab
½ tsp cinnamon
⅓ tsp salt
½ cup fresh orange juice
½ cup olive oil
½ cup avocado oil
⅓ cup honey
2 tbsp water
1 tbsp orange blossom water

Filling

4 cups walnut pieces (400 g)
⅓ cup flaxseeds (47 g)
½ tsp cinnamon
½ cup honey
1 tbsp orange blossom water

INSTRUCTIONS

1. For the dough, measure out the flour, baking powder, mahlab, cinnamon, and salt into a bowl. Mix gently and set aside.
2. In a separate bowl, mix the oils and honey, then pour over the dry ingredients. Add the orange juice, water, and orange blossom water, then mix well until a uniform dough is formed. Knead the dough for a few minutes, then cover the bowl with a plate or towel and let rest for an hour.
3. For the nut filling, place the walnuts in a food blender to coarsely chop. Empty out into a small bowl.
4. Process the flaxseeds in the food blender until flax powder is obtained. Empty out over the walnuts, then add the cinnamon, honey, and orange blossom water. Stir well to mix.
5. Grease a baking pan (recommended dimensions: 29 cm x 35 cm or similar) with some olive oil, then divide the dough in half.
6. Using a coarse cheese grater, grate one half of the dough onto the pan. Press down with one's hands to flatten the surface and bind the grated dough together until the surface is even and the base of the pan is completely covered (this process takes some time and patience).
7. Drop the nut filling onto the dough in small batches. Spread the filling over the dough, patting down well until the whole surface is covered.
8. Preheat the oven to 325 °F.

Instructions continued on the next page »

NUTRITION FACTS PER SLICE

257.5 Kcal	6 g Protein	17 g Fat	23 g Carbs	5 g Fiber	8.5 g Sugar

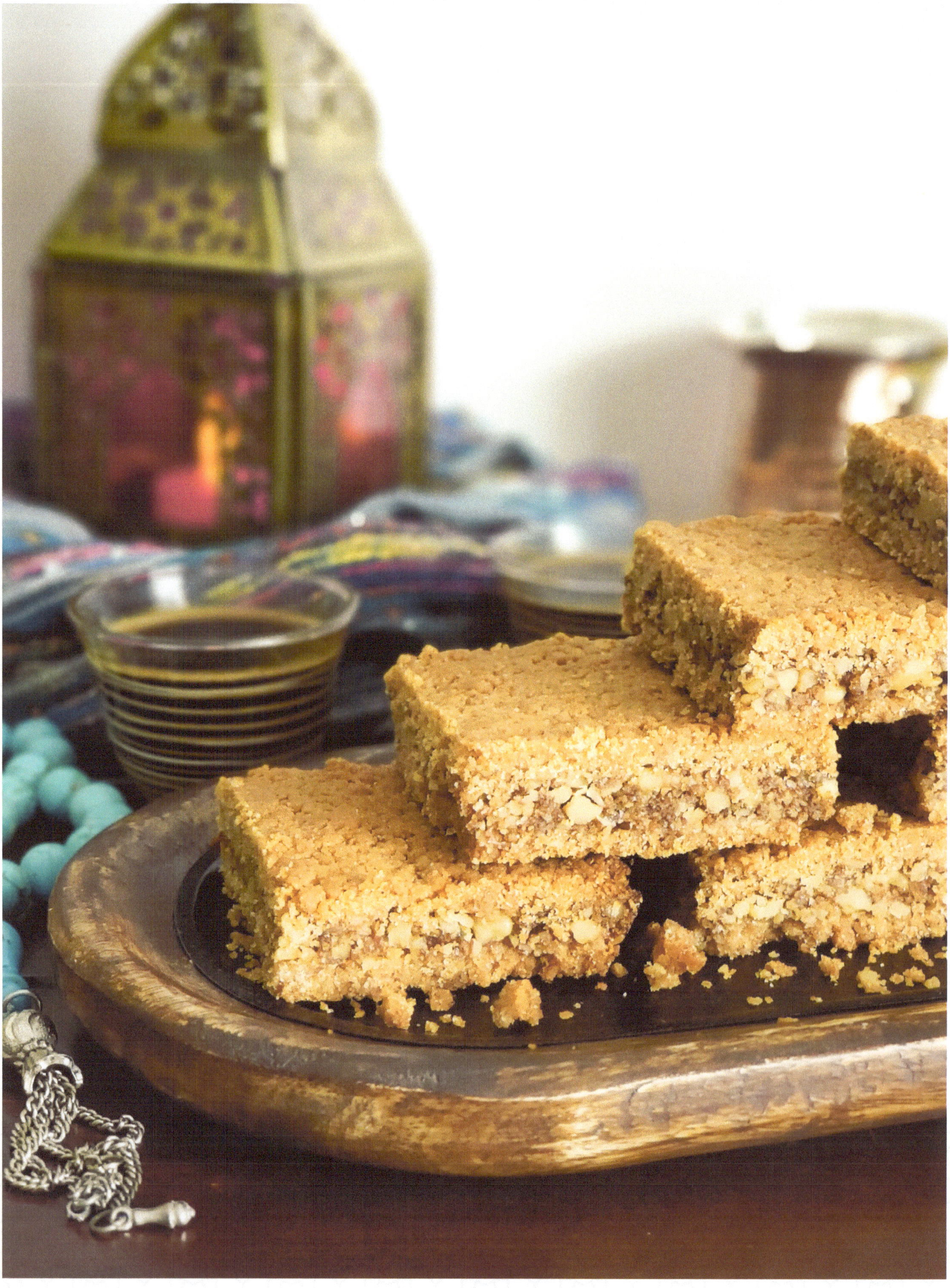

INGREDIENTS

Crust Dough
4 cups whole wheat flour (520 g)
1 tbsp baking powder
2 tsp mahlab
½ tsp cinnamon
⅓ tsp salt
½ cup fresh orange juice
½ cup olive oil
½ cup avocado oil
⅓ cup honey
2 tbsp water
1 tbsp orange blossom water

Filling
4 cups walnut pieces (400 g)
⅓ cup flaxseeds (47 g)
½ tsp cinnamon
½ cup honey
1 tbsp orange blossom water

NOTE

❁ If a smoother look to the baked crust is desired, one can, in steps 6 and 9, avoid using a cheese grater, and instead, flatten small patches of the dough between the hands and lay out onto the pan or over the filling. Join the patches and mold them together with one's hands, patting down gently, until a uniform surface is formed. One can also use a small roller to smoothen out the look of the surface if desired.

RECIPE ALTERNATIVE

❁ To make pistachio bars, use 450 g raw shelled pistachios instead of the walnuts and flaxseeds, omit the cinnamon, and substitute the orange blossom water with rose water.

INSTRUCTIONS

1. For the dough, measure out the flour, baking powder, mahlab, cinnamon, and salt into a bowl. Mix gently and set aside.

2. In a separate bowl, mix the oils and honey, then pour over the dry ingredients. Add the orange juice, water, and orange blossom water, then mix well until a uniform dough is formed. Knead the dough for a few minutes, then cover the bowl with a plate or towel and let rest for an hour.

3. For the nut filling, place the walnuts in a food blender to coarsely chop. Empty out into a small bowl.

4. Process the flaxseeds in the food blender until flax powder is obtained. Empty out over the walnuts, then add the cinnamon, honey, and orange blossom water. Stir well to mix.

5. Grease a baking pan (recommended dimensions: 29 cm x 35 cm or similar) with some olive oil, then divide the dough in half.

6. Using a coarse cheese grater, grate one half of the dough onto the pan. Press down with one's hands to flatten the surface and bind the grated dough together until the surface is even and the base of the pan is completely covered (this process takes some time and patience).

7. Drop the nut filling onto the dough in small batches. Spread the filling over the dough, patting down well until the whole surface is covered.

8. Preheat the oven to 325 °F.

9. Grate the remainder half of the dough over the nut layer. Press down with one's hands to flatten the surface and bind the grated dough together until the surface is even and the nut filling is completely covered.

10. Score the top layer with a sharp knife to define the 30 slices.

11. Bake for 40 minutes (one can then broil the surface until light brown and crisp if desired).

12. Let cool for at least an hour before slicing and serving.

13. Store, covered, at room temperature or in the refrigerator.

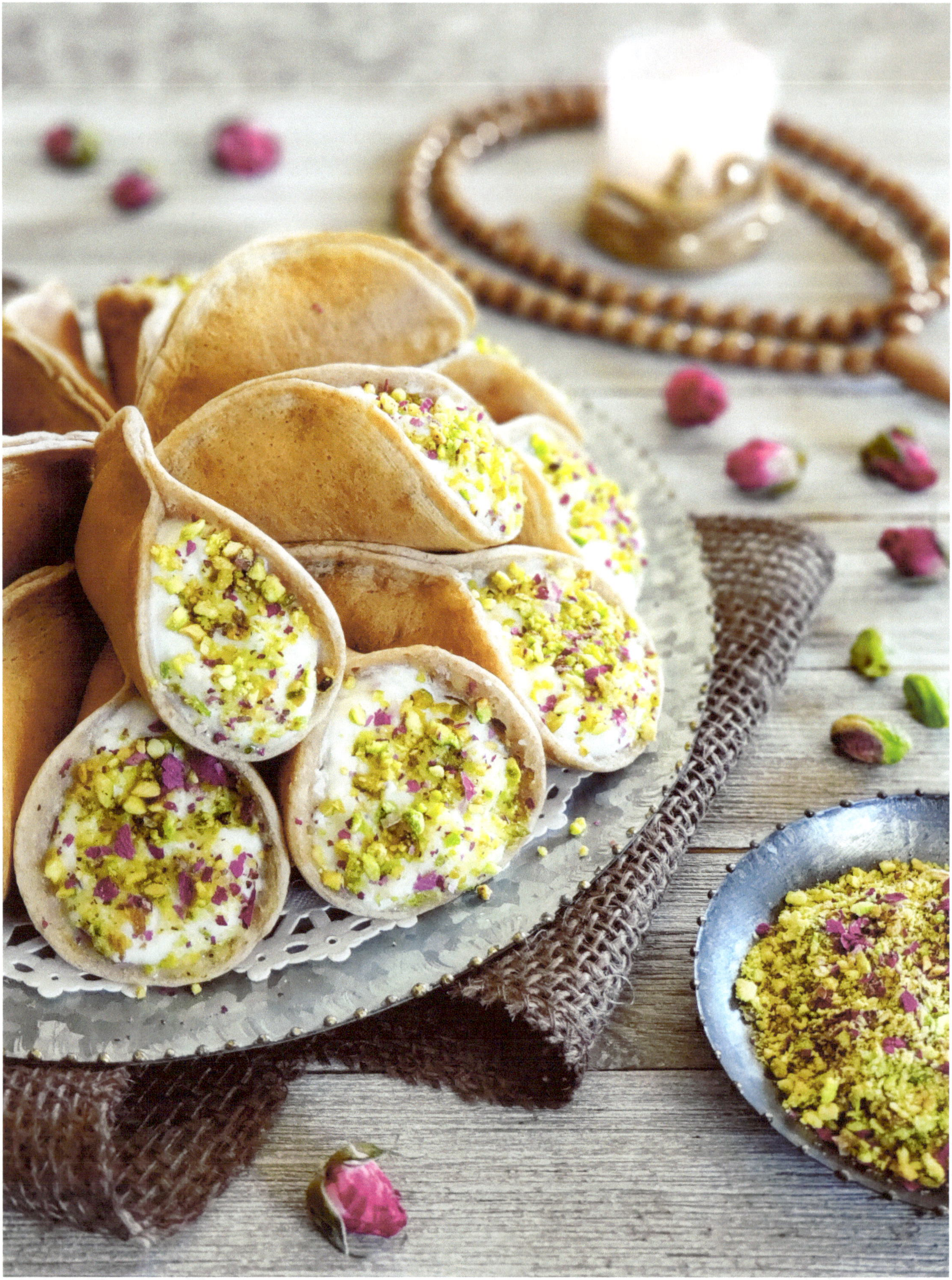

RICOTTA-STUFFED ARABIAN PANCAKES

Qatayef bi Qashta قطايف بقشطة

Qatayef are Middle Eastern folded pancakes, commonly served during the holy month of Ramadan. This smaller version of *qatayef* is traditionally filled with a rich Middle Eastern clotted cream (*qashta*), while a bigger-sized *qatayef* are usually filled with walnuts (recipe on next page). Using ricotta cheese is a much healthier and lighter alternative to *qashta*, and my healthy and whole Arabian pancakes are also made with whole wheat flour and are lightly sweetened with honey.

RECIPE YIELD 16 pieces

EF OF Vt

INGREDIENTS

Pancake Dough

1 ½ cups whole wheat flour (195 g)
2 ½ tsp baking powder
1 tsp mahlab
1 ½ cups + 1 tbsp water
1 tbsp honey
½ tsp rose water

Filling

1 cup part-skim ricotta cheese (230 g)
2 tsp honey
½ tsp rose water

Topping

1 tbsp ground pistachios
¼ tsp crushed dry rose petals

INSTRUCTIONS

1. Combine the filling ingredients in a small bowl, then cover and set aside in the refrigerator.

2. Measure out the flour, baking powder, and mahlab into a medium bowl, then add the water, honey, and rose water. Stir well to mix.

3. Heat a non-stick pan or skillet for 1 to 2 minutes on high heat, then turn down to medium heat, and pour 2 tbsp of the batter to form the first *qatayef* pancake.

4. Turn the heat down to medium-low, then let the pancake cook for 1 to 2 minutes. Once the surface is fully covered with bubbles, turn the heat down to low and continue cooking for an extra minute or so until all the bubbles have lost their shine and have just dried up.

5. Transfer the prepared *qatayef* pancake to a dry towel, and place an extra one over it to keep the pancakes moist and prevent them from drying up as they cool.

6. To form a second *qatayef* pancake, turn up the heat back to medium-low, then pour 2 tbsp of the batter. Once the surface gets covered in bubbles, turn down to low, and continue cooking for an extra minute or so until all the bubbles have dried up. Transfer to the towel, place next to the formed *qatayef* pancake, then cover.

Instructions continued on the next page »

NUTRITION FACTS PER PIECE

74 Kcal	4 g Protein	1.5 g Fat	11 g Carbs	2 g Fiber	2 g Sugar

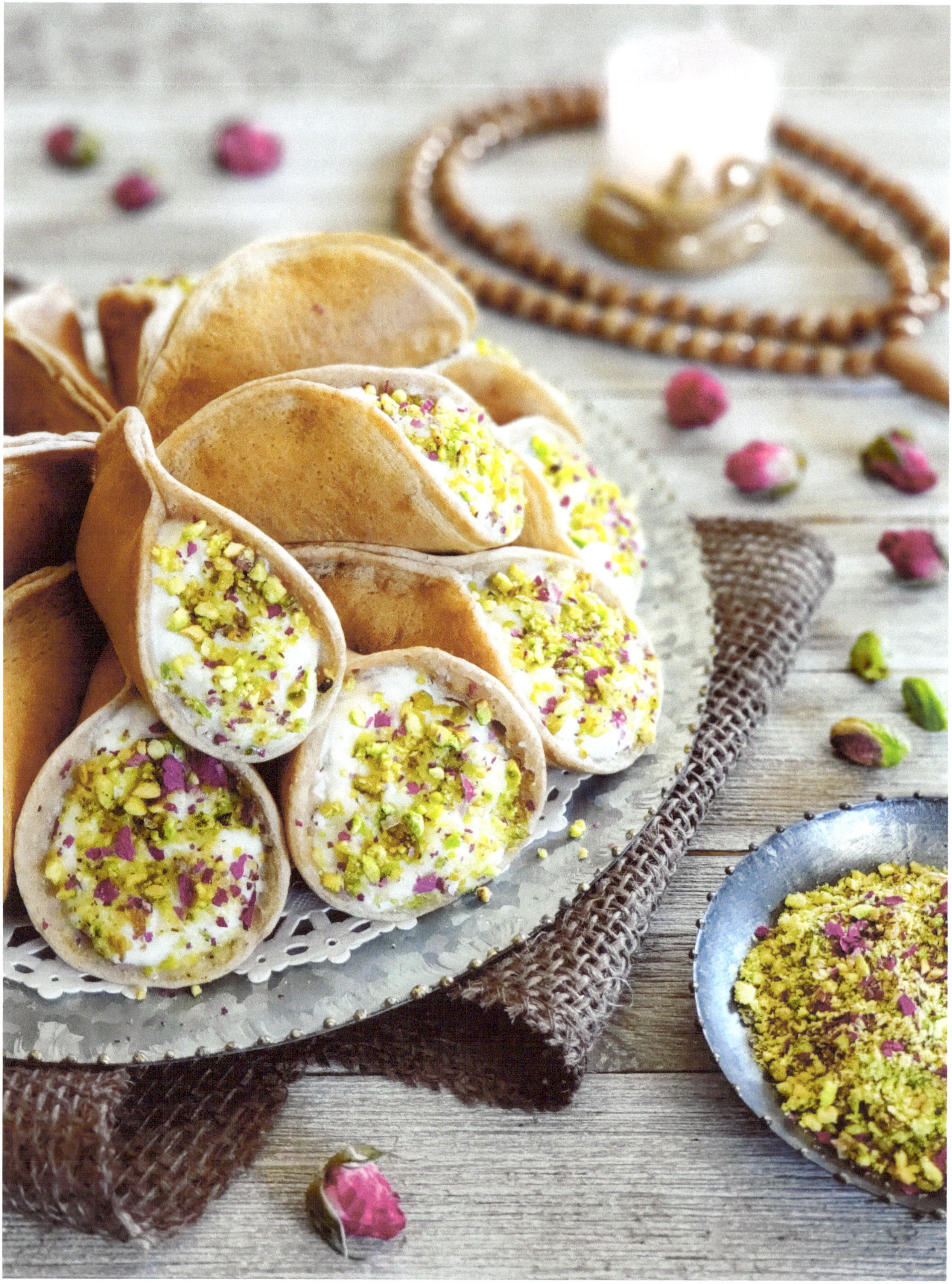

INGREDIENTS

Pancake Dough

1 ½ cups whole wheat flour (195 g)

2 ½ tsp baking powder

1 tsp mahlab

1 ½ cups + 1 tbsp water

1 tbsp honey

½ tsp rose water

Filling

1 cup part-skim ricotta cheese (230 g)

2 tsp honey

½ tsp rose water

Topping

1 tbsp ground pistachio

¼ tsp crushed dry rose petals

NOTE

I like making each *qatayef* pancake one at a time in the pan to better monitor the outcome of each with the back and forth changing of the stove heat (for shorter preparation time, a griddle can be used for the making of several *qatayef* pancakes at once).

INSTRUCTIONS

1. Combine the filling ingredients in a small bowl, then cover and set aside in the refrigerator.

2. Measure out the flour, baking powder, and mahlab into a medium bowl, then add the water, honey, and rose water. Stir well to mix.

3. Heat a non-stick pan or skillet for 1 to 2 minutes on high heat, then turn down to medium heat, and pour 2 tbsp of the batter to form the first *qatayef* pancake.

4. Turn the heat down to medium-low, then let the pancake cook for 1 to 2 minutes. Once the surface is fully covered with bubbles, turn the heat down to low and continue cooking for an extra minute or so until all the bubbles have lost their shine and have just dried up.

5. Transfer the prepared *qatayef* pancake to a dry towel, and place an extra one over it to keep the pancakes moist and prevent them from drying up as they cool.

6. To form a second *qatayef* pancake, turn up the heat back to medium-low, then pour 2 tbsp of the batter. Once the surface gets covered in bubbles, turn down to low, and continue cooking for an extra minute or so until all the bubbles have dried up. Transfer to the towel, place next to the formed *qatayef* pancake, then cover.

7. Repeat step 6 to make the remaining *qatayef* pancakes (cover the batter bowl during the time of working to prevent any drying out to the batter).

8. Once the formed *qatayef* pancakes are all cooled, pinch the sides of each one very well in order to close the pancake by about 2/3 way. Spoon on some ricotta filling (a little less than 1 tbsp), lightly pushing some into the pocket.

9. Mix the ground pistachios and rose petals together in a small bowl, then sprinkle a little by hand onto the apparent filling of each qatayef.

10. Drizzle extra honey or honey syrup (see page 263) onto the *qatayef* if more sweetness is desired.

11. Store, covered, in the refrigerator.

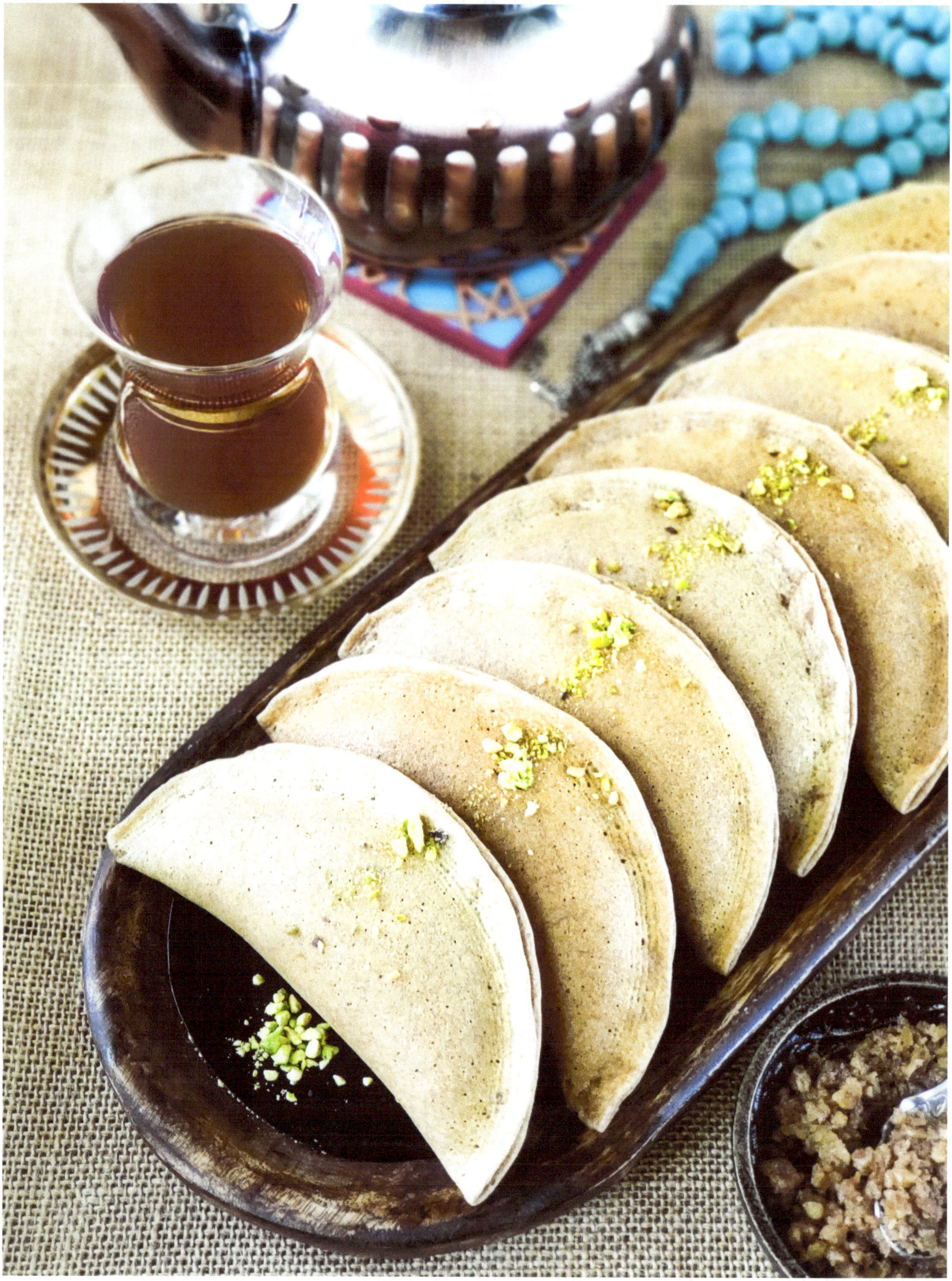

WALNUT-STUFFED ARABIAN PANCAKES

Qatayef bi Joze قطايف بجوز

Middle Eastern folded pancakes, referred to in Arabic as *qatayef*, are commonly served during the holy month of Ramadan. This bigger version of *qatayef* is traditionally filled with walnuts (as compared to a smaller version filled with heavy cream (recipe on previous page)), then fried and dipped into a rich floral-infused sugar syrup (known as *qatir*). My Arabian pancakes are made healthier and more whole by using whole wheat flour, sweetening with honey, baking after being lightly brushed with avocado oil, and then lightly brushing with honey instead of syrup.

RECIPE YIELD 10 pieces

DF EF Vt

INGREDIENTS

Pancake Dough

1 ½ cups whole wheat flour (195 g)
2 ½ tsp baking powder
⅓ tsp cinnamon
¼ tsp mahlab
1 ½ cups + 3 tbsp water
1 tbsp honey
½ tsp rose water

Filling

1 ⅓ cup coarsely chopped walnuts (133 g)
4 tbsp honey
2 tbsp orange blossom water
⅓ tsp cinnamon
⅛ tsp nutmeg

Topping

1 tbsp avocado oil
1 tbsp honey

INSTRUCTIONS

1. Combine the filling ingredients in a small bowl, then cover and set aside in the refrigerator.

2. Measure out the flour, baking powder, cinnamon, and mahlab into a medium bowl, then add the water, honey, and rose water. Stir well to mix.

3. Heat a non-stick pan or skillet for 1 to 2 minutes on high heat, then turn down to medium heat, and pour around ¼ cup of the batter to form the first qatayef pancake.

4. Turn the heat down to medium-low, then let the pancake cook for 1 to 2 minutes. Once the surface is fully covered with bubbles, turn the heat down to low and continue cooking for an extra minute or so until all the bubbles have lost their shine and have just dried up.

5. Transfer the prepared qatayef pancake to a dry towel, then place an extra one over it to keep the pancakes moist and prevent them from drying up as they cool.

6. To form a second qatayef pancake, turn up the heat back to medium-low, then pour ¼ cup of the batter. Once the surface gets covered in bubbles, turn down to low, and continue cooking for an extra minute or so until all the bubbles have dried up. Transfer to the towel, place next to the formed qatayef pancake, then cover.

Instructions continued on the next page »

NUTRITION FACTS PER PIECE

211 Kcal	6 g Protein	10.5 g Fat	26 g Carbs	4.5 g Fiber	11 g Sugar

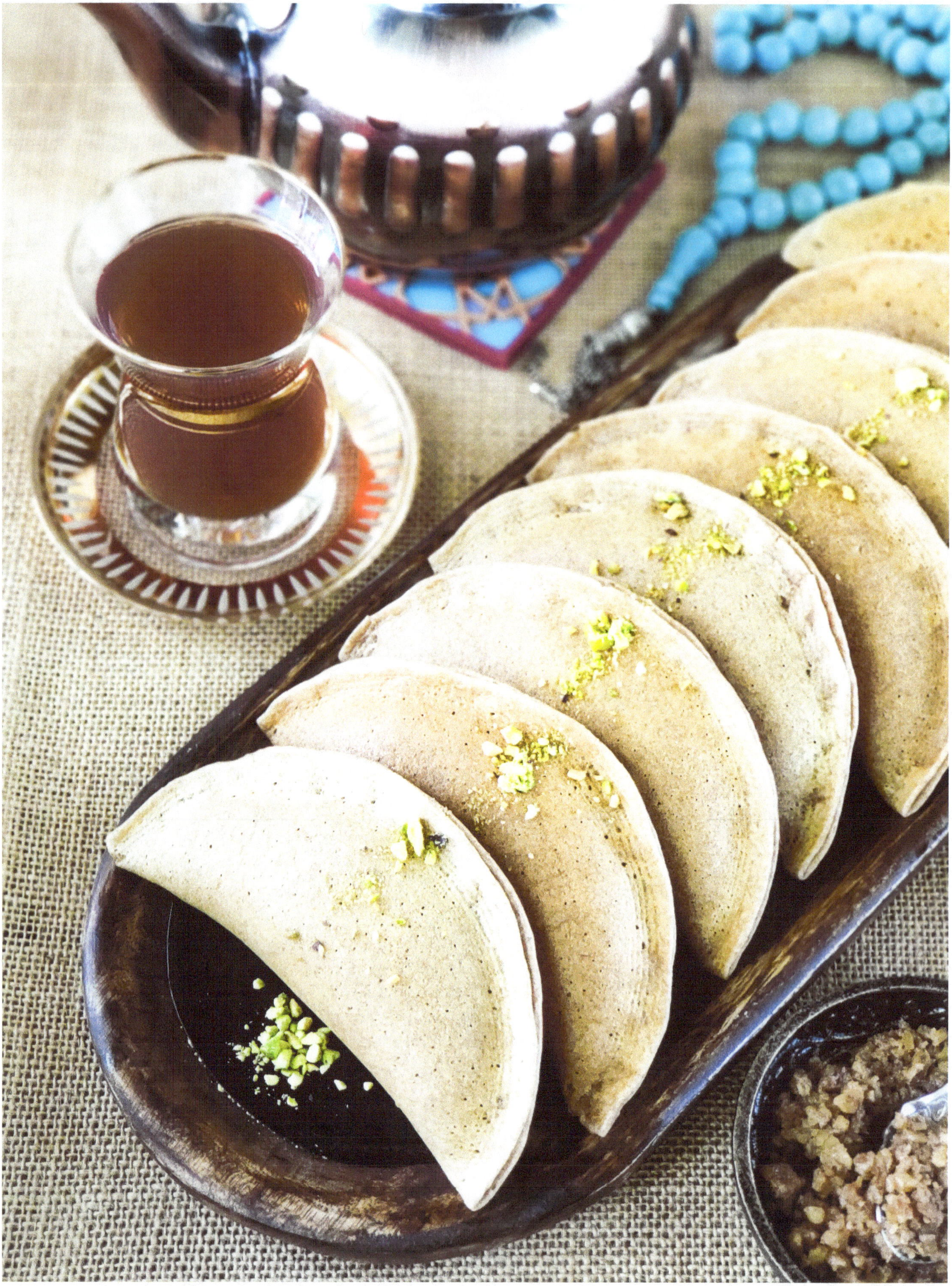

INGREDIENTS

Pancake Dough

1 ½ cups whole wheat flour (195 g)

2 ½ tsp baking powder

1/3 tsp cinnamon

¼ tsp mahlab

1 ½ cups + 3 tbsp water

1 tbsp honey

½ tsp rose water

Filling

1 ⅓ cup coarsely chopped walnuts (133 g)

4 tbsp honey

2 tbsp orange blossom water

⅓ tsp cinnamon

⅛ tsp nutmeg

Topping

1 tbsp avocado oil

1 tbsp honey

NOTES

- I like making each *qatayef* pancake one at a time in the pan to better monitor the outcome of each with the back and forth changing of the stove heat (for shorter preparation time, a griddle can be used for the making of several *qatayef* pancakes at once).
- If the *qatayef* are not going to be all eaten at once, cover and refrigerate them before baking. Brush with oil before baking, then brush with honey, right before serving.

INSTRUCTIONS

1. Combine the filling ingredients in a small bowl, then cover and set aside in the refrigerator.

2. Measure out the flour, baking powder, cinnamon, and mahlab into a medium bowl, then add the water, honey, and rose water. Stir well to mix.

3. Heat a non-stick pan or skillet for 1 to 2 minutes on high heat, then turn down to medium heat, and pour around ¼ cup of the batter to form the first qatayef pancake.

4. Turn the heat down to medium-low, then let the pancake cook for 1 to 2 minutes. Once the surface is fully covered with bubbles, turn the heat down to low and continue cooking for an extra minute or so until all the bubbles have lost their shine and have just dried up.

5. Transfer the prepared qatayef pancake to a dry towel, then place an extra one over it to keep the pancakes moist and prevent them from drying up as they cool.

6. To form a second qatayef pancake, turn up the heat back to medium-low, then pour ¼ cup of the batter. Once the surface gets covered in bubbles, turn down to low, and continue cooking for an extra minute or so until all the bubbles have dried up. Transfer to the towel, place next to the formed qatayef pancake, then cover.

7. Repeat step 6 to make the remaining qatayef pancakes (cover the batter bowl during the time of working to prevent any drying out to the batter).

8. Once the formed qatayef pancakes are all cooled, divide up the nut filling across all of them, placing it along the center of each one, then pinch the sides of each very well until completely closed.

9. Brush each side with a bit of oil, then bake on a sheet pan (recommended dimensions: 25 cm x 35 cm or similar) in a preheated oven at 350 °F for 5 to 10 minutes depending on the desired texture.

10. Brush each side with honey and serve warm.

11. Sprinkle with ground pistachios if desired.

12. Store, covered, at room temperature or in the refrigerator.

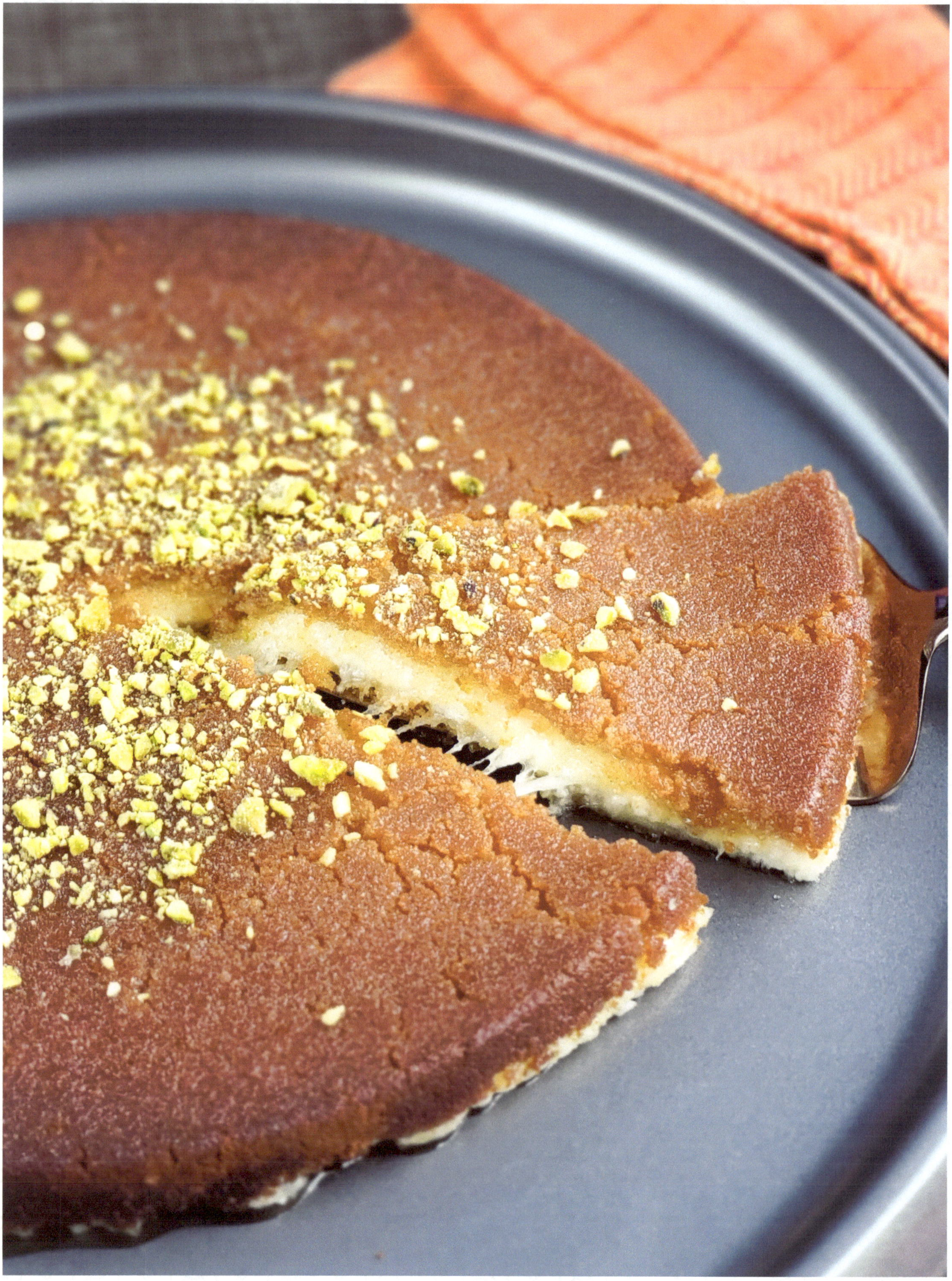

SEMOLINA CHEESE PIE

Knaifeh كنافة

This dessert is also commonly eaten in Lebanon for breakfast, plain or in a pocket of sesame-covered bread. *Knaifeh* is made with two main variations: the Lebanese version which calls for a layer of fine semolina mixed with butter or ghee and the Palestinian version which calls for shredded phyllo dough mixed with either one of the same fats. Under the semolina or shredded phyllo layers comes a layer of either full-fat cheese or *qashta* (a rich Middle Eastern clotted cream) infused with floral waters. *Knaifeh* is then traditionally covered in a rich floral-infused sugar syrup (*qatir*). For my healthy and whole *knaifeh*, I like adding some whole wheat flour to the pie crust, as well as combining low-fat cheese with a light milk pudding for the filling (as a simple and low-fat *qashta* imitation inspired by a friend's recipe). I also opt to cover the *knaifeh* with my healthy honey syrup combined with floral waters.

RECIPE YIELD 8 slices

EF Vt

INGREDIENTS

Pie Crust

¾ cups whole wheat flour (98 g)
1 ½ cups fine semolina flour (225 g)
3 tbsp skim powdered milk
2 tbsp cornstarch
1 tbsp baking powder
1 tsp powdered vanilla
1 cup liquid skim milk
¼ cup avocado oil
2 tbsp honey

Filling

1 cup skim liquid milk
1 tbsp skim powdered milk
1 tbsp fine semolina
¼ tsp rose water
¼ tsp orange blossom water
2 cups coarsely grated low-moisture part-skim mozzarella cheese (200 g)

Honey Syrup

½ cup honey
1 ¼ tsp rose water
1 ¼ tsp orange blossom water

INSTRUCTIONS

1. For the pie crust, measure out the dry ingredients (except for the powdered milk) into a bowl. Mix gently and set aside.
2. Mix the powdered milk and liquid milk in a separate bowl, then stir in the oil and honey.
3. Add the wet ingredients to the dry ingredients, then stir well to mix.
4. Spread the batter onto a lightly greased sheet pan (recommended dimensions: 29 cm x 35 cm or similar), then bake in a preheated oven at 375 °F for 10 minutes.
5. Let cool, then scrape out and break up by hand. Grind in 4 batches using a blender, until a smooth powdery texture is obtained.
6. Divide the obtained crust powder into 3 equal parts, putting one batch aside and freezing the other two (separately) in airtight containers for future use (see note below).
7. For the current batch of crust powder to be used, set aside ¼ cup in a small bowl.
8. Grease a round non-stick baking pan (recommended diameter: 23 cm or similar) very well, then pour the crust powder onto the pan. Spread out and evenly pat down with one's hands. Press down well.

Instructions continued on the next page »

NUTRITION FACTS PER SLICE

240 Kcal	10 g Protein	7.6 g Fat	34.5 g Carbs	1 g Fiber	22 g Sugar

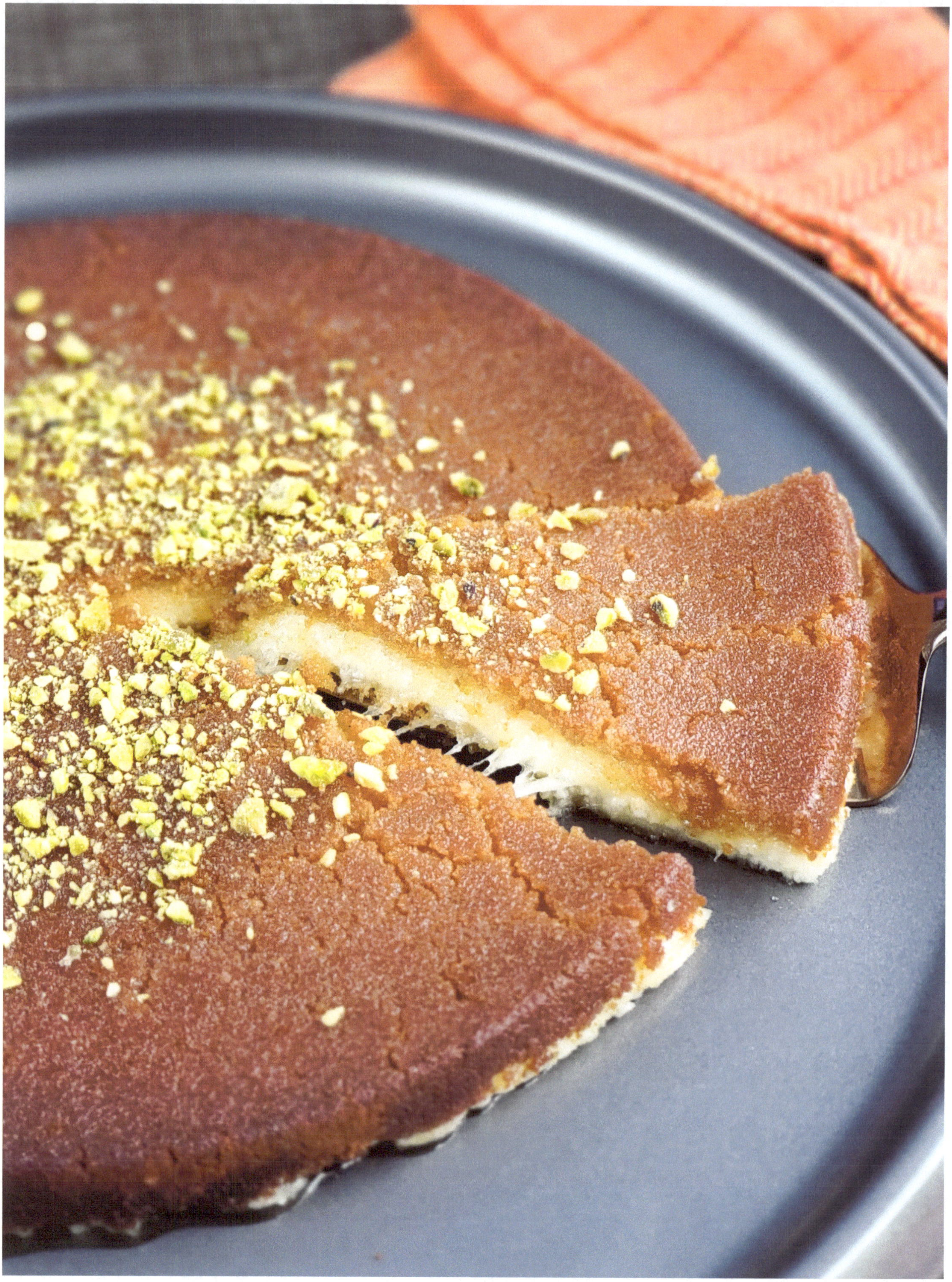

INGREDIENTS

Pie Crust

¾ cups whole wheat flour (98 g)
1 ½ cups fine semolina flour (225 g)
3 tbsp skim powdered milk
2 tbsp cornstarch
1 tbsp baking powder
1 tsp powdered vanilla
1 cup liquid skim milk
¼ cup avocado oil
2 tbsp honey

Filling

1 cup skim liquid milk
1 tbsp skim powdered milk
1 tbsp fine semolina
¼ tsp rose water
¼ tsp orange blossom water
2 cups coarsely grated low-moisture part-skim mozzarella cheese (200 g)

Honey Syrup

½ cup honey
1 ¼ tsp rose water
1 ¼ tsp orange blossom water

NOTES

❁ The pie crust is freezer friendly, and as such, I always make the above big quantity to be able to save 2 batches for later, for a faster preparation of *knaifeh*. If one desires to use up the whole pie crust on the spot, one will need to triple the filling quantities as well as the honey syrup and use a much larger non-stick round pan to yield 24 slices of *knaifeh*.

❁ In step 8, it is vital to generously grease a non-stick pan, or else the knaifeh will most likely stick (I use 2 tsp of coconut oil for the 23 cm diameter pan). To be on the safe side, one could grease the pan, add a round piece of parchment paper, then grease that lightly before adding the crust powder.

INSTRUCTIONS

1. For the pie crust, measure out the dry ingredients (except for the powdered milk) into a bowl. Mix gently and set aside.

2. Mix the powdered milk and liquid milk in a separate bowl, then stir in the oil and honey.

3. Add the wet ingredients to the dry ingredients, then stir well to mix.

4. Spread the batter onto a lightly greased sheet pan (recommended dimensions: 29 cm x 35 cm or similar), then bake in a preheated oven at 375 °F for 10 minutes.

5. Let cool, then scrape out and break up by hand. Grind in 4 batches using a blender, until a smooth powdery texture is obtained.

6. Divide the obtained crust powder into 3 equal parts, putting one batch aside and freezing the other two (separately) in airtight containers for future use (see note below).

7. For the current batch of crust powder to be used, set aside ¼ cup in a small bowl.

8. Grease a round non-stick baking pan (recommended diameter: 23 cm or similar) very well, then pour the crust powder onto the pan. Spread out and evenly pat down with one's hands. Press down well.

9. Bake on the bottom rack of an oven preheated to 350 °F for 15 minutes.

10. In the meantime, measure out the cheese in a separate bowl, then prepare the filling by whisking the liquid milk, powdered milk, and semolina in a small saucepan over medium-high heat. Once it comes to a boil, turn down to medium-low heat and continue whisking well until lightly thickened. Stir in the flower waters once the heat is turned off.

11. Take the pan out of the oven, then evenly sprinkle 2/3 of the cheese, making sure to avoid putting cheese near the pan edges. Pour the milk pudding over the cheese, lightly spreading with a spoon, then evenly scatter the remaining cheese. Sprinkle the remaining ¼ cup of crust powder evenly over the cheese. Spread lightly, then press down gently with one's hands.

12. Return to the bottom rack of the oven, then bake for another 15 minutes.

13. In the meantime, prepare the honey syrup by whisking the honey and flower waters together. Set aside.

14. Switch the oven to a broil setting at 500 °F, then broil the *knaifeh* on the top rack of the oven for 1 minute.

15. Run a knife along the edge between the knaifeh and the pan, then flip over onto a bigger round pan (recommended diameter: 32 cm or similar), so that the pie crust is turned upwards. Pour the honey syrup evenly all over the surface of the crust, spreading gently if needed.

16. Serve warm and garnish with ground pistachios if desired. Store in the refrigerator and enjoy within a week. Store, covered, in the refrigerator.

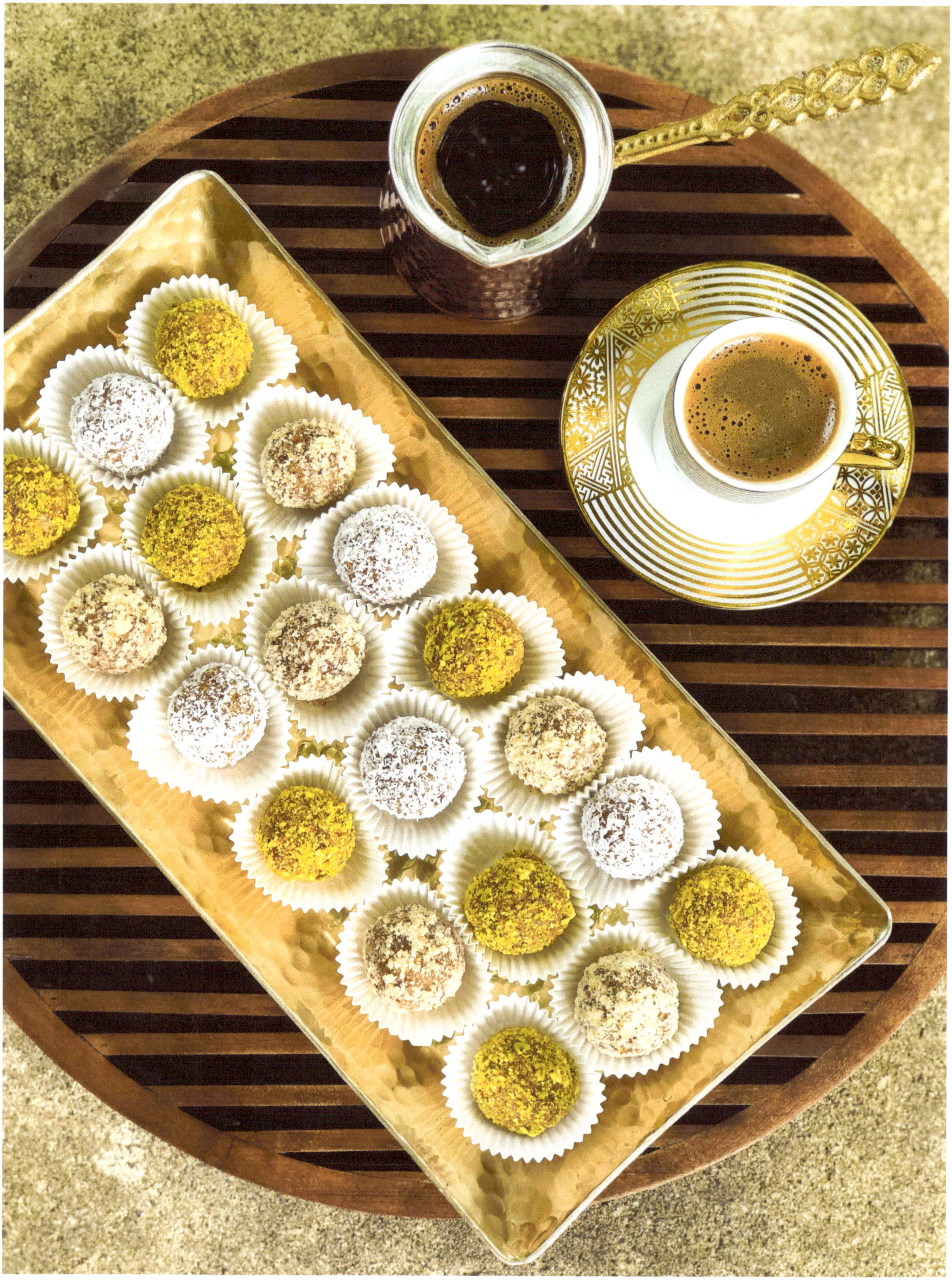

DATE NUT TRUFFLES

Inspired by the Middle Eastern tradition of eating a pitted date stuffed with an almond or a walnut, these delicious and nutritious truffles provide a boost of energy, healthy fat, fiber, and micronutrients, while satisfying a sugar craving with natural sweetness. This recipe is surely one to impress family and friends!

RECIPE YIELD 60 Truffles

DF GF EF OF V FF

INGREDIENTS

Truffle Dough

46 large soft pitted medjool dates (865 g)
1 ½ cups walnut pieces (150 g)
1 cup blanched almonds (150 g)
½ cup finely shredded unsweetened coconut flakes (42 g)
2 tsp orange blossom water

Truffle Coatings

4 tbsp finely shredded unsweetened coconut flakes
4 tbsp ground pistachios
4 tbsp ground blanched hazelnuts

NOTE

Since the coconut, pistachio, and hazelnut-coated truffles have only slight differences in nutritional value, the numbers were averaged between them.

RECIPE ALTERNATIVE

An equally delicious truffle can be made with dried apricots instead of dates. Substitute (in equal quantities by weight) the dates with apricots and the walnuts with pinenuts, keeping the almonds, coconut, and orange blossom water the same. Coat with shredded coconut.

INSTRUCTIONS

1. Grind the walnuts and almonds in a large food processor, scraping down the sides until the nuts are finely ground.
2. Empty into a bowl, then mix in the coconut and orange blossom water.
3. In 2 batches, process the dates and the nut mixture in the food processor, scraping down the sides until well blended and smooth.
4. Empty back into a bowl and knead until a uniform dough is formed.
5. Cover, then place in the refrigerator for an hour to firm up a bit.
6. Divide the dough into three equal parts, then using a tablespoon, scoop level spoonfuls of the dough and round into balls; each third of the dough should yield 20 truffles (if dough is too sticky to work with, lightly grease both hands).
7. Roll each of the truffles in one of the three truffle coatings.
8. Store the truffles in an airtight container for up to a week at room temperature or up to two to three weeks in the refrigerator. Since truffles will harden slightly in the cold of the refrigerator, allow them to soften at room temperature for about 15 minutes before serving.

NUTRITION FACTS PER TRUFFLE

85 Kcal	1.4 g Protein	4 g Fat	12 g Carbs	2 g Fiber	10 g Sugar

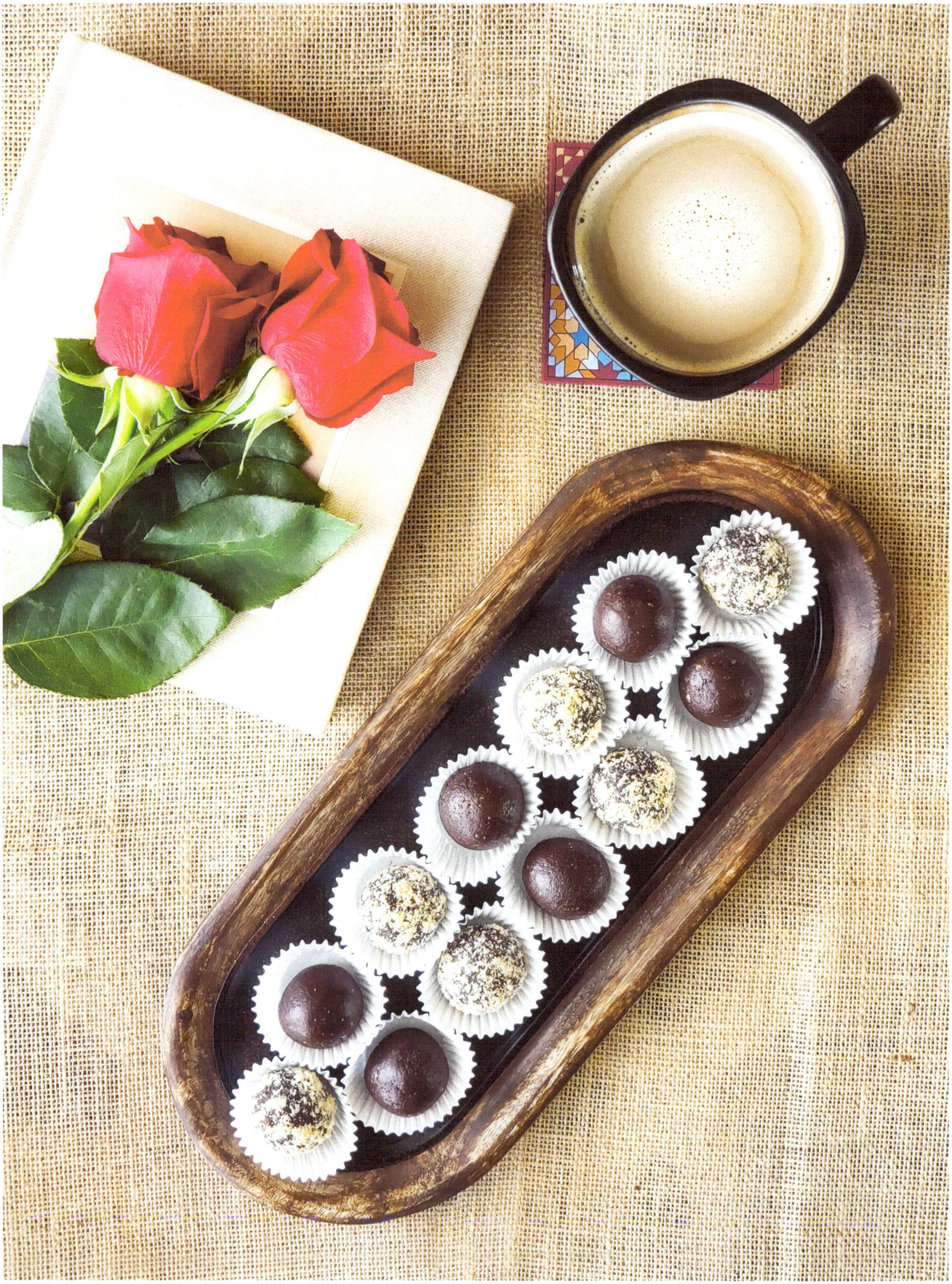

COCOA HAZELNUT TRUFFLES

Inspired by my love for chocolate hazelnut spread, these soft and creamy truffles are packed with healthy calories, protein, fiber, and micronutrients, while being low in fat. They are surely healthy energy balls that can satisfy a chocolate craving as well.

RECIPE YIELD 64 truffles

DF GF EF OF V FF

INGREDIENTS

46 large soft pitted medjool dates (865 g)
1 cup hazelnuts (125 g)
1 cup cashews (135 g)
½ cup unsweetened cocoa powder (45 g)
¼ cup unsweetened creamy peanut butter (55 g)
1 tsp vanilla powder
¼ tsp salt

NOTES

- One could use salted and roasted hazelnuts and cashews instead of the unsalted and raw form of the nuts, but make sure to eliminate the salt from the ingredients.
- One can substitute the peanut butter with cashew or almond butter.
- It is optional to coat half of the truffles in ground hazelnuts. If desired, one will need about 2 tbsp of ground raw blanched hazelnuts.

RECIPE ALTERNATIVE

- For a nut-free version, use ¼ cup raw mashed avocado or *tahini* instead of the peanut butter.

INSTRUCTIONS

1. Grind the hazelnuts and cashews in a large food processor, scraping down the sides until the nuts are finely ground.
2. Add the cocoa, nut butter, vanilla, and salt, then process again until well mixed. Transfer to a bowl.
3. In 2 batches, process the dates and the nut mixture in the food processor, scraping down the sides until well blended and smooth.
4. Empty back into a bowl and knead until a uniform dough is formed.
5. Cover, then place in the refrigerator for an hour to firm up a bit.
6. Using a tablespoon, scoop level spoonfuls of the dough and round into balls (if dough is too sticky to work with, lightly grease both hands).
7. Store the truffles in an airtight container for up to a week at room temperature or up to two to three weeks in the refrigerator. Since truffles will harden slightly in the cold of the refrigerator, allow them to soften at room temperature for about 15 minutes before serving.

NUTRITION FACTS PER TRUFFLE

68 Kcal	1 g Protein	3 g Fat	12 g Carbs	1.5 g Fiber	9 g Sugar

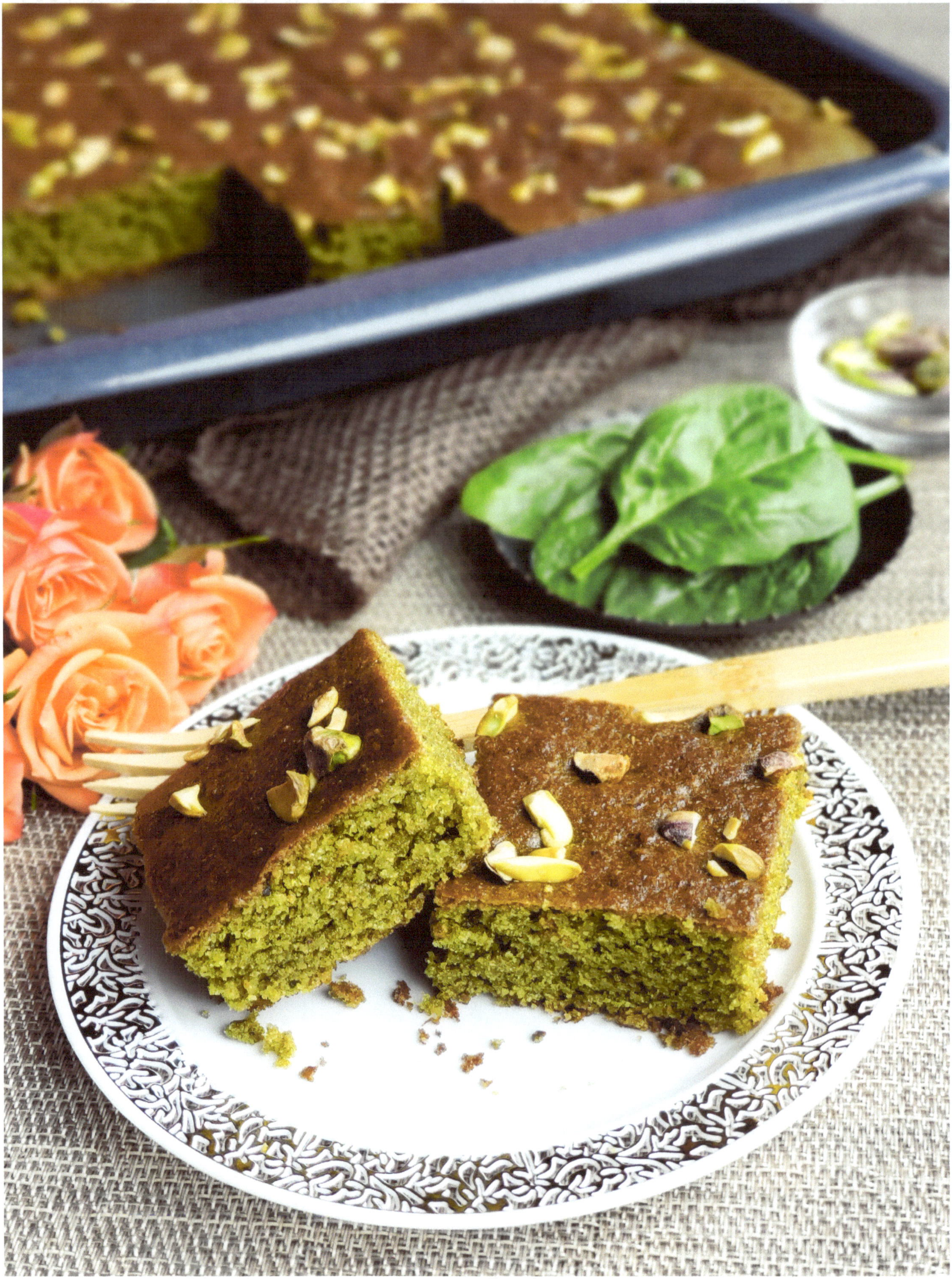

PISTACHIO CAKE

This recipe was inspired by my love for two favorite Middle Eastern ingredients, pistachios and rose water. I add spinach to this recipe to further enhance the green color of the cake while adding much nutritional benefits, without affecting the flavor. Made with nutritious ingredients, this unique cake adds much pleasure to a cup of coffee or tea.

RECIPE YIELD 30 slices

EF Vt

INGREDIENTS

Dry Ingredients

2 ¼ cups pistachios (315 g)
2 cups whole wheat flour (260 g)
2 tsp baking powder
1 tsp baking soda
⅓ tsp salt
¼ cup coarsely chopped pistachios (35 g)

Wet Ingredients

Fresh baby spinach leaves, whole (150 g)
⅔ cup skim yogurt (156 g)
⅓ cup olive oil
1 cup honey
5 tsp rose water

INSTRUCTIONS

1. Break up the spinach by hand, then put in a small saucepan. Over medium heat, cook the spinach for about 3 minutes, stirring frequently, until shriveled up. Let cool.
2. Measure out the dry ingredients (except for the nuts) into a bowl. Mix gently and set aside.
3. In a small food processor, blend the whole pistachios until a paste is formed. Add the rose water then stir to mix. Transfer to a large bowl.
4. Place the spinach in a food blender, then pour in the yogurt, oil, and honey. Blend well.
5. Preheat the oven to 325 °F.
6. Grease a baking pan (recommended dimensions: 29 cm x 35 cm or similar).
7. Combine the spinach mixture with the pistachio mixture in the large bowl.
8. Sift the dry ingredients over the wet ingredients, then mix well.
9. Pour the batter into the pan, then evenly sprinkle on the chopped pistachios.
10. Bake for 25 minutes.
11. Let cool for at least an hour before slicing and serving.
12. Store, covered, at room temperature or in the refrigerator.

NUTRITION FACTS PER SLICE

157 Kcal	4.4 g Protein	8 g Fat	19 g Carbs	3 g Fiber	10.6 g Sugar

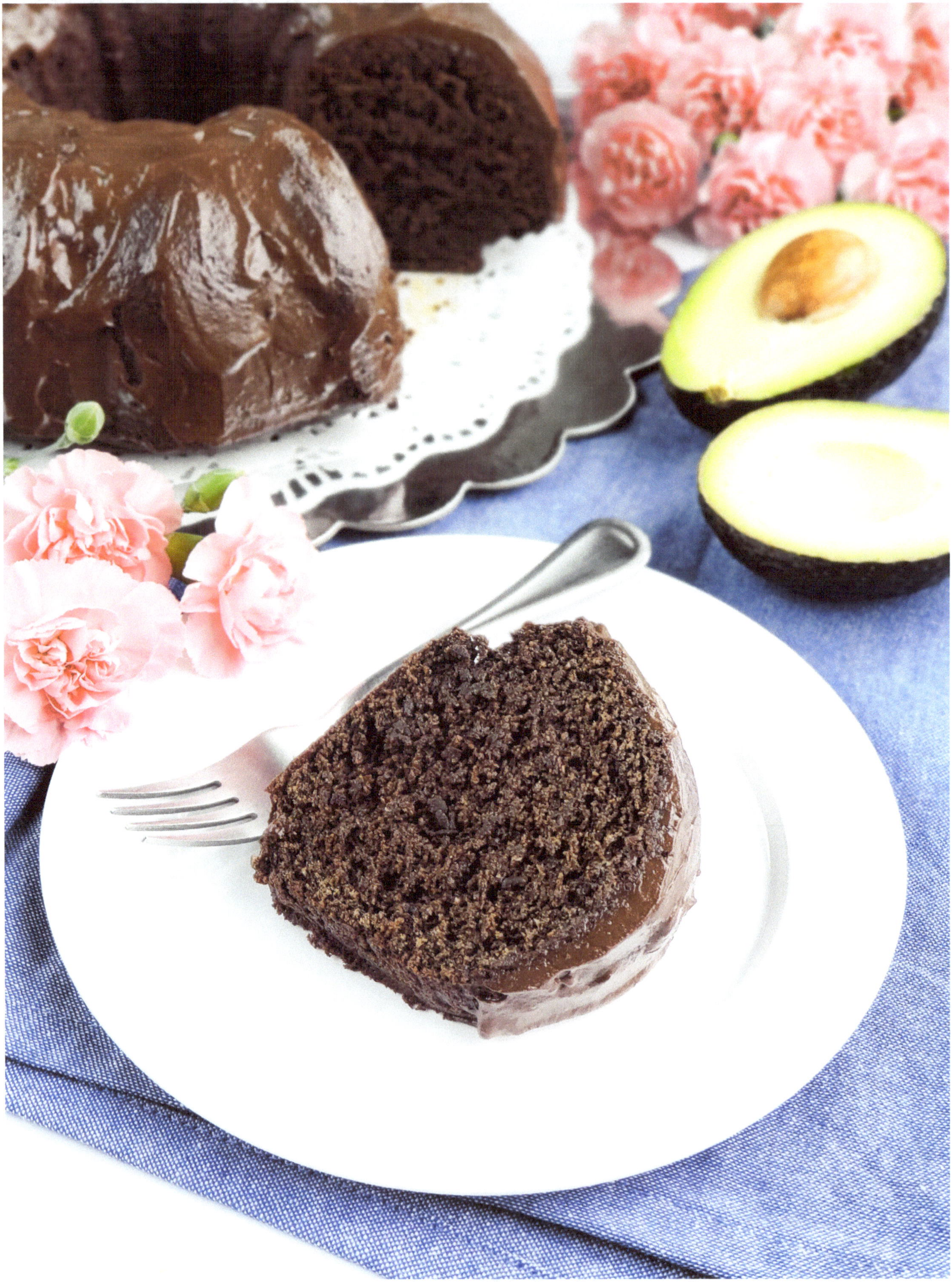

AVOCADO CHOCOLATE CAKE

This cake is a super healthy take on traditional chocolate cakes. It was inspired by my healthy chocolate cake which I adapted from a stove-top cooked chocolate-sauce cake recipe of my mother's, made with traditional unhealthy cake ingredients (butter, refined flour, and refined sugar). To further add nutrition and richness to the cake, I have thrown in an avocado fruit. Although frosting any cake is always optional, I believe the simple but healthy and wholesome cocoa frosting I created goes nicely with the not-so-sweet cake.

RECIPE YIELD 14 slices

Vt

INGREDIENTS

Dry Ingredients

3 cups whole wheat pastry flour (360)
1 cup unsweetened cocoa powder (90 g)
2 ½ tsp baking powder
2 ½ tsp baking soda
1 tsp salt

Wet Ingredients

1 large ripe pitted Hass avocado (no skin) (180 g)
1 ½ cups + 1 tbsp liquid skim milk
⅓ cup avocado oil
1 cup honey
1 tbsp liquid vanilla extract
2 large eggs

Frosting

½ large ripe pitted Hass avocado (no skin) (90 g)
3 large soft pitted medjool dates (57 g)
⅓ cup liquid skim milk
2 tbsp powdered skim milk
5 tbsp unsweetened cocoa powder
1 tsp honey
⅓ tsp vanilla powder
⅛ tsp salt

NOTE

❁ For a reason I don't quite know, my baked avocado-containing desserts tend to taste a bit better after 24 hours.

INSTRUCTIONS

1. For the frosting, put all the ingredients in a small food processor, then blend well until smooth, scraping down the sides as needed. Cover and refrigerate.
2. Measure out the dry ingredients (except for the cocoa) into a bowl. Mix gently and set aside.
3. In a saucepan, pour in the milk, then whisk in the cocoa and 1 egg. Whisk well over medium-high heat just until lightly thickened. Set aside to cool.
4. Put the remaining egg in a blender, then add the avocado, oil, honey, and vanilla. Blend well.
5. Pour out the avocado mixture into a big bowl, then mix in the cooled cocoa sauce.
6. Lower the middle oven rack to one level lower and preheat the oven to 315 °F.
7. In 2 batches, sift the dry ingredients over the wet ingredients, then mix until just blended.
8. Pour the batter into a greased Bundt pan (recommended diameter: 25.4 cm or similar), then bake for 45 minutes.
9. Time 15 minutes for the cake to cool inside the pan before gently flipping out onto a cooling rack. Let cool to room temperature before applying the frosting.
10. Store, covered, in the refrigerator.

NUTRITION FACTS PER SLICE

307 Kcal	8 g Protein	10.6 g Fat	51.6 g Carbs	7 g Fiber	25 g Sugar

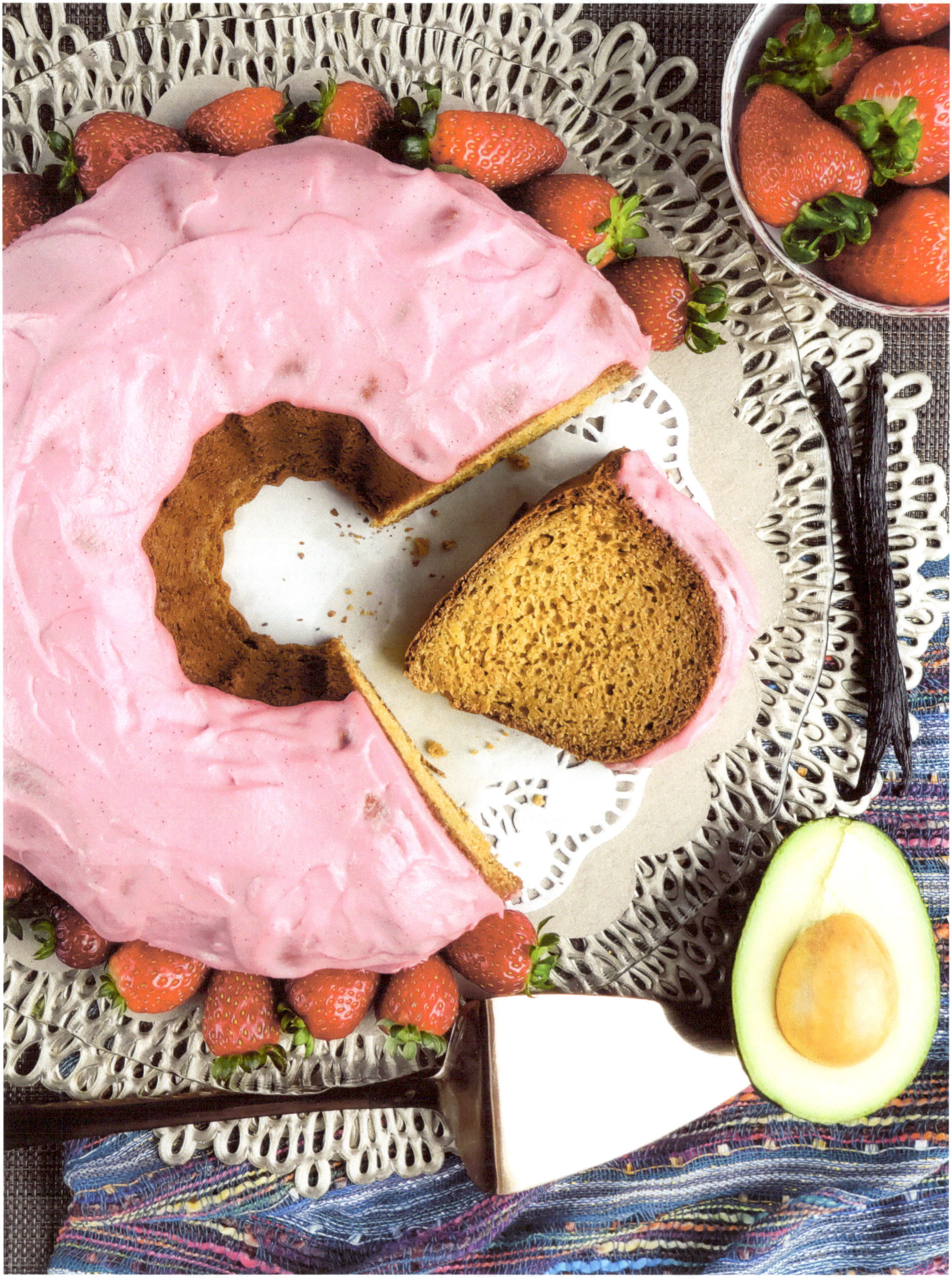

AVOCADO VANILLA CAKE

This cake is a super healthy twist on traditional vanilla white cakes. Inspired by my simple but healthy vanilla cake (recipe below) which I adapted from traditional white cakes made with butter or shortening as well as refined flour and sugar, this recipe includes an avocado, bumping up the nutritional content and rich texture and flavor. Although frosting the cake is optional, I believe the simple but healthy and wholesome vanilla bean frosting I created adds sweetness and moistness to the not-so-sweet cake.

RECIPE YIELD 14 slices

Vt

INGREDIENTS

Dry Ingredients

4 cups whole wheat pastry flour (480 g)
3 tbsp powdered skim milk
2 ½ tsp baking powder
3 tsp baking soda
⅔ tsp salt

Wet Ingredients

1 large ripe pitted Hass avocado (no skin) (180 g)
1 cup + 2 tbsp liquid skim milk
4 tbsp white vinegar
⅓ cup avocado oil
¾ cup honey
2 ½ tbsp liquid vanilla extract
2 large eggs

Frosting

1 ⅓ cups cashews (180 g)
¼ cup + 2 tbsp liquid skim milk
2 tbsp honey
1 whole vanilla bean, scraped
⅛ tsp salt
few drops of beet juice, optional (for pink color)

INSTRUCTIONS

1. For the frosting, soak the cashews in water for 8 hours, then drain, rinse, and pat dry. Put in a blender with the rest of the ingredients, then blend well until smooth, scraping down the sides as needed. Cover and refrigerate.
2. Measure out the dry ingredients (except for the powdered milk) into a bowl. Mix gently and set aside.
3. Mix the powdered milk and liquid milk in a separate bowl. Stir in the vinegar then let sit.
4. Put the eggs and vanilla in a blender, then blend until fluffy.
5. Add the oil, honey, and avocado, then continue blending well.
6. Pour into a big bowl, then stir in the milk mixture.
7. Lower the middle oven rack to one level lower and preheat the oven to 315 °F.
8. In 2 batches, sift the dry ingredients over the wet ingredients, then mix just until blended.
9. Pour the batter into a greased Bundt pan (recommended diameter: 25.4 cm or similar), then bake for 45 minutes.
10. Time 15 minutes for the cake to cool inside the pan before gently flipping out onto a cooling rack. Let cool to room temperature before applying the frosting.
11. Garnish with fresh strawberries if desired.
12. Store, covered, in the refrigerator.

See next page for notes »

NUTRITION FACTS PER SLICE

360 Kcal	9 g Protein	14 g Fat	50.6 g Carbs	5 g Fiber	20 g Sugar

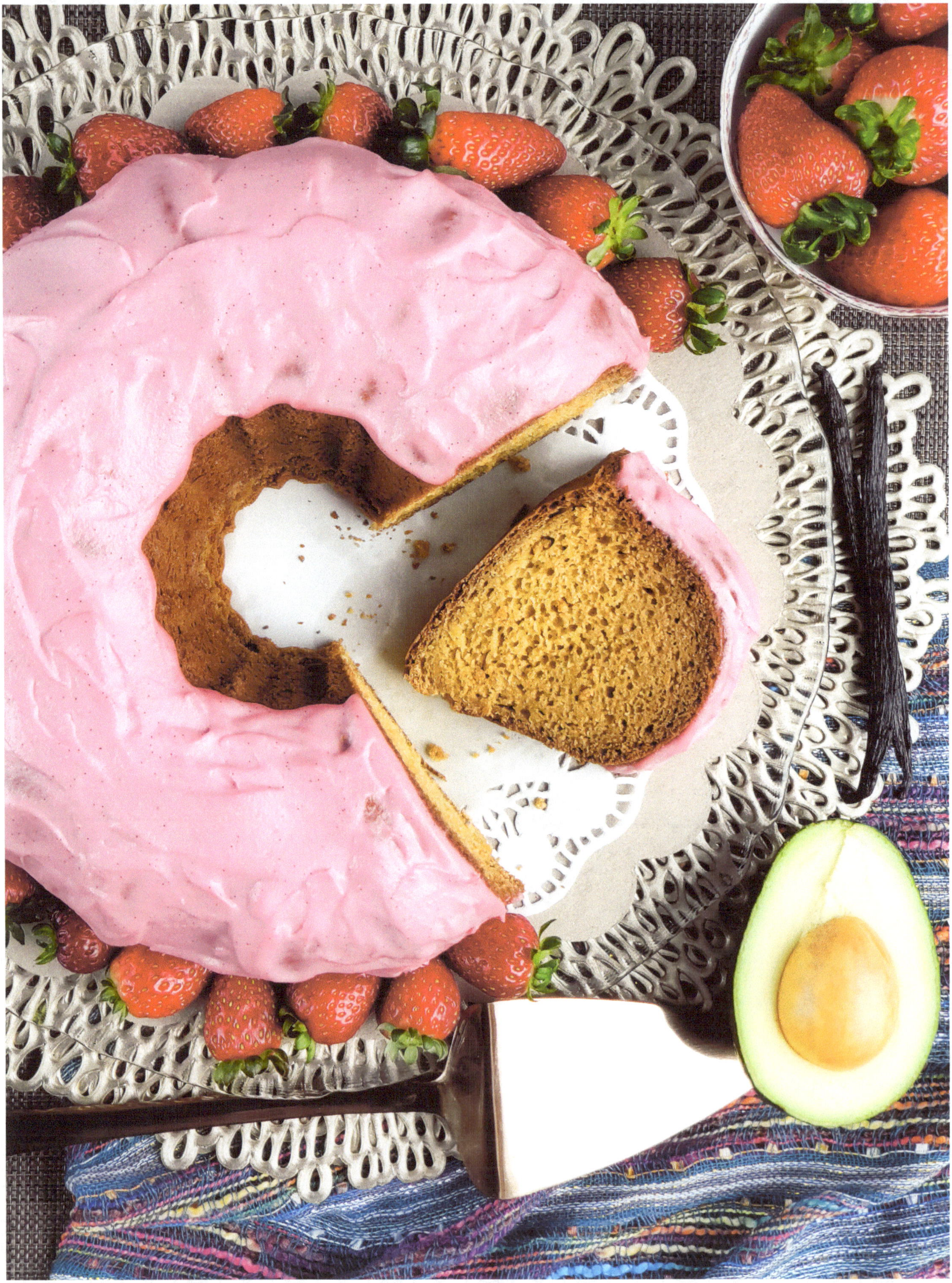

INGREDIENTS

Dry Ingredients
4 cups whole wheat pastry flour (480 g)
3 tbsp powdered skim milk
2 ½ tsp baking powder
3 tsp baking soda
⅔ tsp salt

Wet Ingredients
1 large ripe pitted Hass avocado (no skin) (180 g)
1 cup + 2 tbsp liquid skim milk
4 tbsp white vinegar
⅓ cup avocado oil
¾ cup honey
2 ½ tbsp liquid vanilla extract
2 large eggs

Frosting
1 ⅓ cups cashews (180 g)
¼ cup + 2 tbsp liquid skim milk
2 tbsp honey
1 whole vanilla bean, scraped
⅛ tsp salt
few drops of beet juice, optional (for pink color)

NOTE

For a reason I don't quite know, my baked avocado-containing desserts tend to taste a bit better after 24 hours.

RECIPE ALTERNATIVE

For a lighter and whiter vanilla cake, omit the avocados and follow these ingredients: 3 cups whole wheat pastry flour, 2 tbsp baking powder, 3 tbsp powdered skim milk, ½ tsp salt, 1 cup liquid skim milk, ½ cup avocado oil, 2/3 cup honey, 2 tbsp liquid vanilla extract, and 6 egg whites. Bake the same as above.

INSTRUCTIONS

1. For the frosting, soak the cashews in water for 8 hours, then drain, rinse, and pat dry. Put in a blender with the rest of the ingredients, then blend well until smooth, scraping down the sides as needed. Cover and refrigerate.

2. Measure out the dry ingredients (except for the powdered milk) into a bowl. Mix gently and set aside.

3. Mix the powdered milk and liquid milk in a separate bowl. Stir in the vinegar then let sit.

4. Put the eggs and liquid vanilla in a blender, then blend until fluffy.

5. Add the oil, honey, and avocado, then continue blending well.

6. Pour into a big bowl, then stir in the milk mixture.

7. Lower the middle oven rack to one level lower and preheat the oven to 315 °F.

8. In 2 batches, sift the dry ingredients over the wet ingredients, then mix just until blended.

9. Pour the batter into a greased Bundt pan (recommended diameter: 25.4 cm or similar), then bake for 45 minutes.

10. Time 15 minutes for the cake to cool inside the pan before gently flipping out onto a cooling rack. Let cool to room temperature before applying the frosting.

11. Garnish with fresh strawberries if desired.

12. Store, covered, in the refrigerator.

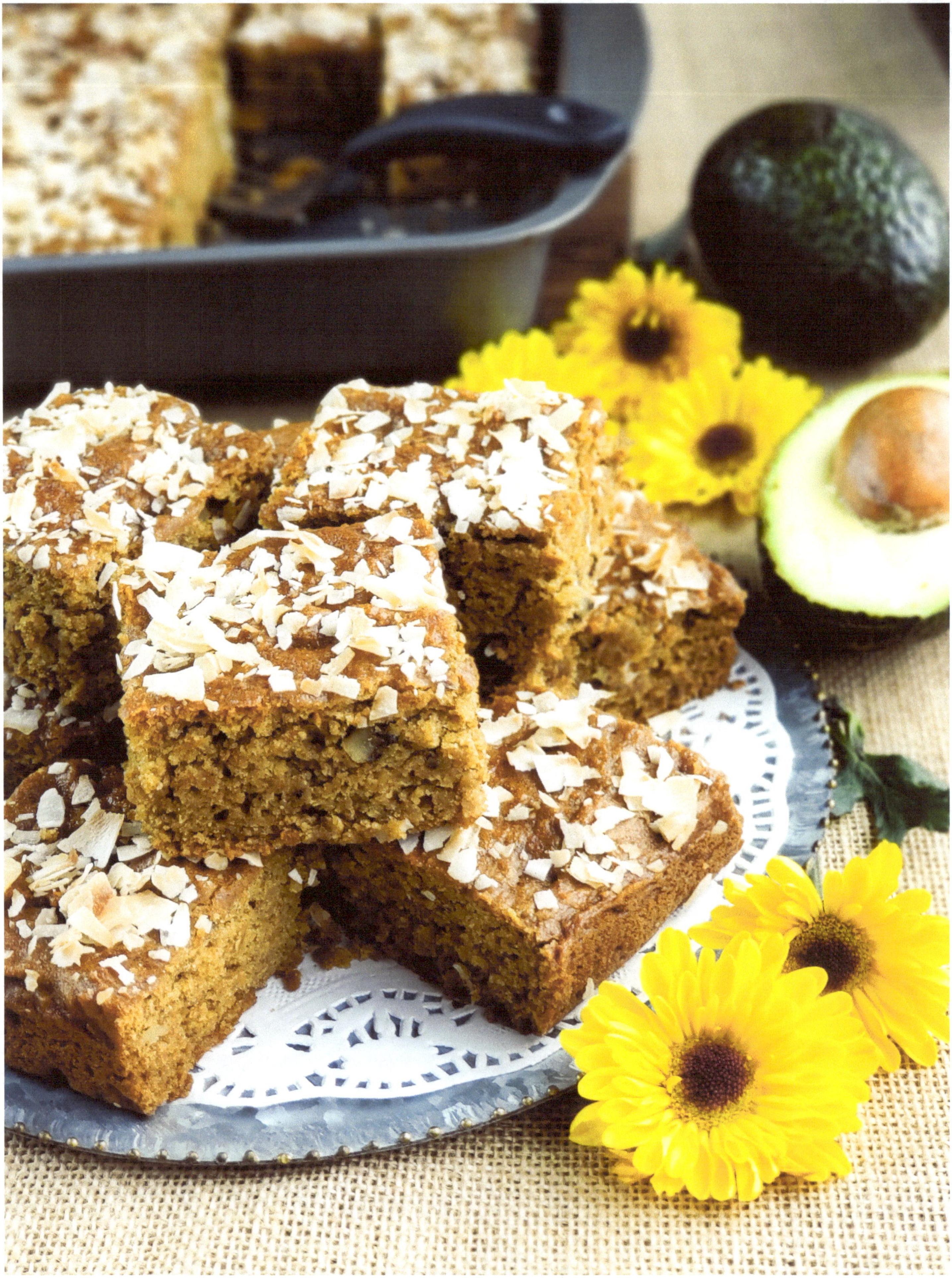

AVOCADO OATMEAL CAKE

This cake recipe was adapted from an oatmeal cake recipe handed down to my mother from a friend, which was originally made with traditional cake ingredients and topped with a rich butter frosting containing sweetened coconut. I made this recipe healthier and more whole by using whole wheat flour, honey, avocado oil, by adding an avocado to the batter, and by eliminating the butter frosting and simply substituting it with unsweetened coconut flakes.

RECIPE YIELD 24 slices

DF Vt

INGREDIENTS

Dry Ingredients

3 cups whole wheat flour (390 g)
2 cups dry quick oats (176 g)
1 tbsp cinnamon
2 ½ tsp baking powder
2 ½ tsp baking soda
1 tsp salt
½ cup coarsely chopped walnuts (60 g)
⅓ cup coarsely grated unsweetened coconut flakes (20 g)

Wet Ingredients

1 large ripe pitted Hass avocado (no skin) (180 g)
2 cups hot water
½ cup avocado oil
1 cup honey
1 tbsp liquid vanilla extract
2 large eggs

NOTE

- For a reason I don't quite know, my baked avocado-containing desserts tend to taste a bit better after 24 hours.

INSTRUCTIONS

1. In a small bowl, add the hot water to the oats. Stir to mix, then let sit to cool.
2. Put the remaining wet ingredients in a blender, and process well until smooth, scraping down the sides as needed. Pour into a bowl.
3. Measure out the remaining dry ingredients (except for the nuts and coconut flakes) into a separate bowl. Mix gently and set aside.
4. Preheat the oven to 320 °F.
5. Grease a baking pan (recommended dimensions: 25 cm x 35 cm or similar).
6. Add the oatmeal mixture to the wet ingredients, then stir to mix.
7. Sift in the dry ingredients, then stir the batter until well blended. Fold in the nuts.
8. Pour the batter into the pan, then evenly sprinkle on the coconut.
9. Bake for 35 minutes.
10. Let cool to room temperature before slicing and serving.
11. Store, covered, at room temperature or in the refrigerator.

NUTRITION FACTS PER SLICE

217 Kcal	5 g Protein	9 g Fat	30 g Carbs	5 g Fiber	12 g Sugar

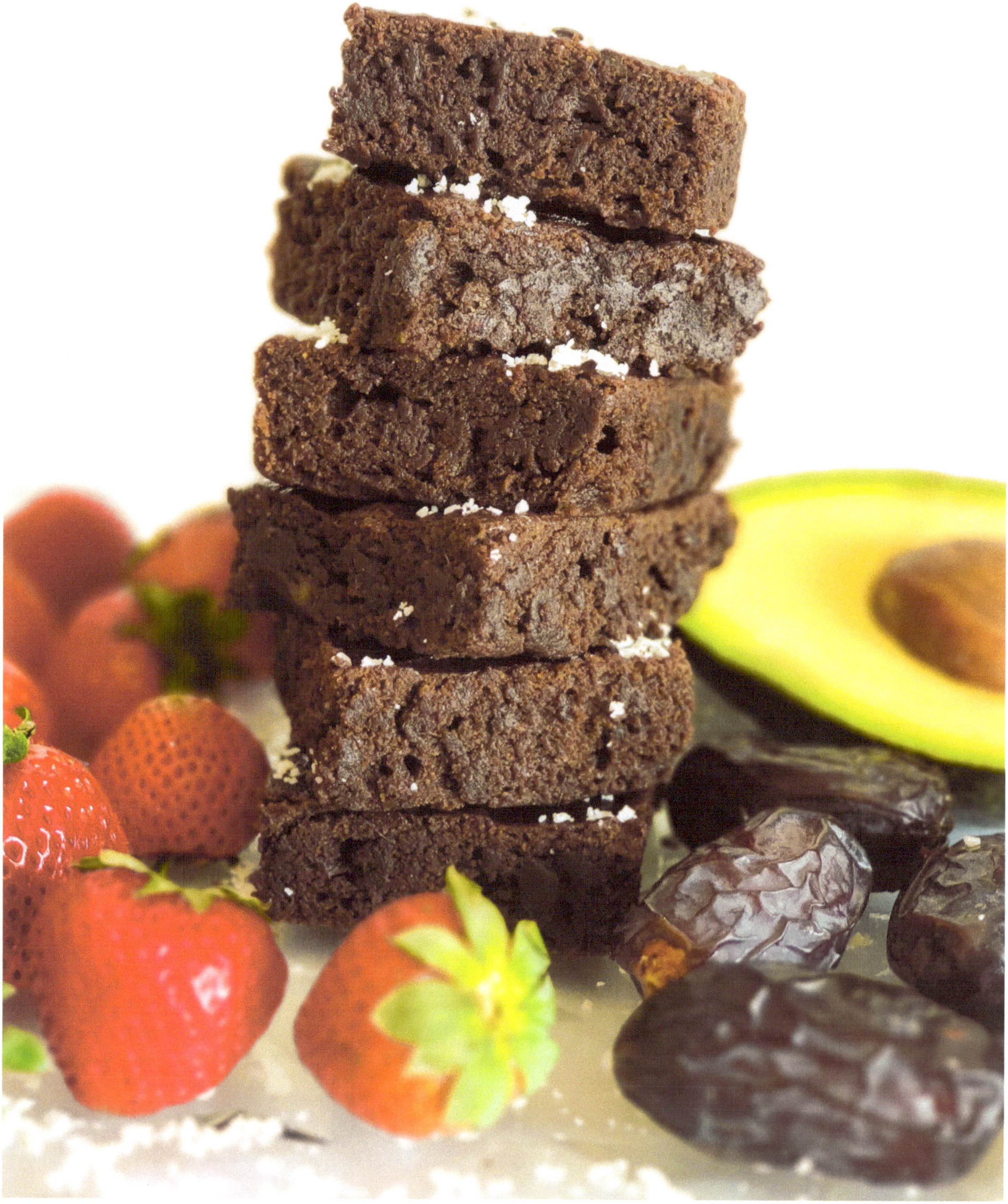

AVOCADO CHOCOLATE BROWNIES

Traditional chocolate brownies have always been a favorite dessert of mine. However, being so rich in butter and eggs, not to mention being full of refined flour and sugar, they have always made me feel so guilty when eating them! My love for brownies pushed me to create a delicious but healthier version, adapted from a recipe of my maternal great-grandmother. Meet my healthy and whole brownies made with olive oil, avocados, dates, honey, whole wheat pastry flour, and just a couple of eggs. While traditional brownies have a unique flaky outside, mine don't - but the goodness they offer on the inside simply surpasses the missing outer crunch!

RECIPE YIELD 16 slices

DF Vt

INGREDIENTS

Dry Ingredients

1 ¼ cups whole wheat pastry flour (150 g)
¾ cup unsweetened cocoa powder (68 g)
2 tsp baking powder
½ tsp salt

Wet Ingredients

½ large ripe pitted Hass avocado (no skin) (90 g)
10 large soft pitted medjool dates (190 g)
⅓ cup hot water
½ cup olive oil
¼ cup honey
2 large eggs
2 tsp liquid vanilla extract

NOTE

For a reason I don't quite know, my baked avocado-containing desserts tend to taste a bit better after 24 hours.

INSTRUCTIONS

1. Place the dates and water in a small food processor and blend well until smooth, scraping down the sides as needed.
2. Add the avocado to the date paste and blend well. Set aside to cool.
3. Measure out the dry ingredients into a bowl. Mix gently and set aside.
4. Preheat the oven to 320 °F.
5. Grease a square pan (recommended dimensions: 23 cm x 23 cm or similar).
6. In a large bowl, whisk the eggs until fluffy.
7. Mix in the oil, honey, and vanilla.
8. Add the date and avocado paste, then stir to mix well.
9. Sift the dry ingredients over the wet ingredients, then stir the batter until well blended.
10. Pour the batter into the pan and bake for 25 minutes.
11. Let cool for at least 30 minutes before slicing and serving.
12. Store, covered, at room temperature or in the refrigerator.

NUTRITION FACTS PER SLICE

172 Kcal	3 g Protein	9 g Fat	23.4 g Carbs	3.6 g Fiber	12.4 g Sugar

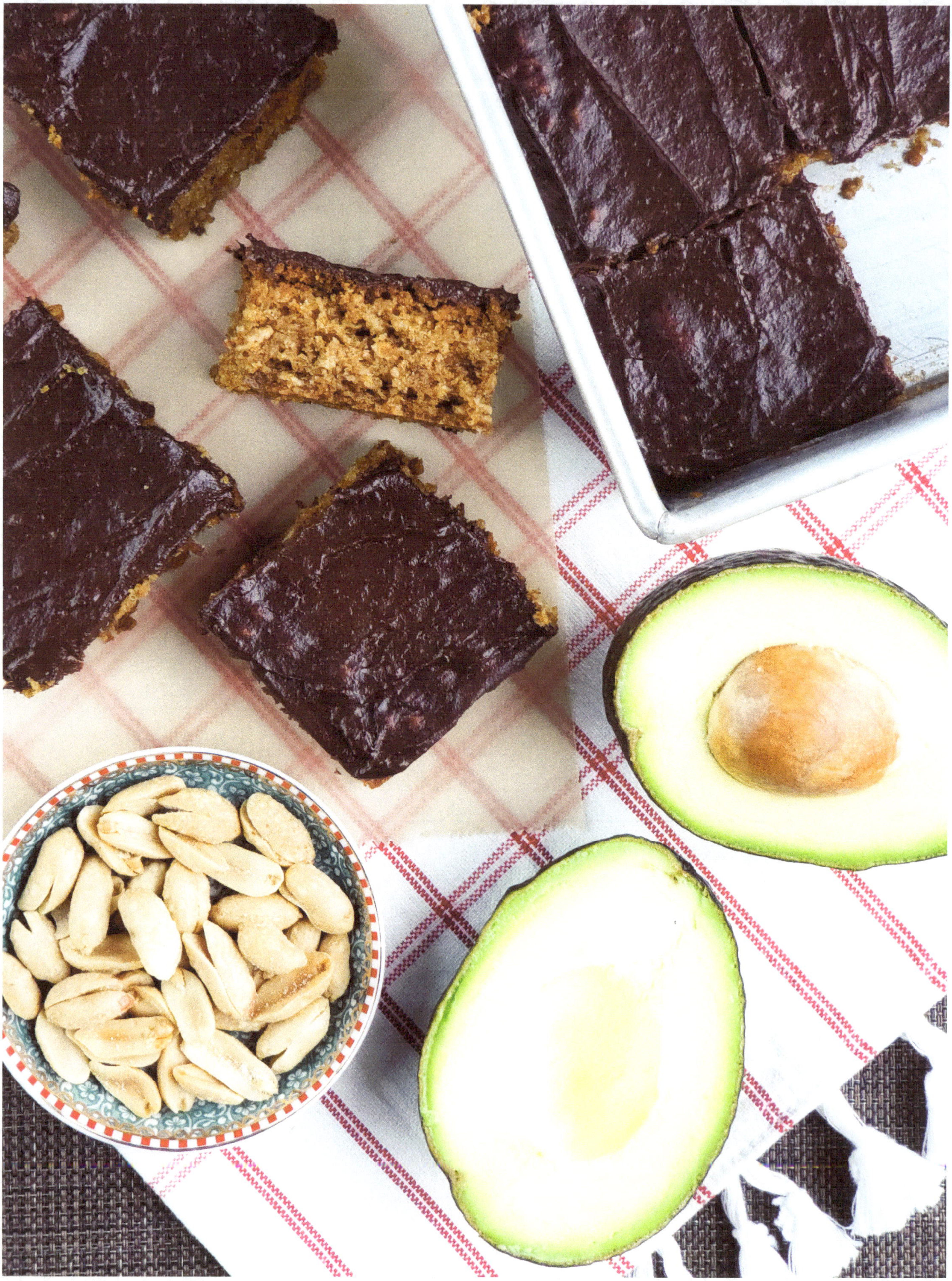

AVOCADO PEANUT BUTTER BROWNIES

For lovers of peanut butter and chocolate, this is the best healthy treat! Adapted from a peanut butter brownie recipe handed down to my mother from a friend of hers years ago, I turned this recipe into a healthier and more whole one by the use of whole wheat flour, honey, and avocado oil, as well as by adding an avocado to the batter and frosting. The healthy frosting I created for these not-too-sweet brownies really complements the flavor and sweetness, and avoids using butter and refined sugar.

RECIPE YIELD 16 slices

Vt

INGREDIENTS

Dry Ingredients

¼ cup whole wheat flour (33 g)
1 cup dry quick oats (88 g)
1 tsp baking soda
½ tsp salt

Wet Ingredients

½ large ripe pitted Hass avocado (no skin) (90 g)
¾ cup unsweetened creamy peanut butter (165 g)
¼ cup avocado oil
½ cup honey
1 large egg
1 ½ tsp liquid vanilla extract

Frosting

¼ large ripe pitted Hass avocado (no skin) (45 g)
2 large soft pitted medjool dates (38 g)
½ tsp avocado oil
2 tbsp liquid skim milk
2 tbsp powdered skim milk
3 tbsp unsweetened cocoa powder
¼ tsp vanilla powder
pinch of salt

NOTE

For a reason I don't quite know, my baked avocado-containing desserts tend to taste a bit better after 24 hours.

INSTRUCTIONS

1. For the frosting, put all ingredients in a small food processor, then blend well until smooth, scraping down the sides as needed. Cover and refrigerate.
2. Measure out the dry ingredients into a bowl. Mix gently and set aside.
3. Put the wet ingredients in a blender, then process well until smooth, scraping down the sides as needed. Pour into a separate bowl.
4. Preheat the oven to 320 °F.
5. Grease a square pan (recommended dimensions: 23 cm x 23 cm or similar).
6. Sift the dry ingredients over the wet ingredients, then stir the batter until well blended.
7. Pour the batter into the pan and bake for 30 minutes.
8. Let cool to room temperature before applying the frosting.
9. Return to the refrigerator and let sit for at least an hour before slicing and serving.
10. Sprinkle the top with ground peanuts if desired.
11. Store, covered, in the refrigerator.

NUTRITION FACTS PER SLICE

187 Kcal	5 g Protein	11 g Fat	20 g Carbs	3 g Fiber	11.5 g Sugar

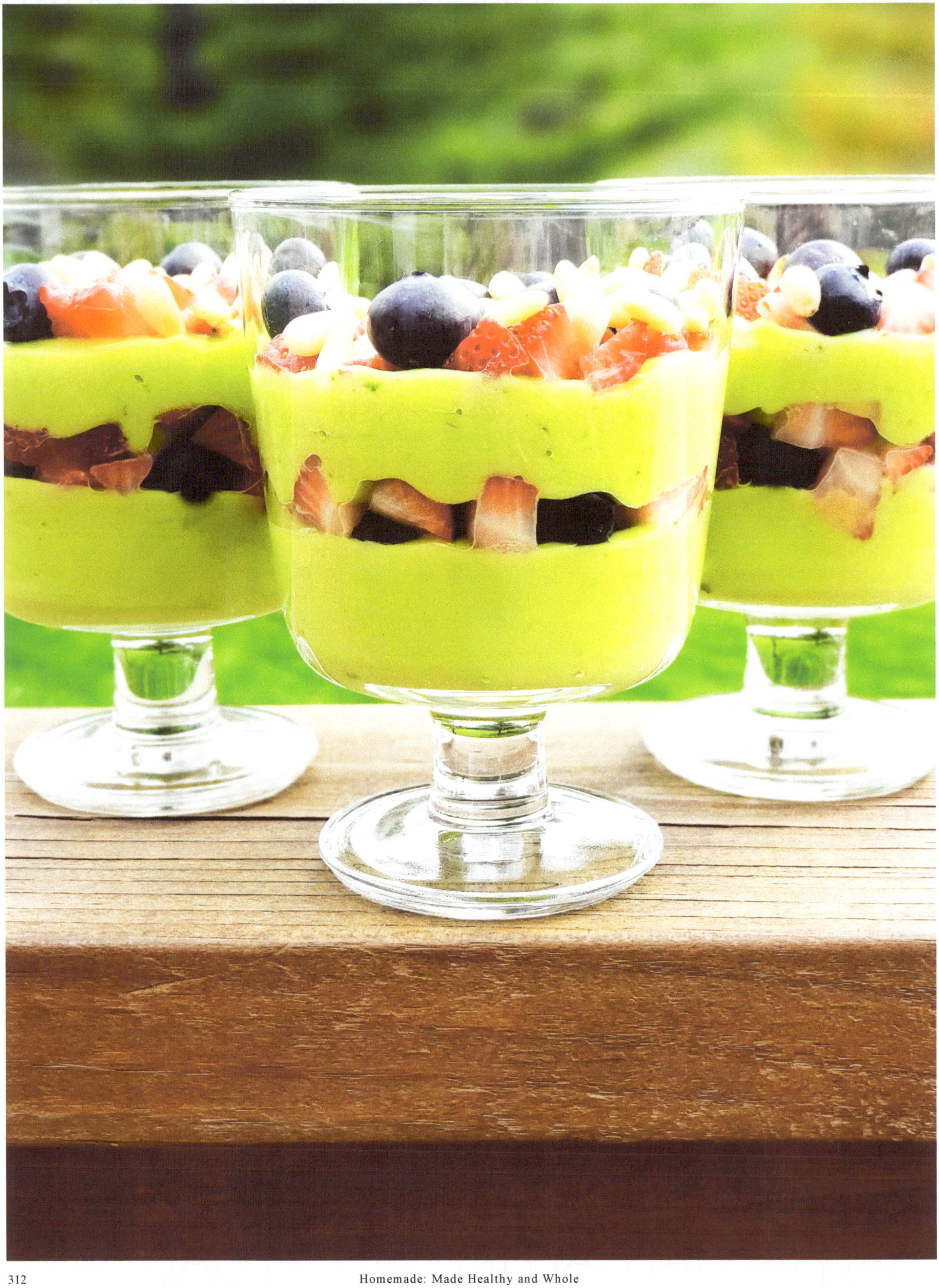

AVOCADO FRUIT PUDDING

This light and refreshing avocado fruit pudding topped with nuts was adapted from a friend's recipe that he made up from scratch. It is a healthy and delicious pudding calling for simple ingredients. This naturally sweetened and nutritious pudding is great for sweet-tooth cravings year-round!

RECIPE YIELD 7 ⅔ cups (11 bowls)

GF EF OF Vt

INGREDIENTS

Pudding

8 medium ripe pitted Hass avocados (no skin) (1,240 g)
4 medium mint leaves (middle vein removed), chopped
1 cup liquid skim milk
2 tbsp powdered skim milk
⅔ cup honey
1 tbsp lemon juice
⅓ tsp salt

Nut and Fruit Layers

⅔ cup pine nuts (90 g)
15 medium strawberries, diced (350 g)
2 cups blueberries (270 g)

NOTE

- Each bowl contains ⅔ cup pudding.

INSTRUCTIONS

1. Place the avocados in a large bowl and mash up a bit with an avocado masher or fork. Add the lemon juice, mint, and salt.
2. In a separate bowl, mix the liquid milk and powdered milk, then pour in the honey and stir to mix.
3. Blend the two mixtures lightly, then in two batches, process in a large food processor, scraping down the sides as needed, and processing until all the ingredients are well blended and smooth.
4. Pour both batches back into a bowl and combine well using a whisk.
5. Pour the pudding into an airtight container and store in the refrigerator for at least 30 minutes before serving.
6. For each bowl to be served, measure out a bit more than ⅓ cup of the pudding and place inside the bowl. Add a small handful of blueberries, strawberries, and pine nuts, then cover with another ⅓ cup of pudding. Add another small handful of fruit and nuts on the top. Repeat the same for all bowls.
7. Best consumed within 48 hours (despite the presence of lemon juice, the avocado pudding will brown slightly on the surface as time passes).

NUTRITION FACTS PER BOWL

340 Kcal	5 g Protein	22 g Fat	36 g Carbs	10 g Fiber	23 g Sugar

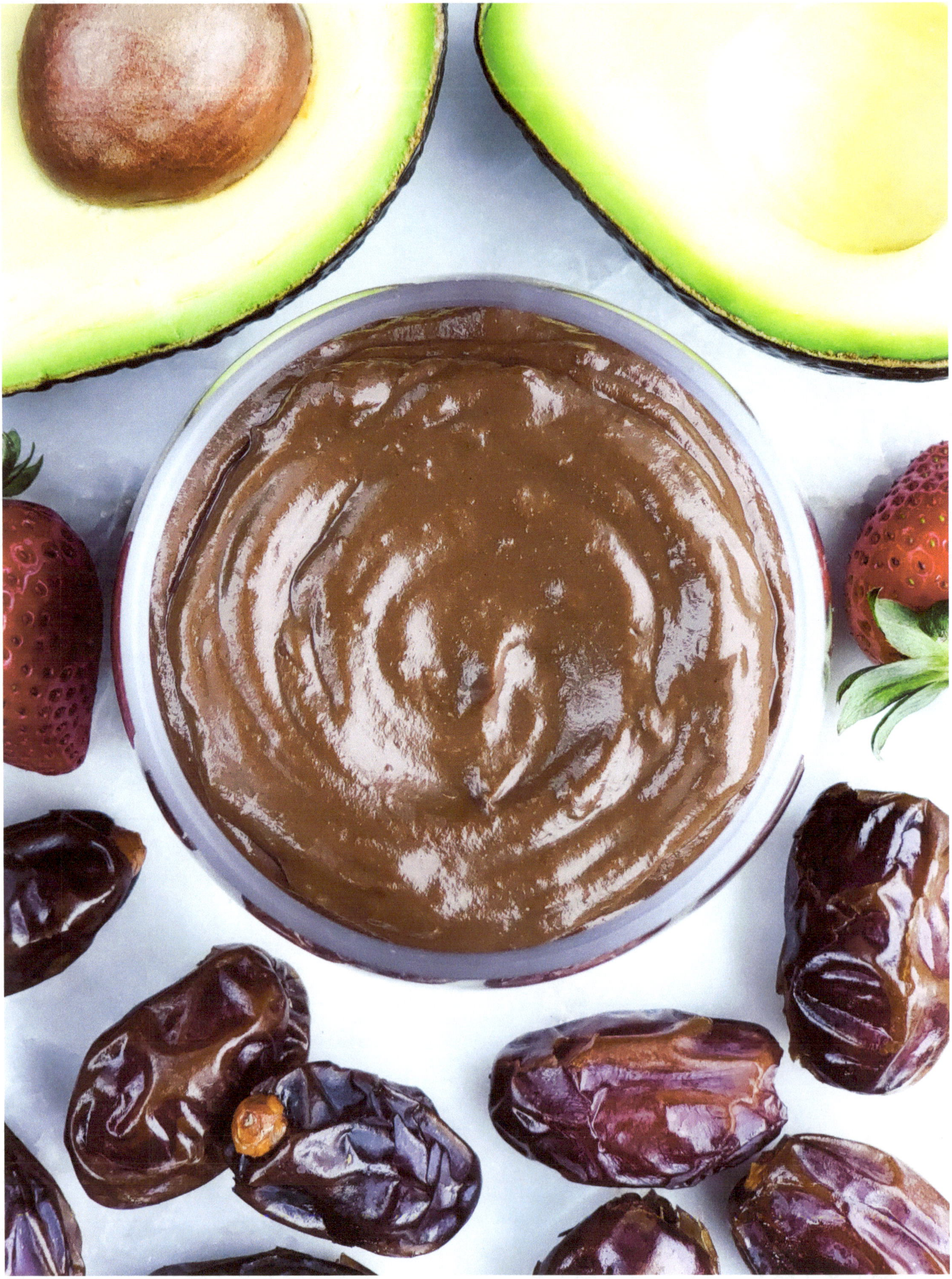

AVOCADO CHOCOLATE PUDDINNG

This nutritious no-cook avocado chocolate pudding is rich, creamy, and super delicious. Made with only avocados as the main fat source, this pudding contains no butter, hydrogenated oil, or full-fat dairy products, as most traditional chocolate puddings may have. It is also egg-free and is naturally sweetened with dates and honey, with no added refined sugar. Vegans can enjoy this pudding by simply substituting the cow milk called for in the recipe with any of their favorite plant-based milks (but the flavor and texture may not be as rich and thick since the recipe also calls for powdered cow milk which helps in adding some richness and thickness).

RECIPE YIELD 9 cups (12 bowls)

GF EF OF Vt

INGREDIENTS

7 medium ripe pitted Hass avocados (no skin) (1,085 g)
14 large soft pitted medjool dates (265 g)
1 ½ cups unsweetened cocoa powder (135 g)
2 cups skim liquid milk
6 tbsp skim powdered milk
⅓ cup honey
½ tsp vanilla powder
⅓ tsp salt

NOTES

- If the dates are not very soft, make sure to warm up the milk, then blend the milk and dates together until a smooth paste is formed, before proceeding with the remaining steps.
- For a stronger cocoa flavor, one can add more cocoa and adjust the sweetness with additional honey if desired.
- Each bowl contains ¾ cup pudding.

INSTRUCTIONS

1. Place the avocados in a large bowl and mash up a bit with an avocado masher or fork.
2. Add the pitted dates, then mash and mix. Set aside.
3. In a separate bowl, sift the cocoa powder, then mix in the powdered milk, vanilla, and salt.
4. Pour in the liquid milk and honey, then whisk well.
5. Blend the two mixtures lightly, then in two batches, process in a large food processor, scraping down the sides as needed, and processing until all the ingredients are well blended and smooth.
6. Pour both batches back into a bowl and whisk well to combine.
7. Pour the pudding into an airtight container or spoon out into individual bowls and cover well (add ¾ cup of the pudding to each bowl served).
8. Refrigerate the pudding for at least 12 hours before serving (this helps the flavors of the avocado and cocoa to set).
9. Can be served as a dessert topped with strawberries (or any other fruit) or eaten as a breakfast mixed in with oats, flaxseeds, chia seeds, or nuts. Best consumed within a few days.

NUTRITION FACTS PER BOWL

284 Kcal	6 g Protein	14 g Fat	45 g Carbs	11 g Fiber	30 g Sugar

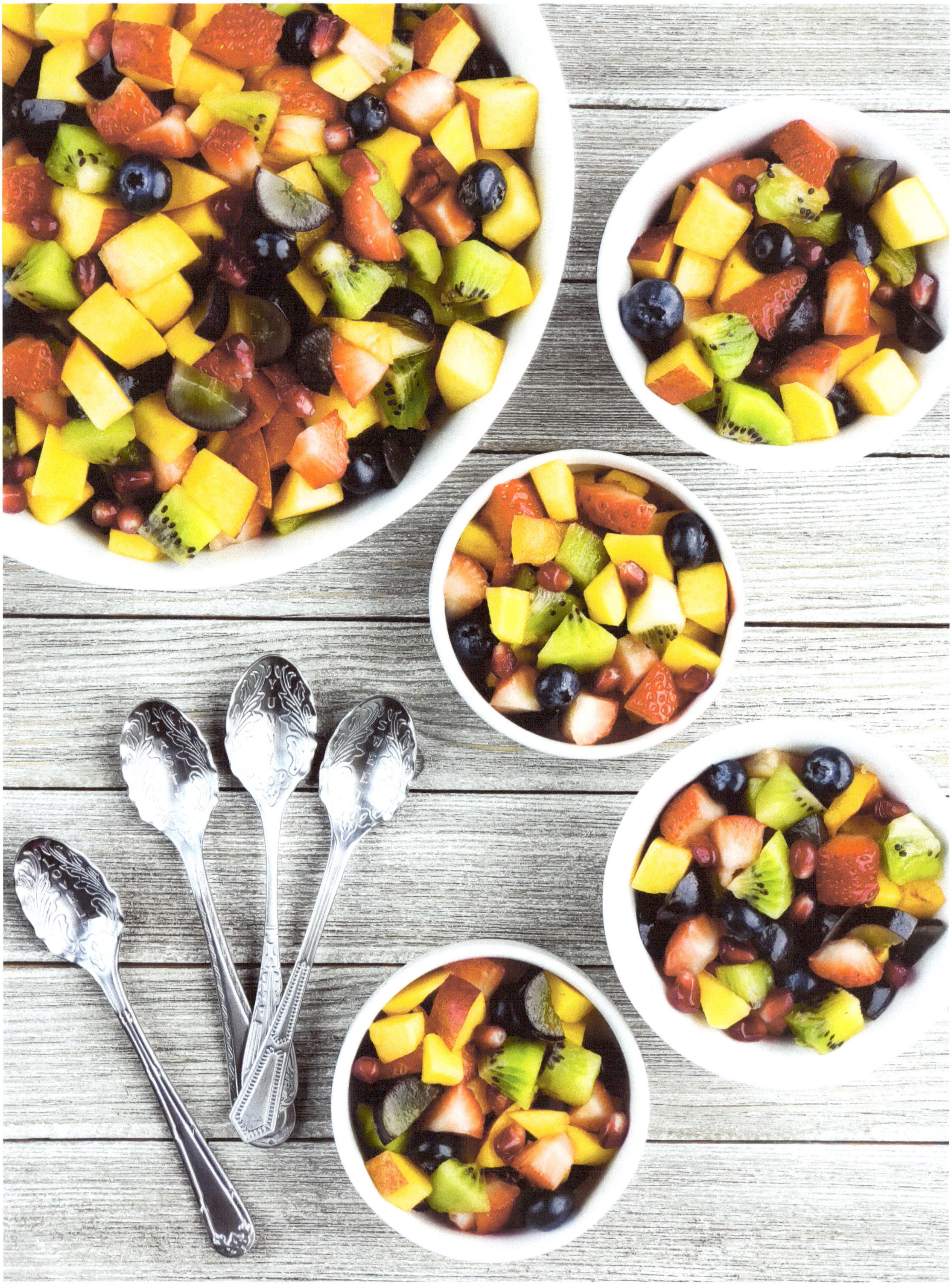

FRUIT SALAD

A healthy fruit salad in my opinion is a salad made with any and every seasonal fruit, in whichever quantities one desires, and guided by one's fruit preferences! I vary my fruit salad combination every time I make one, depending on the mood and the season. I was inclined not to include any quantities for this recipe, but for standardization purposes, here is an example of a simple yet healthy and super colorful and flavorful fruit salad made with a Middle Eastern twist.

RECIPE YIELD 17 cups

DF GF EF OF V

INGREDIENTS

1 medium pitted mango (no skin), diced (345 g)
2 large pitted nectarines (or peaches), diced (470 g)
6 medium-large kiwis (no skin), diced (455 g)
40 medium-large black seedless grapes, sliced (315 g)
22 medium strawberries, diced (515 g)
2 cups blueberries (270 g)
⅔ cup pomegranate seeds (94 g)
⅓ cup fresh orange juice
1 tbsp rose water

NOTES

- I usually avoid adding fruit that brown easily (like bananas, apples, and pears) to my fruit salad, but one can always chop and toss some in just before serving. Also, pouring extra orange juice will help minimize fruit browning.
- If some of the fruit are not super ripe/sweet, one can drizzle some honey or maple syrup over the fruit salad if desired.

INSTRUCTIONS

1. Place all the prepared fruit together in a large bowl.
2. Add the orange juice and rose water, then gently fold.
3. Add more rose water and/or orange blossom water if desired.
4. Garnish with pistachios, pine nuts, or almond slivers if desired.
5. Store, covered, in the refrigerator.

NUTRITION FACTS PER CUP

78 Kcal	1 g Protein	0.5 g Fat	19 g Carbs	3 g Fiber	14.4 g Sugar

BIBLIOGRAPHY

Acrylamide and Cancer Risk. American Cancer Society (ACS). 2016. Accessed December 2018.

Advanced Glycation End-Products: A Biological Consequence of Lifestyle Contributing to Cancer Disparity. Turner DP. *Cancer Research.* 75(10): 1925–1929. 2015.

Advice about Eating Fish. U.S. Food and Drug Administration (FDA) and Environmental Protection Agency (EPA). 2017. Accessed March 2019.

An Avocado a Day May Help Keep Bad Cholesterol at Bay. American Heart Association (AHA) News. 2015. Accessed April 2019.

Are Eggs Risky for Heart Health? Harvard Health Publishing. Harvard Medical School. 2017. Updated 2019. Accessed December 2019.

Arsenic in Rice and Rice Products. Questions and Answers. Metals. Food Borne Illnesses and Contaminants. Food. U.S Food and Drug Administration (FDA). 2018. Accessed February 2019.

Avocado. Fruit and Tree. Encyclopaedia Britannica. 2019. Accessed April 2019.

Bisphenol A (BPA). Health and Education. National Institute of Environmental Health Sciences. National Institute of Health (NIH). 2018. Accessed February 2019.

Canada's Dietary Guidelines. Health Canada. 2019. Accessed November 2019.

Cinnamon. Diet and Weight Management. WebMD. 2017. Accessed April 2019.

Cinnamon. US Department of Health and Human Services. National Institute of Health. National Center for Complementary and Integrative Health. 2017. Accessed April 2019.

Coconut Oil. Food Features. The Nutrition Source. Harvard T.H. Chan School of Public Health. Updated 2020. Accessed July 2020.

Cooking Utensils and Nutrition. Medical Encyclopedia. U.S National Library of Medicine. National Institute of Health (NIH). 2017. Accessed February 2019.

Common Questions about Diet and Cancer. American Cancer Society Guidelines on Nutrition and Physical Activity for Cancer Prevention. American Cancer Society (ACS). 2016. Accessed January 2019.

Cuts of Beef: A Guide to the Leanest Selections. Healthy Lifestyle. Nutrition and Healthy Eating. Mayo Foundation for Medical Education and Research (MFMER). 2018. Accessed October 2018.

Dairy Products - Milk, Yogurt, and Cheese. Healthy Living. American Heart Association (AHA). 2018. Accessed November 2018.

Date Fruits (Phoenix dactylifera Linn): An Emerging Medicinal Food. Vayalil PK. *Crit Rev Food Sci Nutr.* 2012;52(3):249-71.

Date Palm. Plant. Encyclopaedia Britannica. 2019. Accessed May 2019.

Definition and Facts for Lactose Intolerance. National Institute of Diabetes and Digestive and Kidney Diseases. National Institute of Health. 2018. Accessed November 2019.

Diabetes Treatment: Can Cinnamon Lower Blood Sugar? Patient Care and Health Info. Mayo Clinic. 2019. Accessed April 2019.

Dietary Guidelines for Americans 2015 - 2020. U.S. Department of Health and Human Services (USDHHS) and U.S. Department of Agriculture (USDA). 8th Edition. 2015. Accessed June 2018.

Dietary Guidelines for Americans 2020 - 2025. U.S. Department of Health and Human Services (USDHHS) and U.S. Department of Agriculture (USDA). 9th Edition. 2020. Accessed January 2021.

Dioxins and Their Effects on Human Health. News. Fact Sheets. Detail. World Health Organization (WHO). 2016. Accessed February 2019.

Ditch the Gluten, Improve Your Health? Health Topics. Harvard Health Publishing. Harvard Medical School. Updated 2019. Accessed December 2019.

Does Cinnamon Help Diabetes? Diabetes. WebMD. 2019. Accessed April 2019.

Fats. Healthy Living. American Heart Association (AHA). 2018. Accessed November 2018.

Food Composition Tables for Use in the Middle East. Pellet PL and Shadarevian S. American University of Beirut. Lebanon. Second Edition. 1970.

FoodData Central. Agricultural Research Service. U.S. Department of Agriculture. 2019. Accessed 2019, 2020, and 2021.

Food Safety in Your Kitchen. U.S. Food and Drug Administration. 2018. Accessed October 2019.

Garlic. Plant. Encyclopaedia Britannica. 2019. Accessed May 2019.

Garlic. Vitamins and Supplements. WebMD. 2018. Accessed May 2019.

Gluten-Free Diet. Nutrition and Healthy Eating. Healthy Lifestyle. Mayo Clinic. 2017. Accessed December 2019.

Health Benefits of Walnuts. Harvard Health Publishing. Harvard Medical School. 2018. Accessed September 2019.

Health Benefits of Walnuts. Food and Recipes. WebMD. 2019. Accessed September 2019.

Healthy Diet. Fact Sheet N°394. World Health Organization. 2018. Accessed February 2019.

Healthy Eating Plate. The Nutrition Source. Harvard T.H. Chan School of Public Health. 2011. Accessed January 2019.

How to Make Your Own Aromatic Vinegar Spray for All-Purpose Cleaning. Green Cleaning Tips. The Spruce. Updated 2019. Accessed December 2019.

Human Health Implications of Organic Food and Organic Agriculture: A Comprehensive Review. Mie A et al. *Environmental Health*. 16(1):111. 2017.

If Olive Oil Is High in Fat, Why Is It Considered Healthy? Healthy Lifestyle. Nutrition and Healthy Eating. Mayo Clinic. 2016. Accessed August 2019.

Iron. Fact Sheet for Consumers. Health Information. National Institute of Health. Office of Dietary Supplements. Updated 2019. Accessed December 2019.

Is Butter Really Back? Clarifying the Facts on Fats. Magazine of the Harvard T.H. Chan School of Public Health. Harvard Public Health. 2014. Accessed June 2020.

I've Heard That Salmon is High in Dangerous PCBs. So What Are PCBs and What Risk Do They Pose? Nutrition and Healthy Eating.

Healthy Lifestyle. Mayo Clinic. 2019 Accessed November 2019.

Joy of Cooking. Rombauer IS, Becker MR, and Becker E. Scribner. NY. 75th Anniversary Edition. 2006.

Mayo Clinic Minute: Are There Health Benefits to Taking Turmeric? Mayo Clinic. 2018. Accessed September 2019.

Mercury Guide. Natural Resources Defense Council. 2016. Accessed December 2019.

New "Guidelines" Say Continue Red Meat Consumption Habits, But Recommendations Contradict Evidence. The Nutrition Source. Harvard T.H. Chan School of Public Health. 2019. Accessed October 2019.

Nutritional and Functional Properties of Dates: A Review. Al-Farsi MA and Lee CY. *Crit Rev Food Sci Nutr.* 2008;48(10):877-87.

Olive. Vitamins and Supplements. WebMD. 2019. Accessed August 2019.

Olive Oil. Food Product. 2018. Encyclopaedia Britannica. Accessed August 2019.

Olive Oil: What Are the Health Benefits. The Mayo Clinic Diet. Mayo Foundation for Medical Education and Research. 2019. Accessed August 2019.

Onion. Plant. Encyclopaedia Britannica. 2019. Accessed September 2019.

Onion. Vitamins and Supplements. WebMD. 2018. Accessed September 2019.

Onions: Full of Nutrients. Diet and Weight Management. Feature Stories. WebMD. 2006. Accessed September 2019.

Oats. Food Features. The Nutrition Source. Harvard T.H. Chan School of Public Health. 2020. Accessed January 2020.

Pantry, Fridge, Countertop: Where to Store Your Food. WebMD. 2019. Accessed December 2019.

Parmesan Cheese. Encyclopaedia Britannica. 2008. Accessed January 2020.

Pesticide Residues in Food. News. Fact Sheets. Detail. World Health Organization (WHO). 2018. Accessed February 2019.

Polyvinyl Chloride (PVC). Chemicals and Contaminants. U.S National Library of Medicine. National Institute of Health (NIH). 2017. Accessed February 2019.

Pure Vanilla Extract vs Imitation. Peggy Trowbridge Filippone. The Spruce Eats. Updated 2019. Accessed December 2019.

Red and Processed Meat Still Pose Cancer Risk, Warn Global Health Experts. World Cancer Research Fund International. Accessed October 2019.

Shopper's Guide to Pesticides in Produce. Environmental Working Group (EWG). 2021. Accessed March 2021.

Should You Go Organic? Harvard Health Letter. Harvard Health Publishing. Harvard Medical School. 2015. Accessed March 2019.
Sodium. Healthy Living. American Heart Association (AHA). 2018. Accessed October 2018.

Squash. Plant. Encyclopaedia Britannica. 2019. Accessed December 2019.
Sumac. Nutrition Facts. Nutritionix Database. Syndigo. 2020. Accessed April 2020.

Teflon and Perfluorooctanoic Acid (PFOA). American Cancer Society (ACS). 2016. Accessed March 2019.

The Eatwell Guide- A Revised Healthy Eating Model. The British Nutrition Foundation. 2018. Accessed November 2019.

The Facts about Bisphenol A. Children's Health. WebMD. 2017. Accessed February 2019.

Therapeutic Effects of Date Fruits (Phoenix dactylifera) in the Prevention of Diseases Via Modulation of Anti-Inflammatory, Anti-Oxidant and Anti-Tumor Activity. Rahmani AH et al. *Int J Clin Exp Med.* 2014; 7(3):483–491.

Turmeric. Plant. Encyclopaedia Britannica. 2019. Accessed September 2019.

Turmeric. Vitamins and Supplements. Therapeutic Research Faculty. WebMD. 2018. Accessed September 2019.

<u>Understanding Food. Principles and Preparation</u>. Amy Brown. Thomson Wadsworth. Third Edition. 2008.

Vanilla. Plant and Flavoring. Encyclopedia Britannica. 2017. Accessed December 2019.

Walnut. Tree and Nut. Encyclopaedia Britannica. 2019. Accessed September 2019.

Want to Stay Hydrated? Drink Before You're Thirsty. Mayo Clinic. 2018. Accessed January 2020.

Water. The Nutrition Source. Harvard T.H. Chan School of Public Health. 2020. Accessed January 2020.

What Are Ultra-Processed Foods and Are They Bad for Our Health? Harvard Health Blog. Harvard Medical School. Harvard Health Publishing. 2020. Accessed January 2020.

What Is BPA, and What Are the Concerns About BPA. Healthy Lifestyle. Nutrition and Healthy Eating. Bauer BA. Mayo Clinic. 2016. Accessed January 2019.

What You Can Use in Place of Vanilla Beans. Erin Huffstetler. The Spruce Eats. Updated 2019. Accessed December 2019.

What You Need to Know About Mercury in Fish and Shellfish. U.S. Food and Drug Administration (FDA) and Environmental Protection Agency (EPA) Advisory ("Online Advisory"). 2004. Accessed March 2019.

Which Type of Oil Should I Use For Cooking With High Heat. Healthy Lifestyle. Nutrition and Healthy Eating. Mayo Clinic. 2019. Accessed April 2019.

Whole Grains. What Should I Eat? The Nutrition Source. Harvard T.H. Chan School of Public Health. 2020. Accessed March 2018.

Why Are Walnuts Good For Me. WebMD. 2019. Accessed September 2019.

Wild Caught vs. Farm Raised Seafood. Kendall Reagan Nutrition Center. College of Health and Human Sciences. 2018. Accessed November 2019.

Yogurt. Food Features. The Nutrition Source. Harvard T.H.Chan School of Public Health. 2019. Accessed December 2019.

You Can't Always Trust Measuring Cups, But Here's What You Can Do About It. Voraciously. The Washington Post. 2019. Accessed July 2019.

Zucchini. Squash Subspecies. Encyclopaedia Britannica. 2019. Accessed December 2019

INDEX

SUBJECT INDEX

(Page numbers in italics indicate photos)

RECIPE INDEX

(Page numbers in italics indicate photos)

To good health
and happiness,
always!
Warmest regards,
Sara

صحّة و هنا!
مع أطيب تمنّياتي،
سارة

www.ingramcontent.com/pod-product-compliance
Lightning Source LLC
LaVergne TN
LVHW072326150926
848178LV00014B/180
* 9 7 8 1 7 3 7 7 5 3 0 7 0 *